Exercise and the Heart

Edition 2

Cardiovascular Clinics Series

Brest	1/1	Hypertensive Cardiovascular Disease
Brest	1/2	Coronary Heart Disease
Brest	1/3	Cardiovascular Therapy
Downing	2/1	Congenital Heart Disease
Dreifus	*2/2	Arrhythmias
White	2/3	International Cardiology
Gifford	3/1	Peripheral Vascular Disease
Harken	*3/2	Cardiac Surgery 1
Harken	*3/3	Cardiac Surgery 2
Burch	*4/1	Cardiomyopathy
Edwards	*4/2	Clinical-Pathological Correlations 1
Engle	4/3	Pediatric Cardiology
Edwards	*5/1	Clinical-Pathological Correlations 2
Likoff	*5/2	Valvular Heart Disease
Fisch	*5/3	Complex Electrocardiography 1
Fisch	*6/1	Complex Electrocardiography 2
Melmon	*6/2	Cardiovascular Drug Therapy
Fowler	6/3	Diagnostic Methods in Cardiology
Vidt	7/1	Cleveland Clinic Cardiovascular Consultations
Brest et al.	7/2	Innovations in the Diagnosis and Management of Acute Myocardial Infarction
Spodick	7/3	Pericardial Diseases
Corday	8/1	Controversies in Cardiology
Rahimtoola	8/2	Coronary Bypass Surgery
Rios	8/3	Clinical Electrocardiographic Correlations
Onesti, Brest	9/1	Hypertension
Kotler, Segal	9/2	Clinical Echocardiography
Wenger	*9/3	Exercise and the Heart
Roberts	*10/1	Congenital Heart Disease in Adults
Willerson	*10/2	Nuclear Cardiology
Brandenburg	10/3	Office Cardiology
Castellanos	11/1	Cardiac Arrhythmias: Mechanisms and Management
Engle	11/2	Pediatric Cardiovascular Disease
Rackley	11/3	Critical Care Cardiology
Noble, Rothbaum	12/1	Geriatric Cardiology
Vidt	12/2	Cardiovascular Therapy
McGoon	12/3	Cardiac Surgery
Rahimtoola	13/1	Controversies in Coronary Artery Disease
Spittell	13/2	Clinical Vascular Disease
Fowler	13/3	Noninvasive Diagnostic Methods in Cardiology
Goldberg	14/1	Coronary Artery Spasm and Thrombosis
Dreifus	14/2	Pacemaker Therapy
Conti	14/3	Cardiac Drug Therapy
Schroeder	15/1	Invasive Cardiology

*Not Available

Exercise and the Heart
Edition 2

Nanette K. Wenger, M.D. | Editor

Professor of Medicine (Cardiology)
Emory University School of Medicine
Director, Cardiac Clinics
Grady Memorial Hospital
Atlanta, Georgia

CARDIOVASCULAR CLINICS

Albert N. Brest, M.D. | Editor-in-Chief

James C. Wilson Professor of Medicine
Director, Division of Cardiology
Jefferson Medical College
Philadelphia, Pennsylvania

 F. A. DAVIS COMPANY, PHILADELPHIA

Cardiovascular Clinics, 15/2, Exercise and the Heart, edition 2

Copyright © 1985 by F. A. Davis Company

Printed in the United States of America

NOTE: As new scientific information becomes available through basic and clinical research, recommended treatments and drug therapies undergo changes. The author(s) and publisher have done everything possible to make this book accurate, up-to-date, and in accord with accepted standards at the time of publication. However, the reader is advised always to check product information (package inserts) for changes and new information regarding dose and contraindications before administering any drug. Caution is especially urged when using new or infrequently ordered drugs.

Library of Congress Cataloging in Publication Data

Cardiovascular clinics. 1-
    Philadelphia, F. A. Davis, 1969-
        v. ill. 27 cm.
    Editor: v. 1- A. N. Brest.
    Key title: Cardiovascular clinics, ISSN 0069-0384.
    1. Cardiovascular system—Diseases—Collected works. I. Brest, Albert N., ed.
    [DNLM: W1 CA77N]
RC681.A1C27   616.1   70-6558
ISBN 0-8036-9227-7   MARC-S

Library of Congress   75[8307]

Preface

In all cardiac cases that are fit to walk about, outdoor exercise is beneficial, for it encourages health of mind and body. The principle . . . for these patients is that they live strictly within the limits set by their symptoms. Patients who suffer from breathlessness may take exercise that makes them breathe a little rapidly from time to time, so that they begin to be conscious of the breathlessness; but there must be no pressing on to a point of distress, or to a point where the sense of breathlessness is not lost almost as soon as rest is taken. So, too, with anginal pain . . . In neither one case nor the other must so much exercise be taken as subsequently to bring about unpleasant fatigue . . . Exactly the same principle applies to work . . . It is often better to curtail the hours than to attempt to change the work . . . Occupation of mind and body banishes anxiety and cultivates contentment.*

So wrote Sir Thomas Lewis half a century ago, presaging the current era of the increased application of exercise testing and exercise training to the management of patients with a variety of cardiovascular disorders.

In the intervening years, considerable precision has been added to his recommendations for exercise, aided by a wide spectrum of technologic advances; and more detailed documentation has been obtained of the multidimensional beneficial and potentially adverse effects of physical activity in selected subsets of patients of all ages with differing cardiovascular problems. Significantly more is known about the response to exercise both in health and in disease, and extrapolation of these data has enabled the additional diagnostic and therapeutic uses of exercise.

The considerable expansion of our information base since 1978 and its relevance to the clinical practice of medicine suggested that it was appropriate to prepare a second edition of *Exercise and the Heart*. In so doing, the interdependence of the spheres of the scientist and the clinician has become increasingly prominent. I would like to express my appreciation to the chapter authors for their lucid and authoritative presentations, which often encompass personal research contributions. I am also indebted to Dr. Albert Brest and the staff at F. A. Davis for their expertise and efficiency.

Nanette K. Wenger, M.D.
Guest Editor

*Lewis, Sir Thomas. *Diseases of the Heart*. Macmillan and Company Limited, 1933.

Editor's Commentary

The initial Cardiovascular Clinics issue of *Exercise and the Heart* was published in 1978. Subsequently, interest in exercise testing and exercise training has continued to expand. Patients are enthusiastic about exercise generally as a self-help technique. Physicians have embraced the clinical use of exercise in the prevention, diagnosis, and treatment of heart disease. In addition to broadening the base of information covered in the earlier volume, this book explores new topics, such as distance running, effects of exercise in the elderly, upper extremity testing and training, effects of cardiovascular drugs on exercise testing and training, supervised versus nonsupervised exercise rehabilitation, exercise training of patients with ventricular dysfunction and heart failure, and exercise testing and training in noncoronary heart disease, and other topics as well. I hope the reader will find this book a worthy successor to the initial offering. I am extremely grateful to the individual authors for their exemplary contributions. I am indebted again to Dr. Nanette K. Wenger for her invaluable guidance in the re-formulation of this issue.

Albert N. Brest, M.D.
Editor-in-Chief

Contributors

Ezra A. Amsterdam, M.D.
Professor of Internal Medicine (Cardiology), Chief, Division of Cardiovascular Medicine, University of California-Davis School of Medicine; Director, Coronary Care Unit, University of California-Davis Medical Center, Sacramento, California

Harvey J. Berger, M.D.
Director, Nuclear Medicine Division and Magnetic Resonance Research, Emory University School of Medicine, Atlanta, Georgia

C. Gunnar Blomqvist, M.D.
Professor of Internal Medicine and Physiology; Weinberger Laboratory for Cardiopulmonary Research, Southwestern Medical School, University of Texas Health Science Center, Dallas, Texas

Jane Chappelear, B.S.
Northside Cardiology, Inc., Indianapolis, Indiana

Myrvin H. Ellestad, M.D.
Clinical Professor of Medicine, University of California-Irvine School of Medicine; Director, Division of Cardiology, Memorial Hospital Medical Center of Long Beach, Long Beach, California

W. Doyle Gentry, Ph.D.
Clinical Professor, Department of Behavioral Medicine and Psychiatry, University of Virginia Medical School, Charlottesville, Virginia

Diane Goforth, M.D.
Fellow, Pediatric Cardiology, Division of Cardiology, Children's Hospital Medical Center, Cincinnati, Ohio

L. Howard Hartley, M.D.
Associate Professor of Medicine, Harvard Medical School, Director, Cardiac Rehabilitation, Brigham and Women's Hospital, Boston, Massachusetts

Herman K. Hellerstein, M.D.
Professor of Medicine, Case Western Reserve University School of Medicine, University Hospitals of Cleveland, Cleveland, Ohio

Frederick W. James, M.D.
Professor of Pediatrics, University of Cincinnati College of Medicine; Director, Cardiovascular Exercise Physiology Laboratory, Children's Hospital Medical Center, Cincinnati, Ohio

Ronald J. Landin, M.D.
Cardiovascular Consultant, Northside Cardiology, Inc. and St. Vincent Hospital and Health Care Center; Associate Clinical Professor of Medicine, Indiana University School of Medicine, Indianapolis, Indiana

Lawrence J. Laslett, M.D.
Assistant Professor of Internal Medicine, University of California-Davis School of Medicine; Director, Cardiac Catheterization Laboratory, Director, Cardiac Rehabilitation, University of California-Davis Medical Center, Sacramento, California

Thomas J. Linnemeier, M.D.
Cardiovascular Consultant, Northside Cardiology, Inc. and St. Vincent Hospital and Health Care Center, Indianapolis, Indiana

Jerre F. Lutz, M.D.
Associate Professor of Medicine (Cardiology), Emory University School of Medicine; Director, Cardiac Catheterization/Cardiac Function Laboratories, Grady Memorial Hospital, Atlanta, Georgia

Jay L. Meizlish, M.D.
Research Fellow, Nuclear Cardiology, Yale University School of Medicine, New Haven, Connecticut

Henry S. Miller, Jr., M.D.
Professor of Medicine/Cardiology, Section of Cardiology, Bowman Gray School of Medicine, Winston-Salem, North Carolina

T. William Moir, M.D.
Professor of Medicine, Case Western Reserve University School of Medicine, and University Hospitals of Cleveland, Cleveland, Ohio

John Naughton, M.D.
Professor of Medicine, Dean, School of Medicine, Interim Vice President for Health Sciences, State University of New York at Buffalo, Buffalo, New York

R. Joe Noble, M.D.
Clinical Professor of Medicine, Indiana University School of Medicine, Cardiovascular Consultant, Northside Cardiology, Inc. and St. Vincent Hospital and Health Care Center, Indianapolis, Indiana

Michael L. Pollock, Ph.D.
Director, Cardiac Rehabilitation Program, University of Wisconsin Medical School (Milwaukee Clinical Campus)-Mount Sinai Medical Center, Milwaukee, Wisconsin

Donald A. Rothbaum, M.D.
Associate Clinical Professor of Medicine, Indiana University School of Medicine, Cardiovascular Consultant, Northside Cardiology, Inc. and St. Vincent Hospital and Health Care Center, Indianapolis, Indiana

Roy J. Shephard, M.D. (Lond), Ph.D.
Director, School of Physical and Health Education, University of Toronto; Consultant to the Toronto Rehabilitation Centre, Toronto, Ontario, Canada

Martha A. Stewart, B.A.
Graduate Program, Department of Psychology, Wake Forest University, Winston-Salem, North Carolina

Bruce F. Waller, M.D.
Associate Professor of Pathology and Medicine, Indiana University School of Medicine; Research Associate, Krannert Institute of Cardiology, Director, Cardiovascular Pathology Division, Indianapolis, Indiana

John G. Weg, M.D.
Professor of Internal Medicine, University of Michigan Medical School; Physician-in-Charge, Pulmonary and Critical Care Medicine Division, University of Michigan Medical Center, Ann Arbor, Michigan

Donald A. Weiner, M.D.
Associate Professor of Medicine, Boston University School of Medicine, Boston, Massachusetts

Nanette K. Wenger, M.D.
Professor of Medicine (Cardiology), Emory University School of Medicine; Director, Cardiac Clinics, Grady Memorial Hospital, Atlanta, Georgia

R. Sanders Williams, M.D.
Assistant Professor of Medicine and Physiology, Duke University Medical Center, Durham, North Carolina

Barry L. Zaret, M.D.
Professor of Medicine and Diagnostic Radiology, Chief, Cardiology Section, Yale University School of Medicine, New Haven, Connecticut

Contents

The Role of Exercise in the Primary and Secondary Prevention of Atherosclerotic
Coronary Artery Disease 1
  L. Howard Hartley, M.D.

Exercise-Related Sudden Death in Young (Age $\leq$ 30 Years) and Old (Age $>$ 30
Years) Conditioned Subjects 9
  Bruce F. Waller, M.D.

Distance Running in the 1980s: Cardiovascular Benefits and Risks 75
  Herman K. Hellerstein, M.D. and T. William Moir, M.D.

Effects of Exercise on the Myocardium: Echocardiographic Studies 87
  Ezra A. Amsterdam, M.D. and Lawrence J. Laslett, M.D.

Predischarge Exercise Testing after Myocardial Infarction: Prognostic and
Therapeutic Features 95
  Donald A. Weiner, M.D.

Exercise Nuclear Imaging for the Evaluation of Coronary Artery Disease 105
  Jay L. Meizlish, M.D., Harvey J. Berger, M.D., and Barry L. Zaret, M.D.

Exercise-Induced Arrhythmias and Hypotension: Significance and Clinical
Management 125
  Myrvin H. Ellestad, M.D.

Cardiovascular Drugs: Effects on Exercise Testing and Exercise Training of the
Coronary Patient 133
  Nanette K. Wenger, M.D.

Exercise Regimens after Myocardial Infarction: Rationale and Results 145
  Roy J. Shephard, M.D. (Lond), Ph.D.

Exercise Regimens after Myocardial Revascularization Surgery: Rationale and
Results 159
  Michael L. Pollock, Ph.D.

Upper Extremity Exercise Testing and Training 175
   C. Gunnar Blomqvist, M.D.

Cardiac Rehabilitation: Current Status and Future Possibilities 185
   John Naughton, M.D.

Supervised versus Nonsupervised Exercise Rehabilitation of Coronary Patients.... 193
   Henry S. Miller, Jr., M.D.

Exercise Testing and Training of the Elderly Patient 201
   Ronald J. Landin, M.D., Thomas J. Linnemeier, M.D., Donald A. Rothbaum,
   M.D., Jane Chappelear, B. S., and R. Joe Noble, M.D.

Exercise Training of Patients with Ventricular Dysfunction and Heart Failure 219
   R. Sanders Williams, M.D.

Use of Exercise Testing in Noncoronary Heart Disease 233
   Jerre F. Lutz, M.D. and Nanette K. Wenger, M.D.

Exercise Training in Noncoronary Heart Disease 243
   Diane Goforth, M.D. and Frederick W. James, M.D.

Psychologic Effects of Exercise Training in Coronary-Prone Individuals and in
Patients with Symptomatic Coronary Heart Disease........................ 255
   W. Doyle Gentry, Ph.D. and Martha A. Stewart, B.A.

Therapeutic Exercise in Patients with Chronic Obstructive Pulmonary Disease.... 261
   John G. Weg, M.D.

Index 277

The Role of Exercise in the Primary and Secondary Prevention of Atherosclerotic Coronary Artery Disease

L. Howard Hartley, M.D.

Exercise conditioning has the potential to prevent disease and improve life expectancy by several mechanisms (Table 1). Systolic pressure and circulating levels of catecholamines are reduced at rest and during exercise.[1] These two adjustments to conditioning would be expected to lessen stresses on the arterial wall and hence decrease the rate of atheroma formation. Blood lipids also are changed in a direction that is favorable for prevention of coronary disease. Cholesterol and triglycerides are usually reduced, but a change that is probably more important is an increase of high-density lipoproteins. That lipid fraction is believed to protect the arteries from developing atherosclerosis.[2]

The cross-sectional area of the coronary arterial tree has been said to increase after exercise conditioning. Eckstein reported that canine coronary collateral formation was increased by regular exercise in animals with experimentally induced coronary arterial narrowing.[3] More recently, collateral formation was increased by exercise in nonhuman primates with extensive diet-induced atheromatous disease.[4] Also the caliber of the coronary arteries is said to increase in dogs as a result of vigorous exercise.[5] These and other studies support the concept that collateral formation can be induced by exercise in experimental animals. However, whether these changes occur in man is not known. Tremendously enlarged coronary arteries have been reported in the hearts of top athletes.[6] Still other studies report reductions in ST segment depression and angina on the exercise test,[7,8] which strongly suggests that an improved arterial supply can accompany increased physical activity in patients with coronary disease. However, because other explanations cannot be excluded, the actual effects of exercise on the coronary circulation of man are uncertain.

The behavioral aspects of exercise conditioning are undoubtedly important, but their mechanisms are not well understood. Lessening of depression scores and development of a sense of well being have been repeatedly demonstrated.[9] A number of neurohormonal factors have been implicated in the behavioral aspects of exercise conditioning. It is not certain that these changes have any importance in protecting persons from the development of coronary disease. However, the potential preventive value seems clear, and virtually all investigators and clinicians with extensive experience in the field of cardiac rehabilitation are impressed with the obvious benefits to patients because of their improved sense of well being and lessened proneness to depression.

In addition to these primary actions of exercise conditioning, certain secondary effects are potentially important. Individuals who regularly exercise have more healthful behaviors than their sedentary counterparts, as shown in Table 2.[10,11] In the study of Hickey,[10] significant negative associations between leisure activity and relative weight and cigarette smoking were found in men under 60. In the observations that Hartley[11] made of apparently normal indi-

Table 1. Exercise conditioning effects that are potentially beneficial for preventing atheromatous arterial disease

Reduction of systolic pressure
Lowering of circulating catecholamines
Reduction of blood clotting tendencies
Reduction of serum cholesterol, triglycerides
Increase of HDL lipoproteins
Augmentation of coronary arterial bed
Improved psychological profile

viduals in New England, fewer participants in heavy activity were overweight or smoked. Also individuals who are more fit have a greater likelihood of obtaining regular medical checkups and of complying with medical advice.[11]

Epidemiologic studies that have examined the relationship of exercise to the genesis of coronary disease can be categorized as retrospective, prospective, or interventional. These studies carry increasing power for detecting a causal relationship. Many retrospective studies are reported, but they will not be discussed; such studies are badly flawed because of biases inherent in the selection of the study population. However, several prospective studies are worth reviewing because they clearly indicate an association of physical activity with athero-sclerotic coronary disease, even though the association has not been proven to be causal. These prospective studies characterize populations initially for known risk factors and activity habits. This approach permits an assessment of the independent association of physical activity with the development of coronary disease during a period of followup. Interventional studies are better because they randomly allocate individuals of similar characteristics into either an exercise or a no-exercise group. This could prove whether exercise directly affects health and life expectancy. However, no interventional studies have been (or are likely to be) performed because costs are prohibitive. Prospective studies are designed to demonstrate a difference, if one exists. However, the statistical techniques address a null hypothesis and failure to demonstrate an effect certainly does not mean that an effect does not exist. Hence, this chapter will review only the studies that have shown an effect. Several review articles extensively discuss both negative and positive studies, and the reader is referred to them for an exhaustive bibliography of the subject.[12]

Table 2. Relationship of leisure time physical activity and coronary risk factors in normal men with sedentary occupations

		Minimal Activity	Heavy Activity
cholesterol (mg/dl)	1.	232	206
	2.	222	222
blood pressure (mm Hg)	1.	139/85	125/80
	2.	125/80	125/80
% overweight	1.	7.2	4.2
	2.	35	22
cigarette (number per day)	1.	9.4	5.7
(percent)	2.	9%	5%

1. Hickey: 15,721 men.
2. Hartley: 473 men

Of course, demonstration of an association between physical activity and the development of atherosclerotic coronary disease is not necessarily cause and effect. However, because it is unlikely that more definitive studies will be performed in our lifetime, this article will review the best studies available on the subject in an effort to deduce the amount of activity that seems to protect from coronary disease. More studies are necessary to determine whether these assumptions are correct. Experience with other risk factors, such as hypertension, suggests that this approach is completely reasonable.

PRIMARY PREVENTION OF ATHEROSCLEROTIC CORONARY DISEASE

One of the earliest and most extensive prospective studies to be performed in relationship to coronary disease is the Framingham Study.[13] In the Framingham Study the cohort was carefully characterized in many ways including histories, physical examinations, blood tests, and questionnaires. Questionnaires concerning physical activity were administered at the time of entry. Based upon indices generated from their responses, individuals were categorized for activity habits into one of three groups: least, intermediate, and most active. The scoring system was simple. Individuals were asked to specify activities for each hour of their usual day, and the activities were judged to be resting, standing, slight, moderate, or heavy activities. These variables were assigned weighting values that were multiples of resting energy requirements.

sleep	1.0
standing	1.1
slight (walking)	1.5
moderate	2.4
heavy	5.0

Hence, an individual who spent all day and night in bed would have a total score of 24. The subjects were distributed into three groups of physical activity scores: <29, 29–36, >37. At 10 years of followup, significant differences existed between the incidence of coronary disease (death, angina pectoris, heart attack) and the level of physical activity at entry. The most significant changes were in incidence rates between the least active groups and the moderate groups. Significant differences could not be detected between moderate and heavy activity.

The least amount of exercise that seems to protect persons from the development of coronary disease is that performed by the moderate activity group. In order to determine activities that would generate an intensity equal to the moderate group, the amount of time available for exercise must be known. Although physical effort is quite heavy in some jobs, we will restrict our attention to individuals whose jobs are basically sedentary. A certain amount of time is required for activities of daily living: sleeping, eating, working, traveling to and from work, and engaging in leisure time. If we assign certain reasonable values for the daily activities (sleeping—8 hours, eating—3 hours, working—8 hours, traveling—2 hours), we find that 3 hours remain for allocation to leisure time. Since we are assuming a sedentary occupation, all of the physical activity must come during these 3 hours. The individual needs approximately 8 or more MET-hours of activities to enter the lower incidence group. One hour of brisk walking would provide most of the activity needed to meet the requirements of low coronary incidence of the Framingham Study. It certainly would be enough if it were combined with 1 hour of walking during daily work. A useful formula would be to walk briskly for 8 hours per week according to the following: 1 hour per working day during leisure time and the remaining 3 hours disbursed throughout the working day. Also the same amount of activity could be provided by half as much time if more vigorous activity such as jogging (10 MET-hours × 5) was used. Also, of course, physical activity on weekends could contribute to the overall activity profile.

The studies of Paffenbarger also prospectively examined the relationship between physical activity and incidence of coronary disease. The earliest study[14] determined that longshoremen with occupations that had low or moderate energy requirements (under 5 kcal per min) had 1.8 times (p < .001) the risk of dying from coronary heart disease compared with those who had jobs that required substantial exertion (5.2 to 7.5 kcal per min). No differences could be detected between those individuals who had job activity levels of 2.4 to 5 kcal per min (moderate) and those who had levels of under 2.4 (light). Jobs in the heavy category were extremely laborious[15] and are largely mechanized now so that very few longshoremen perform work at such intensities at this time. Hence, for practical purposes, occupational classifications for coronary risk are of little value; most are less than the heavy work group of Paffenbarger.

The second study guided by Paffenbarger is more germane to the question of deciding how much activity is necessary to provide protection from disease.[16] In that study he related energy expenditure to the risk of a first heart attack in 16,936 male college alumni. Risk of heart attack was related to the reported incidence of certain activities. Individuals who reported climbing fewer than 5 flights of stairs per day were at 25 percent increased risk of heart attack compared with those who climbed more than 5. Also individuals who walked fewer than 5 city blocks had 23 percent more heart attacks than those who walked more. Men who reported not playing any sports or only light sports had 38 percent greater risk of heart attack than those who engaged in vigorous activities. When strenuous sports were qualified by hours per week of participation, men who played less than 3 hours per week or not at all had an age-adjusted rate of heart attack that was 54 percent higher than that of men who played 3 or more hours per week. When all activities were considered, individuals who had an index indicating that they participated in exercise that consumed less than 2000 kcal per week were at 64 percent increased risk of heart attack compared with their more energetic counterparts.

The final study of coronary disease prevention via physical activity that will be examined in this chapter was performed in London to examine the relationship between vigorous leisure time exercise and the incidence of coronary heart disease.[17] In that study, 16,882 male executive grade civil servants in Britain recorded their activities for a Friday and Saturday and completed questionnaires on habits and personal history. Activities were considered vigorous if the energy expenditures were believed likely to reach peaks of 7.5 kcal per minute. Individuals who had heart attacks reportedly engaged in such activities only half as often as individuals who were similar in all characteristics but did not have a heart attack. The types of activities are defined in some detail, but little can actually be gained from this article for making specific recommendations because the sampling technique does not provide knowledge of amounts of usual activities. It is interesting that brisk walking and climbing stairs were two common forms of activity. This finding again points out that vigorous sports are not the only acceptable forms of activity.

A summary of the epidemiologic data relating exercise to coronary disease is reviewed in Table 3. Each study provides unique data that help us to understand the profile of physical activity associated with low risk for coronary disease. The Framingham Study indicates that the level of activity that is necessary to enter into low-risk classification is actually quite low. The study of college alumni suggests that the level of activity associated with low risk is also low, but that larger amounts of activity may be associated with even less risk. A summary of the profile for low risk is developed in the summary of this review.

SECONDARY PREVENTION OF CORONARY DISEASE AND REHABILITATION

Exercise is now used routinely in coronary rehabilitation programs. However, because medical interventions are used with exercise, it is difficult to separate the effects of these interventions from the effects of physical activity. The physiologic changes of exercise conditioning that were discussed in the beginning of this chapter also apply to coronary disease. This portion of the discussion will focus on health outcomes.

Table 3. Epidemiologic studies that have examined the relationship of exercise to the occurrence of coronary artery disease

Study	Findings
Framingham	Moderate physical activity is associated with less coronary disease.
San Francisco Longshoremen	Very vigorous activity on the job that would require heavy lifting or carrying loads is associated with low risk.
College Alumni	Risk profile can be reduced by: climbing 5 flights of stairs per day; walking more than 5 city blocks per day; engaging in vigorous sports; engaging in strenuous sports at least 3 hours/week; performing 2000 kcal/week or more (all activities considered).
London Civil Servants	Fewer individuals who had heart attacks engaged in vigorous leisure time activity than counterparts who did not have such an event.

As in the case of primary prevention, many studies have suggested a relationship between physical activity and morbidity and mortality for patients with atherosclerotic coronary disease. However, in contrast to primary prevention, randomized and controlled trials of the usefulness of such programs have been performed. Although the results of these studies are not conclusive, they do allow us to make certain generalizations concerning the use of physical activity in coronary rehabilitation.

The value of early mobilization for patients who have had a myocardial infarction has only recently been recognized. The first randomized controlled trial comparing early mobilization with prolonged bed rest was reported less than 10 years ago.[18] In that study, patients who had survived acute myocardial infarction were randomly assigned to either an early mobilization group or prolonged bed rest. The group that was mobilized early had shorter durations of hospitalization and greater abilities to return to work. No complications occurred as a result of the early activity.

In 1975 a controlled trial of physical training after myocardial infarction was performed by Swedish investigators.[19] All patients born in 1913 or later were included in the study, and 158 were randomized into the training group and 157 into the controls. During 4 years of followup, 28 patients died in the training group and 35 in the control group, a difference that did not reach statistical significance. However, individuals who complied had lower mortality than those who did not. Also those who attended the program had lower mortality than matched controls.

The National Exercise and Heart Disease Project was reported in 1981.[20] This multicenter study enrolled 651 men with myocardial infarctions and randomly assigned them to one of two groups—exercise or control. The patients were screened 2 to 36 months after their infarction, and for 2 months they participated in a preliminary program designed to enhance compliance. Hence, these patients started in the program rather late after myocardial infarction. The three-year mortality was 7.3 percent for the control group and 4.6 percent for the intervention group. Recurrent myocardial infarctions occurred in 7 percent and 5.3 percent, respectively, of control and exercise groups. Again, the trend toward improved prognosis in the exercise group could not be supported statistically. Fewer individuals who had a myocardial infarction died (0.3 percent) in the exercise compared with the control group (2.4 percent), a finding that was statistically significant ($p < .05$). The fact that statistical significance was not reached in regard to recurrent infarction was hardly surprising, inasmuch as the study had been designed as a pilot to determine if a definitive experiment should be performed. Although a trend toward the benefits of exercise was present, performance of a definitive study was not recommended largely on economic grounds.

Another controlled trial was conducted in Canada in which 733 patients who had recovered from a myocardial infarction were allocated to either a low intensity exercise group (LIE) or a high intensity exercise group (HIE) by a stratified random allocation.[21] The HIE group exercised at a walking or jogging pace requiring between 65 and 85 percent of maximal oxygen uptake. The patients came to the center twice per week and were encouraged to exercise at least two other times per week on their own. The LIE subjects met once per week for relaxation and supervised activities such as volleyball, bowling, or swimming, and attempts were made to keep the activity at an intensity not greater than 50 percent of maximal. The recurrence rates for myocardial infarctions and death rates were not significantly different between the two groups. Although the HIE group improved working capacity more than LIE, both did, in fact, improve. This finding strongly suggests that a training effect was induced even in the LIE group. This could obscure differences between groups because both had good prognoses. Indeed, examination of the mortality rates strongly suggests low values for both groups. The only conclusion that can be drawn is that HIE does not seem to confer any more protection than LIE. Unfortunately, no control subjects were studied.

Perhaps one of the most important studies is that of Kallio and coworkers[22] from Finland. In that study, 375 patients were randomized into either a control or an intervention group at the time of discharge from the hospital and were followed in one of two groups for 3 years. The mortality was significantly less in the intervention (rehabilitation) compared with the control group (18 vs 29 percent) and was in large part due to fewer sudden deaths (6 vs 14 percent). The reduction was greatest in the first 6 months. This intervention was multifactorial, consisting of medical examinations and counselling by social workers, psychologists, dietitians, and physiotherapists. Antismoking, dietary, and lifestyle advice was given. The exercise component of the program was based upon working capacity and was started under supervision. Followup was most intensive during the first 3 months and tapered to trimonthly. The intervention started early, about 1 month after infarction.

In order to summarize our experiences to date in epidemiologic studies of secondary prevention for coronary disease, attention is called to Table 4. The first two studies listed (Wilhelmsen and NEHDP) have the most similar experimental techniques, including the use of controls. Both studies suggest a benefit of exercise for both fewer nonfatal reinfarctions and deaths. The Canadian study does not show the same tendency, but the death rates are so low that one suspects either a protective effect in both groups or patient selection techniques that resulted in unusually hardy subjects. The higher death rates in the Wilhelmsen and Kallio studies reflect randomization at a much earlier stage of the illness than the other studies.

Table 4. Studies of secondary prevention of coronary disease

Study	Reinfarction	Coronary Deaths
Wilhelmsen (4 yrs)		
control	28 (18%)	35/157 (22%)
exercise	25 (16%)	28/158 (18%)
National Exercise and Heart Disease Program (3 yrs)		
control	23 (7%)	24/328 (7%)
exercise	17 (5%)	15/323 (5%)
Canadian Exercise and Rehabilitation Study (4 yrs)		
LIE	33 (9%)	13/354 (4%)
HIE	39 (10%)	15/379 (4%)
Kallio (3 yrs)		
control	21 (11%)	55/187 (29%)
intervention	34 (18%)	35/188 (19%)

SUMMARY

Although exact definitions of exercise requirements for primary and secondary prevention of coronary disease cannot be stated with certainty on the basis of currently available information, we can make some general conclusions.

The characteristics associated with lowered risk from coronary disease in apparently normal populations are:

8 MET-hours of activity during leisure time or job:

walking briskly during leisure time (1 hour = 1 MET-hour)

walking at job (same as above)

jogging during leisure time (30 minutes of activity = 1 MET-hour)

walking to and from work (same as walking above)

performing very heavy work in occupational pursuits (few jobs today have those energy requirements)

regularly climbing 5 flights or more of stairs (10 steps per flight)

regularly walking 5 city blocks per day (12 blocks per mile)

regularly engaging in strenuous sports (basketball, running, mountaineering, skiing, swimming, or tennis)

accumulating activities that use 2000 or more kcal per week

Conclusions concerning the prevention of reinfarction in patients who are recovering from a first heart attack include:

Exercise is helpful in hastening the recovery process after myocardial infarction and should be started early in the recovery period.

Exercise helps to reduce mortality when used in conjunction with a multifactorial program.

REFERENCES

1. HARTLEY, LH, MASON, JW, HOGAN, RP, ET AL: *Multiple hormonal response to graded exercise in relation to physical training.* Appl Physiol 33:601, 1972.

2. GORDON, DJ, WITZTUM, JL, HUNNINGHAKE, D, ET AL: *Habitual physical activity and high-density lipoprotein cholesterol in men with primary hypercholesterolemia.* Circulation 67:512, 1983.

3. ECKSTEIN, RW: *Effect of exercise and coronary artery narrowing on coronary collateral circulation.* Circ Res 5:230, 1957.

4. KRANSCH, DM, ASPEN, AJ, ABRAMOWITZ, BM, ET AL: *Reduction of coronary atherosclerosis by moderate conditioning exercise in monkeys on an atherogenic diet.* N Engl Med 305:1483, 1981.

5. WYATT, HL AND MITCHELL, J: *Influences of physical conditioning and deconditioning on coronary vasculature in dogs.* J Appl Physiol 45:619, 1978.

6. BROWN, CE, HUANG, TC, AND McCAY, CM: *Observations on blood vessels and exercise.* Gerontol 11:292, 1956.

7. EHSANI, AA, HEATH, GW, HAGBERG, JM, ET AL: *Effects of 12 months of intense exercise training on ischemic ST-segment depression in patients with coronary artery disease.* Circulation 64:1116, 1981.

8. SIM, D AND NEILL, W: *Investigation of the physiological basis for increased exercise threshold for angina pectoris after physical conditioning.* J Clin Invest 54:763, 1974.

9. HARTLEY, LH: *Post myocardial infarction.* In HERD JA (ED): *Behavior and Atherosclerosis.* Plenum Press, New York, 1983, pp 111–116.

10. HICKEY, N, MULCAHY, R, BOURKE, GJ, ET AL: *Study of coronary risk factors related to physical activity in 15,721 men.* Br Med J 3:507, 1975.

11. HARTLEY, LH: Personal observations, 1982.

12. COHEN, LS, MOCK, MB, AND RINGQVIST, I: *Physical Conditioning and Cardiovascular Rehabilitation.* John Wiley & Sons, New York, 1981.

13. KANNEL, WB, GORDON, T, SORLIE, P, ET AL: *Physical activity and coronary vulnerability: The Framingham Study.* Cardiology Digest 6:28, 1971.

14. PAFFENBARGER, RS AND HALE, WE: *Work activity and coronary heart mortality.* N Engl J Med 292:545, 1975.

15. GORDON, EE: *The use of energy costs in regulating physical activity in chronic disease.* Arch Industrial Health 16:437, 1957.

16. PAFFENBARGER, RS, WING, AL, AND HYDE, RT: *Physical activity as an index of heart attack risk in college alumni.* Am J Epidemiol 108:161, 1978.

17. MORRIS, JN, ADAM, C, CHAVE, SPW, ET AL: *Vigorous exercise in leisure time and the incidence of coronary heart disease.* Lancet 1:333, 1973.

18. BLOCH, A, MAEDER, J-P, HAISSLY, J-C, ET AL: *Early mobilization after myocardial infarction.* Am J Cardiol 34:152, 1974.

19. WILHELMSEN, L, SANNE, H, ELMFELDT, D, ET AL: *A controlled trial of physical training after myocardial infarction.* Prev Med 4:491, 1975.

20. SHAW, L: *Effects of a prescribed supervised exercise program on mortality and cardiovascular morbidity in patients after a myocardial infarction.* Am J Cardiol 48:39, 1981.

21. RECHNITZER, PA, CUNNINGHAM, DA, ANDERW, GM, ET AL: *Relation of exercise to the recurrence rate of myocardial infarction in men.* Cardiol 51:65, 1983.

22. KALLIO, V, HAMALAINEN, H, HAKKILA, J, ET AL: *Reduction in sudden deaths by a multifactorial intervention programme after acute myocardial infarction.* Lancet 2:1091, 1979.

Exercise-Related Sudden Death in Young (Age ≤ 30 Years) and Old (Age > 30 Years) Conditioned Subjects

Bruce F. Waller, M.D.

Each year in the United States the popularity of exercise performed on a regular basis increases in allegedly healthy individuals as well as in those with known cardiovascular disease. This popularity expresses itself in many forms of regular exercise including running (jogging), tennis, swimming, football, basketball, baseball, and wrestling. Current data indicate that the number of adult runners or joggers increased from several hundred in 1960 to nearly 6 million in 1972.[1-6] In 1975 there were about 11 million runners, and 3 years later there were 17 million runners. Tennis has also increased in popularity and currently involves about 10 million players. Racquetball has grown from 50,000 players in 1972 to about 3 million participants in 1978.

The intensity of exercise as well as the number of persons exercising competitively has also risen with the increased number of individuals involved in exercise. Nearly 1 of every 6 adult Americans invests an average of 300 minutes per week in vigorous exercise.[4] There are more than 200 marathon races in the United States each year, and more than 50,000 Americans have successfully completed at least one marathon.[6] It is estimated that more than 4000 (8 percent) of these runners have completed the marathon distance in less than 3 hours. In the United States the Boston Marathon attracts more than 3000 runners and the New York City Marathon more than 14,000 runners. In Britain the *Sunday Times* National Fun Run has over 11,000 entries. Exercise participation appears higher in younger age groups, but nearly 40 percent of Americans 50 years and older exercise regularly.[5,6] Several reasons are given for this epidemic interest in regularly performed exercise: improved cardiovascular fitness, weight reduction, feeling better, positive effects on mental health, increases in leisure time and affluence, and intense efforts by public and private agencies to promote exercise and sports.

With increasing participation in exercise have come several reports of cardiovascular complications and sudden deaths during or following vigorous exercise.[7-39] Opie[7] estimated 1 death per 50,000 player-hours of rugby football, and Vuori and coworkers[33] estimated 1 death per 13,000–26,000 man-hours of cross-country skiing. Recently, Thompson and associates[39] found the incidence of death during jogging for men aged 30 to 64 years was 1 per 7620 joggers or 1 death per 396,000 man-hours of jogging. It has been argued that no proof exists that exercise is dangerous for anyone, inasmuch as there is a per-hour risk of sudden death from occult coronary atherosclerotic disease (CAD), and that sudden death during exercise is a chance event and not a causal occurrence. Koplan[40] has estimated that about 100 deaths per year should occur during jogging, simply by chance alone. Although this argument has statistical validity, Thompson and associates[39] found the rate of death from CAD during jogging in Rhode Island was seven times the estimated death rate from CAD during more sedentary activities. These data suggest that exercise contributes to sudden death in susceptible persons.

Although a number of reports[7–39] have described exercise-related causes of sudden death, there has been no systematic compilation and analysis of these data. This chapter summarizes personal and previously reported necropsy observations[7–33] in 185 conditioned subjects dying suddenly, most of whom had no symptoms of cardiovascular disease when they began exercising regularly. Furthermore, 7 additional individuals are described in whom nonfatal heart disease was unmasked by exercise, and 3 other subjects are discussed who had previously recognized heart disease and who died suddenly during vigorous exercise.

SUDDEN DEATH IN CONDITIONED SUBJECTS AGED ≤ 30 YEARS

Although young conditioned persons engaged in vigorous competitive or noncompetitive sports or exercise epitomize the healthy segment of society, sudden death occurs in such persons and is traumatic for family members and training or coaching staffs.

Personal Series

The 15 subjects who constitute the study group (Tables 1A and 2; Figs. 1 through 5) died suddenly and unexpectedly during or shortly after vigorous exercise. For inclusion in this series, each subject must have been conditioned (defined as exercise performed daily or several times per week) for at least 1 year before death. Ten of the 15 subjects were considered competitive athletes, in that each was an active and well-conditioned member of an organized athletic team (high school [7 subjects], college [1], or professional [1]). It also was necessary that a complete necropsy examination be performed in each patient to exclude traumatic causes of death.

Demographic Data

The 15 conditioned subjects (Table 1A) ranged in age from 13 to 29 years (mean 20) and 13 (87 percent) were males. Types of exercise included running (10), football (4), basketball (4), cross-country track (2), baseball (2), tennis (1), soccer (1), and wrestling (1). Symptoms suggesting heart disease (chest pain and syncope) were, in retrospect, present in 4 subjects (number 1 and numbers 11 through 13, Table 1A), and sudden death was the first manifestation of cardiac disease in the remaining 11 subjects. Four subjects had family histories of ischemic heart disease, but no other family members of victims with hypertrophic cardiomyopathy are known to have the disease.

Necropsy Findings and Causes of Death

The heart weights in the 15 subjects ranged from 280 to 530 grams (mean 401), and only 1 (number 14) had transmural myocardial necrosis or fibrosis. All of the subjects had epicardial coronary arteries free of atherosclerotic plaques. Structural cardiovascular alterations were identified in 14 of the 15 (93 percent) subjects. The remaining subject (number 10, Table 1A), a 21-year-old male who participated in noncompetitive soccer and wrestling, had a normal heart by gross and histologic examination. The 14 subjects with structural alterations had 1 or more congenital coronary, valvular, or myocardial abnormalities (Tables 1A and 2, Figs. 1 through 5). Of the 14 subjects, 7 had cardiac disease that almost certainly caused sudden death: 2, congenital coronary anomalies (origin of the right coronary artery from left sinus of Valsalva [number 4, Table 1A, Fig. 1], hypoplastic coronary arteries [number 6, Table 1A, Fig. 3[37]]), 3, hypertrophic cardiomyopathy (numbers 3, 11, and 14,

Table 1A, Fig. 4), and 2, valvular disease (2 floppy mitral valves [numbers 7 and 12, Table 1A]). Subject number 12 (Table 1A) also had hyperthermia at necropsy. The remaining 7 subjects had cardiac structural alterations *which probably* represent cardiac disease. Of these 7 subjects, 6 had gross and histologic evidence of left ventricular hypertrophy (LVH), 1 had Ebstein's anomaly of the tricuspid valve (number 12, Table 1A, Fig. 5), and 1 had a myocardial bridge over the left anterior descending coronary artery (number 8, Table 1A). Of the 6 subjects with idiopathic LVH, in 5 it was the only structural alteration and none of these 5 individuals had clinical symptoms of cardiac dysfunction.

Thus, of 15 conditioned subjects aged 30 years and younger, 14 (93 percent) had cardiac structural alterations, which almost certainly caused sudden death in 7.

Previously Reported Subjects

Several previous studies[10,14,15,17,20–21,24–32,34] have reported exercise-related sudden death in 72 subjects 30 years and younger (Tables 2 and 3; Figs. 6 through 10). Their ages ranged from 11 to 30 years (mean 19) and 65 (90 percent) were males. Clinically relevant data are scant in most of these reports. The largest series, by Maron and colleagues,[17] reports the causes of sudden and unexpected death in 29 highly conditioned, competitive athletes aged 13 to 30 years (Table 3, Figs. 6 through 9). Sudden death occurred during or just after severe exertion on the athletic field in 22 (76 percent) athletes. Structural cardiovascular abnormalities were identified at necropsy in 28 (97 percent) of the 29 athletes. The most common cause of death in this series was hypertrophic cardiomyopathy, present in 14 (48 percent) athletes (Figs. 6 and 7). Six of the 29 athletes had probable cardiovascular disease, including 6 (21 percent) with idiopathic LVH. Other causes of cardiovascular sudden death were congenital coronary anomalies (3 athletes, Fig. 8), atherosclerotic coronary disease (3 athletes), and ruptured aorta in 2 athletes with Marfan syndrome.

Of 8 conditioned subjects aged 11 to 25 years with exercise-related sudden death reported by Jokl and McClellan[25] (Table 3, Fig. 10), 5 had congenital coronary anomalies, and 1 each had myocarditis, discrete subaortic stenosis, and aortic dissection (non-Marfan). Thus, in this smaller series, congenital coronary anomalies were the most common structural cardiac abnormality found at necropsy in conditioned subjects aged ≤ 30 years dying suddenly during or shortly after exercise.

Of 7 subjects under age 30 years with nontraumatic sudden death reported by Virmani and colleagues,[14] 1 had valvular heart disease (floppy mitral valve), 1 had severe coronary atherosclerosis with acute myocardial infarction, and the remaining 5 had no cardiovascular abnormality identified and had uncertain causes of death.

Thus, of 72 previously reported conditioned subjects (aged 30 years and younger) dying suddenly during exercise, the most common (39 percent) structural cardiac abnormality found at necropsy was congenital coronary anomalies (Table 2). Of the 28 subjects with congenital coronary anomalies, 20 (71 percent) had origin of the left main coronary artery from the right sinus of Valsalva and passage between the aorta and pulmonary trunk (Fig. 8); 3 (11 percent) had origin of the right coronary from the left sinus of Valsalva and passage between the aorta and pulmonary trunk (Fig. 1); 2 (7 percent) subjects had a single epicardial coronary artery; 2 (7 percent) had origin of the left coronary artery from the pulmonary trunk; and 1 had hypoplastic epicardial coronary arteries (Figs. 3, 10). The second most common structural cardiac abnormality causing exercise-related sudden death was hypertrophic cardiomyopathy (including discrete subaortic stenosis), which was observed in 22 percent (Figs. 4 and 7). Other cardiovascular abnormalities (Table 2) included atherosclerotic heart disease (6 percent), floppy mitral valves (3 percent), idiopathic dilated cardiomyopathy, and myocarditis (1 percent each). The remaining 17 subjects (17 percent) had traumatic or undetermined causes of exercise-related sudden death.

Table 1A. Certain clinical and morphologic observations in 15 conditioned athletes dying suddenly during or shortly after exercise (age at death ≤ 30 years)

	Case 1 (LL)	Case 2 (JE)	Case 3 (JW)	Case 4 (TB)	Case 5 (CJ)	Case 6 (RB)[37]	Case 7 (KR)	Case 8 (GP)	Case 9 (RV)	Case 10 (JT)	Case 11 (BK)	Case 12 (BM)	Case 13 (KB)	Case 14 (LG)	Case 15 (JN)	Subtotal
Age (yr)	13	15	16	17	17	17	17	17	18	21	23	24	26	29	29	m = 20
Sex	F	M	M	M	M	F	M	M	M	M	M	M	M	M	M	13M 2F
Race	W	W	W	B	B	B	W	W	W	W	W	W	B	W	W	11W 4B
Type E	T, R, So, BB	R, CC	R, FB	BkB	R	R	R, CC, Bkb	BB	R, FB	Wr, So, H	Bkb	R	BKb	FB, R	R	
Yrs E	—	many	many	—	—	3	several	—	several	—	several	—	several	several	several	
Running HX Yrs	—	—	—	—	several	3	—	—	—	—	—	5	—	—	several	
Wkly Mi	—	—	—	—	—	65	—	—	—	—	—	70	—	—	—	
C/NC	C^b	C^b	C^b	C^b	NC	C^b	C^b	C^b	C^g	NC	NC	C	NC	C^i	NC	10C 5NC
FH HD	+	+	0	0	0	0	+	0	0	0	—	0	0	+	—	4/13
CP	+^a	0	0	0	0	0	0	0	0	0	—^h	0^h	0^h	0	0	1/14
Int. from last PE	67 da	—	—	17 mo	—	75 da	4 yr	2 yr	—	—	—	—	4 mo	—	—	
SAP (mm Hg)	—	—	—	140/80	—	110/70	145/70	—	N	—	—	—	N	—	—	
TC (mg/dl)	—	—	—	—	—	—	—	—	—	—	—	—	—	—	—	
Abn ECG Re	0	—^c	—	—^c	—	0	—	—	—	—	—	—^c	—	—	—	0/2
Abn ECG E	—	—	—	—	—	—	—	—	—	—	—	—	—	—	—	

12

BW (lb)	Ht (in)	HW (g)	LV Tm (N)	(Fi)	No. 3 CA ↓ >75% XSA	No. 5 mm CA segments ↓ >75% XSA	COR	VALVE	PRIM MYO	Other	Cause of Death
120	67	340	0	0	0	—	0	0	0	ILVH	Uncertain
175	70	430	0	0	0	—	0	0	0	ILVH	Uncertain
185	74	440	0	0	0	—	0	0	+	0	HC
180	74	440	0	0	0	—	+ (cong)	0	0	0	R From L[a]
158	68	405	0	0	0	—	0	0	0	ILVH[e]	Uncertain
147	66	280	0	0	0	—	+ (cong)	0	0	0	Hypoplastic CA[f]
190	72	530	0	0	0	—	0	+	0	ILVH	FMV
144	71	350	0	0	0	—	0	0	0	ILVH	Uncertain[f]
225	70	330	0	0	0	—	0	0	0	ILVH	Uncertain
140	70	350	0	0	0	—	0	0	0	0	Uncertain
190	75	400	0	0	0	—	0	0	+	0*	HC
130	69	450	0	0	0	—	0	+	0	0	FMV + HS
170	77	380	0	0	0	—	0	0	0	ILVH	Uncertain
—	—	550	0	+	0	—	0	+[k]	+	0	HC
150	69	340	m = 401	0	1	0	2 (cong)	3	3	0	7

Please note: The following abbreviations apply to Tables 1A and 1B; footnotes at end of Table 1B apply to both Tables.

Abbreviations: Abn = abnormal/abnormality; ACHD = atherosclerotic coronary heart disease; AMI = acute myocardial infarction; B = black; BB = baseball; Bkb = basketball; BW = body weight; C = competitive; CA = epicardial coronary artery; CAD = coronary atherosclerotic disease; CC = cross country track; Cong = congenital; COR = coronary; CP = chest pain; CV = cardiovascular; da = days; E = exercise; ECG = electrocardiogram; F = female; FB = football; FH HD = family history of heart disease; Fi = fibrosis (scar); FMV = floppy mitral valve (mitral valve prolapse); g = grams; H = hiking; HC = hypertrophic cardiomyopathy; HS = heat stroke; Ht = height; HW = heart weight; ILVH = idiopathic left ventricular hypertrophy; in = inches; int = interval; lb = pounds; LV = left ventricular; M = male; Mi = miles; mo = months; N = necrosis; NC = non-competitive; No. = number; PE = physical exam; PRIM MYO = primary cardiomyopathy (excludes secondary effects of CAD); R = running; Re = rest; R → L = right Ca arising from left sinus of Valsalva; SAP = systemic arterial pressure; So = soccer; T = tennis; TC = total serum cholesterol; Tm = transmural; W = white; Wkly = weekly; Wr = wrestling; XSA = cross-sectional area narrowing; yr = year.

13

Table 1B. Certain clinical and morphologic observation in 12 conditioned athletes dying suddenly during or shortly after exercise (age at death > 30 years)

	Case 1 (JH)	Case 2 (PS)[35]	Case 3 (LW)[35]	Case 4 (TV)	Case 5 (DW)[35]	Case 6 RH	Case 7 (GB)[35]	Case 8 (RB)[36]	Case 9 (RH)	Case 10 (JL)	Case 11 (DC)[35]	Case 12 (BS)	Subtotal	Total (n = 27) (Tables 1A + 1B)
Age (yr)	37	40	40	41	46	47	49	51	51	52	53	65	m = 48	13–65 (32)
Sex	M	M	M	M	M	M	M	M	M	M	M	M	12 M	25 M / 2 F
Race	W	W	W	W	W	W	W	W	W	W	W	W	12 W	23 W / 4 B
Type E	R	R	R	R, BB	R	R	R	R	R	R, T	R	R		
Yrs E	8	5	1	10	3	5	10	5	1	several	5	12	1–12	1–12
Running Hx Yrs	several	5	1	10	3	5	10	5	1	several	5	12	1–12	1–12
Wkly Mi	—	30	69	15	42	10	107	19	4	>10	14	55		
C/NC	NC	NC	NC	NC	C[n]	NC	C[p]	NC	NC	NC	NC	NC[u]	2 C / 10 NC	12 C / 15 NC
FH HD	+	0	+	+	0	0	+	0	0	—	+	+	6/11	10/24 (42%)
CP	+[l]	0	0	0	0	0	+[q]	0	+[r]	+[s]	0	0	4/12	5/26 (19%)
Int. from last PE	1 yr	—	90 da	—	2 da	3 yr	320 da	120 da	33 da	—	45 da	14 da		
SAP (mm Hg)	Sh	140/80	130/80	N	135/100	145/95	160/100	140/95	120/80	N	130/70	120/70		
TC (mg/dl)	↑[m]	—	240	—	310	↑[m]	305	273	278	—	468	345		
Abn ECG Re	0	0	0	0	+	+	+	+	0	0	0	0	4	4/14 (29%)
Abn ECG E	0	—	0	—	0	0	+	—	+	0	0	—	2/8	2/8
BW (lb)	—	180	169	180	172	190	163	163	—	—	174	139		
Ht (in)	—	71	65	70	68	72	68	64	—	—	71	—		

14

HW (g)	430	385	460	450	380	500	480	390	320	380	425	345	m = 412	m = 406
LV Tm (N)	0	0	0	0	0	0	0	0	0	0	0	+	1	1 (4%)
(Fi)	0	+	+	0	+(o)	+	+	+	0	+(t)	0	0	7	8 (30%)
No. 3 CA ↓ >75% XSA	3	3	3	1	3	2	3	2	3	3	3	1	12	12 (44%)
No. 5 mm CA Segments ↓> 75% XSA	14/35 (40%)	27/54 (40%)	10/58 (17%)	—	31/55 (56%)	—	—	9/53 (17%)	15/88 (77%)	—	15/44 (34%)	3/63 (5%)	124/450 (28%)	
Type CV Abn COR	+ (CAD)	+ (CAD)	+ (CAD)	+ (CAD)	+ (CAD)	+ (CAD)	+ (CAD)	+ (CAD)	+ (CAD)	+ (CAD)	+ (CAD)	+ (CAD)	12	14 (52%)
VALVE	0	0	0	0	0	0	0	0	0	0	0	0	0	3 (11%)
PRIM	0	0	0	0	0	0	0	0	0	0	0	0	0	3 (11%)
MYO														
Other	0	0	0	0	0	0	0	0	0	0	0	0	0	7 (26%)
Cause of Death	ACHD	ACHD	ACHD	ACHD	ACHD	ACHD	ACHD	ACHD	ACHD	ACHD	ACHD	ACHD (AMI)		

a Chest pain while playing 8 years before death
b High school competition
c Ventricular fibrillation at resuscitation
d High take-off CA
e LVFW = 16, VS = 17 mm
f Tunneled CA
g College
h History of syncope with exertion
i Professional
j Abnormal intramural coronary arteries + extensive scar
k Mild Ebstein's anomaly of tricuspid valve
l Onset 5 years before death and several years after starting to exercise
m Abnormal lipid plaques in ascending aorta
n Completed one 42-km race
o Posterior LV aneurysm with scarred and atrophied papillary muscle
p Completed 6 Boston 42-km marathon races and 7 JFK 80-km races
q Onset 8 years after beginning running and occurring only during running
r Chest pain while running with onset 1 year after beginning to run
s Onset of chest pain while playing tennis (AMI) and death 45 days later
t Posterior LV aneurysm
u Four YMCA awards for 1000 mile/year club, ran over 3500 miles between 1970-1974. No marathon races. Decreased miles/week because of hip problems

Table 2. Causes of sudden death in 87 necropsy athletes age $\leq$ 30 years dying during or shortly after exercise

Condition	Present Study Ages 13–29 (20) 13 M (87%)	Previous Studies Ages 11–30 (19) 65 M (90%)	Total Ages 11–30 (20) 78 M (90%)
A. Congenital Coronary Anomaly	2 (13%)	28 (39%)	30 (35%)
1. Origin of LM from R sinus of Valsalva	(0)	(20)	(20)
2. Origin of R from L sinus of Valsalva	(1)	(3)	(4)
3. Origin of L from pulmonary trunk	(0)	(2)	(2)
4. Single coronary artery	(0)	(2)	(2)
5. Hypoplastic R, L, or both coronary arteries	(1)	(1)	(2)
B. Atherosclerotic Coronary Heart Disease	0	4 (6%)	4 (5%)
C. Hypertrophic Cardiomyopathy	3 (21%)	16 (22%)[c]	19 (22%)
D. Rupture or Dissection Ascending Aorta	0	3 (4%)	3 (3%)
E. Valvular Heart Disease	2 (13%)	2 (3%)	4 (5%)
1. Floppy mitral valve	(2)	(2)	(4)
F. Idiopathic Dilated Cardiomyopathy	0	1 (1%)	1 (1%)
G. Myocarditis	0	1 (1%)	1 (1%)
H. Trauma	0	1 (1%)	1 (1%)
I. Uncertain	8 (53%)[a]	16 (23%)[b]	24 (27%)
TOTALS:	15 (100%)	72 (100%)	87 (100%)

[a]Of 8 subjects, 6 had idiopathic left ventricular hypertrophy (ILVH).
[b]Of 16 subjects, 4 had ILVH.
[c]Includes 1 subject with discrete subaortic stenosis.

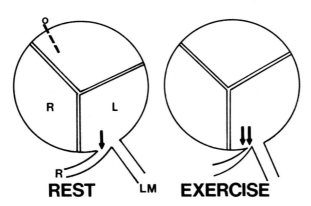

REST   LM   **EXERCISE**

Figure 1. T.B. (number 4), Table 1A. Anomalous origin of the right (R) coronary artery from the left (L) sinus of Valsalva. The R ostium has an acute angle take-off (arrows, *upper*) that becomes slitlike with exercise (arrows, *lower*). Ao = aorta; LM = left main coronary artery.

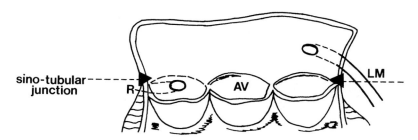

Figure 2. T.B. (number 4), Table 1A. Diagram showing high take-off position of the left main (LM) coronary ostium observed in this athlete. The anomalous origin of the right (R) coronary artery from the left sinus of Valsalva is not depicted. AV = aortic valve.

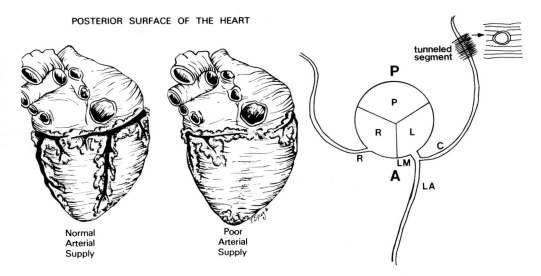

Figure 3. R.B. (number 6), Table 1A. *Left,* Diagram of posterior surface of the heart showing normal and poor arterial supply. Diminished arterial supply to the posterior ventricular surface appeared to result from congenitally hypolastic right (R) and left circumflex (LC) coronary arteries. (From Maron, BJ, Roberts, WC, McAllister, HA, et al[17], with permission.) *Right,* Diagram of the coronary arterial tree depicting a tunneled segment of LC coronary artery. A = anterior; LAD = left anterior descending; LM = left main; P = posterior.

Table 3. Summary of certain clinical and morphologic observations in 158 previously reporte...

First Author	Year Published	Age (Yrs)	Sex	Type(s) Exercise	No. Yrs.	Ma	Wkly	FH HD	AP	Hx AMI	Int. from Last Exam	SH	TC	RS	E
Opie (7)	1975	—	7 M	V	—	+[b]	—	—	—	—	—	—	—	—	—
Opie (8)	1975	—	M	R	—	+[b]	—	—	—	—	—	—	—	—	—
Green (9)	1976	44	M	R	8	+[d]	50	0	0	0	1 da	—	—	0	—
Cantwell (10)	1978	28	M	R	—	—	25	0	0	0	—	—	—	—	—
Noakes (11)	1979	41	M	R	Many[g]	+	—	—	0	0	—	0[h]	—	0	—
Noakes (12)	1979	44	M	R	1.2	+[i]	30–50	—			—	0[h]	296	—	—
		41	M	R	>2	+	—[j]	—	+[j]	+[j]	—[k]	—	265	+	—
		36	M	R	7	+	50[l]	—	0	0	26 mo	0	—	0	0
		27	M	Rug, FB R	1.2[m]	+	—	—	—	—	—	—	—	—	—
		38	M	R	3	+[n]	—	—	—	—	—	—	—	—	—
Thompson (13)	1979	—[o]	17M 1F	R	—	—	—[p]	5/13	0[q]	1[r]	10/13 ≤ 1 yr	(125)[s] (75)	(200)[s]	3	0/4[t]
Virmani (14)	1982	27[x]	M	R	5	+	70	—	+	—	—	+	N[w]	—	—
		33[x]	M	R	1	0	—	+	+	—	—	0	275	—	—
		37[x]	M	R	1	0	—	0	0	+	—	+	214	—	—
		38[x]	M	R	0.5	0	—	—	+	—	—	0	—	—	—
		41[x]	M	R	0.5	0	—	0	0	+	—	+	—	—	—
		41[x]	M	R	12	0	42	0	0	+	—	0	—	—	—
		50[x]	M	R	28	0	14	0	+	0	—	+	274	—	—
		57[x]	M	R	4	0	—	0	+	0	—	+	—	—	—
		18	M	R	0.5	0	—	—	0	0	—	—	—	—	—
		22	M	R	1	0	—	—	0	0	—	+	—	—	—
		22	M	R	0.5	0	—	—	0	0	—	—	—	—	—
		26	M	R	1	0	21	0	0	0	—	0	160	—	—
		27	M	R	2	0	14	0	0	0	—	—	—	—	—
		29	M	R	0.5	0	—	—	0	0	—	—	—	—	—
		31	M	R	2	0	—	—	0	0	—	—	—	—	—
		31	M	R	14	0	84	—	0	0	—	—[y]	—	—	—
		33	M	R	0.5	0	—	0	0	0	—	+	↑	—	—
		38	M	R	3	0	28	+	0	0	—	+	—	—	—
		38	M	R	23	+	105	+	0	0	—	0[y]	—	—	—
		39	M	R	18	0	12	+	0	0	—	0	240	—	—
		40	M	R	16	0	7	0	0	0	—	0	—	—	—
		40	M	R	3.5	0	7	0	0	0	—	0	—	—	—
		42	M	R	3	0	21	+	0	0	—	0	220	—	—
		42	M	R	3	+	50	+	0	0	—	+	242	—	—
		42	M	R	3	0	21	+	0	0	—	0	220	—	—
		42	M	R	3.5	0	7	0	0	0	—	—	—	—	—
		44	M	R	1	0	—	+	0	0	—	+	—	—	—
		45	M	R	5	0	35	0	0	0	—	0	—	—	—
		45	M	R	28	0	21	+	0	0	—	+	—	—	—
		46	M	R	4	0	21	0	0	0	—	0	—	—[bb]	—
Roberts (15)	1982	17	M	Bkb	—	—	—	—	—	0	0	—	—	—	—
Siegel (16)	1982	54	F	R	1	—	14	—	0	0[dd]	—	—	—	—	—
		46	M	R	—	—	—	—	0	0[dd]	—	—	—	—	—
Maron (17)[ee]	1980	13	M	Bkb, FB, R	—	—	—	+	—	—	—	—	—	—	—
		14[ff]	M	W	—	—	—	+	—	—	—	—	—	+[gg]	—
		14[ff]	M	R	—	—	—	+	—	—	—	—	—	+[hh]	—
		17	F	G	—	—	—	+	—	—	—	—	—	—	—
		17	M	R	—	—	—	0	—	—	—	—	—	—[ii]	—
		17[ff]	M	FB	—	—	—	—	—	—	—	—	—	+[ii]	—
		17	M	W	—	—	—	+	—	—	—	—	—	—	—
		17	M	Bkb	—	—	—	+	—	—	—	—	—	—	—
		19	M	R, Bkb	—	—	—	+	—	—	—	—	—	—	—
		20[ff]	M	Bkb	—	—	—	+	—	—	—	—	—	+[jj]	—

HW (g)	LV Tm N	LV Tm Fi	Major CA ↓ >75% in XSA (no.)	Mode of Death	Type Cardiac Abnormality			Cause of Death
					Cor	Valve	Prim Myo	
—	—	—	—[a]	7S	+(CAD)	0	0	7 ACHD
—	—	—	—[c]	S	+(CAD)	0	0	ACHD
350	+[e]	0	0	S	0	0	0	Uncertain
—	0	0	0[f]	S	0	0	0	Uncertain
460	0	0	0	S	0	0	+	HC
357	0	+	(2)	S	+(CAD)	0	0	ACHD
344	0	+	(3)	S[k]	+(CAD)	0	0	ACHD
360	0	0	(1)	S	+(CAD)	0	0	Trauma
350	(SE)	0	0	S	0	0	0	Trauma
—	0	0	0	S	0	0	0	Trauma
—	2	4	13/18 pts[u]	18S	13(CAD)[v]	0	+[l]	13 ACHD (2AMI) 1 Myoc 3Uncert 1HS
420	0	0	0	S	0	+	0	Floppy MV
400	0	0	(2)	S	+(CAD)	0	0	ACHD
600	0	+	(2)	S	+(CAD)	0	0	ACHD
420	0	+	(1)	S	+(CAD)	0	0	ACHD
370	0	+	(2)	S	+(CAD)	0	0	ACHD
550	+	+	(2)	S	+(CAD)	0	0	ACHD(AMI)
450	0	0	severe	S	+(CAD)	0	0	ACHD
350	+	+	(1)	S	+(CAD)	0	0	ACHD(AMI)
345	0	0	0	S	0	0	0	Uncertain
440	0	0	0	S	0	0	0	Uncertain
400	0	0	0	S	0	0	0	Uncertain
400	0	0	0	S	0	0	0	Uncertain
350	+	0	(3)	S	+(CAD)	0	0	ACHD(AMI)
345	0	0	0	S	0	0	0	Uncertain
440	0	0	0	S	0	0	0	Uncertain
480	0	0	(1)	S[z]	+(CAD)	0	0	ACHD
400	0	0	0	S	0	0	0	Uncertain
350	+	0	(1)	S[z]	+(CAD)	0	0	ACHD(AMI)
460	0	0	(4)	S	+(CAD)	0	0	ACHD
480	0	+	(2)	S	+(CAD)	0	0	ACHD
450	+	0	(2)	S[aa]	+(CAD)	0	0	ACHD(AMI)
430	+	0	(1)	S	+(CAD)	0	0	ACHD(AMI)
350	0	0	(1)	S[aa]	+(CAD)	0	0	ACHD
425	+	0	severe	S	+(CAD)	0	0	ACHD
350	0	0	(1)	S[aa]	+(CAD)	0	0	ACHD
430	0	0	(1)	S	+(CAD)	0	0	ACHD
500	0	+	(2)	S	+(CAD)	0	0	ACHD
400	0	0	(2)	S	+(CAD)	0	0	ACHD
510	+	+	(1)	S[z]	+(CAD)	0	0	ACHD(AMI)
375	0	+	(2)[cc]	S	+(CAD)	0	0	ACHD
440	0	0	0	S	+(Cong)	0	0	R from L
—	—	—	—	—	0	0	+	Amyloid
—	—	—	—	—	0	0	+	Amyloid
450	0	0	0	S	0	0	+	HC
390	0	0	0	S	0	0	+	HC
360	0	0	0	S	0	0	+	HC
440	0	0	0	S	0	0	+	HC
530	0	0	0	S	0	0	+	HC
370	0	0	0	S	+(Tun Ca)	0	+	HC
460	0	0	0	S	0	0	+	HC
490	0	0	0	S	+(Cong)	0	+	HC (L from R)
475	0	0	0	S	0	0	+	HC
630	0	0	0	S	0	0	+	HC
500	0	0	0	S	0	0	+	HC

Table 3. Summary of certain clinical and morphologic observations in 158 previously reported

First Author	Year Published	Age (Yrs)	Sex	Type(s) Exercise	Running Hx No. Yrs.	Miles Ma	Miles Wkly	FH HD	AP	Hx AMI	Int. from Last Exam	SH	TC	Abn ECG RS	Abn ECG E
		22	M	Box	—	—	—	+	—	—	—	—	—	—	—
		23[ff]	M	Bkb	—	—	—	0	—	—	—	—	—	+[kk]	+
		24	M	Bab	—	—	—	+	—	—	—	—	—	—	—
		30[ff]	F	T	—	—	—	—	—	—	—	—	—	+[ll]	—
		16	M	Bkb	—	—	—	0	—	—	—	—	—	—	—
		16	M	R	—	—	—	0	—	—	—	—	—	—	—
		17	M	So	—	—	—	0	—	—	—	—	—	—	—
		17	M	Bkb	—	—	—	0	—	—	—	—	—	—	—
		28	M	—	—	—	—	—	—	—	—	—	—	—	—
		17	F	R	—	—	—	—	—	—	—	—	—	—	—
		17	—	—	—	—	—	—	—	—	—	—	—	—	—
		17	—	—	—	—	—	—	—	—	—	—	—	—	—
		22	—	—	—	—	—	—	—	—	—	—	—	—	—
		24	M	—	—	—	—	—	—	—	—	—	—	—	—
		26	M	—	—	—	—	—	—	—	—	—	—	—	—
		28	M	FB	—	—	—	—	—	—	—	—	—	—	—
		18[ff]	M	Bkb	—	—	—	—	—	—	—	—	—	0	—
		21	M	Bab	—	—	—	—	—	—	—	—	—	—	—
		14	M	FB	—	—	—	0	—	—	—	—	—	—	—
Ullyot (18)	1976	—	M	R	many	0	—[mm]	—	—	—	—	—	—	—	—
Warren (19)	1979	28	F	T	many	—	—	+	0[nn]	0	>2 yr	0	—	0[oo]	0
Tsung (20)	1982	17	M	FB	—	—	—	+	0	0	—	0	—	—	—
		14	M	Bkb	—	—	—	—	0	0	—	0	—	—	—
		18	M	FB	—	—	—	—	0	0	—	0	—	—	—
		18	M	FB	—	—	—	—	0	0	—	0	—	—	—
James (21)	1967	18	M	FB	—	—	—	0	0[pp]	0	2.5 yr	—	—	—	—
		15	M	W	—	—	—	0	0	0	9 mo	—	—	—	—
Roberts (22)	1981	—	M	FB	—	—	—	+	0[rr]	0	6 wk	0	350	0	—
Colt (23)	1980	49	M	R	—	+	—	—	—	—	—	—	—	—	—
		49	M	R	—	—	—	—	—[ss]	—	—	—	—	—	—
Hanzlick (24)	1983	26	M	R, WL	—	+	—	—	—[tt]	—	—	—	—	—	—
Jokl (25)	1971	45	M	W	>20	—	—	—	0	0	—	—	—	—	—
		16	M	Bkb	—	—	—	—	—	—	—	—	—	—	—
		25	M	G, R	several	—	several	—	—	—	few da	—	—	—	—
		32	M	R, Rug	—	—	—	—	—	—	—	—	—	—	—
		24	M	R	—	—	—	—	—	—	—	—	—	—	—
		22	F	Sk	—	—	—	—	—	—	—	—	—	—	—
		14	M	R	—	—	—	—	—	—	—	—	—	—	—
		11	M	R	—	—	—	—	—	—	—	—	—	—	—
		16	F	D	—	—	—	—	—	—	—	—	—	—	—
		15	M	WL, W	—	—	—	—	—	—	—	—	—	—	—
Roberts (26)	1947	22	M	H	—	—	—	—	—	—	—	—	—	—	—
Rotter (27)	1952	16	M	V	—	—	—	—	—	—	—	—	—	—	—
Nieod (28)	1952	21	M	—	—	—	—	—	—	—	—	—	—	—	—
Cohen (29)	1967	11	M	R	—	—	—	—	—	—	—	—	—	—	—
Benson (30)	1968	13	M	R	—	—	—	—	—	—	—	—	—	—	—
		13	M	Bkb	—	—	—	—	—	—	—	—	—	—	—
Cheitlin (31)	1974	14	M	—	—	—	—	—	—	—	—	—	—	—	—
		18	M	R	—	—	—	—	—	—	—	—	—	—	—
		17	M	R	—	—	—	—	—	—	—	—	—	—	—
		18	M	R	—	—	—	—	—	—	—	—	—	—	—
		22	M	R	—	—	—	—	—	—	—	—	—	—	—
		20	M	Mar	—	—	—	—	—	—	—	—	—	—	—
		22	M	R	—	—	—	—	—	—	—	—	—	—	—
Liberthson (32)	1979	11	M	—	—	—	—	—	—	—	—	—	—	—	—
		17	M	—	—	—	—	—	—	—	—	—	—	—	—
Vuori (33)	1978	49 (mean)	22 M	2R 16 Ski 4 V	—	—	—	—	—	—	—	—	—	—	—

necropsy subjects dying during or shortly after exercise (*Continued*)

HW (g)	LV Tm N	LV Tm Fi	Major CA ↓ > 75% in XSA (no.)	Mode of Death	Type Cardiac Abnormality			Cause of Death
					Cor	Valve	Prim Myo	
500	0	0	0	S	0	0	+	HC
490	0	0	0	S	0	0	+	HC
530	0	0	0	S	0	0	+	HC
440	0	0	0	S	0	0	(LVH)	Uncertain
420	0	0	0	S	0	0	(LVH)	Uncertain
530	0	0	0	S	0	+(FMV)	0	Uncertain
465	0	0	0	S	0	0	(LVH)	Uncertain
465	0	0	0	S	0	0	(LVH)	Uncertain
280	0	0	0	S	+(Cong)	0	0	Hypoplastic + Tun Ca
—	0	0	0	S	+(Cong)	0	0	L from R
—	0	0	0	S	+(Cong)	0	0	L from R
—	0	0	0	S	+(Cong)	0	0	L from R
—	0	0	(1)	S	+(CAD)	0	0	ACHD
—	0	+	(3)	S	+(CAD)	0	0	ACHD
—	0	+	(3)	S	+(CAD)	0	0	ACHD
—	0	0	0	S	0	+(AR)	0	Rupture AA (Marfan's)
—	0	0	0	S	0	0	0	Rupture AA (Marfan's)
—	0	0	0	S	0	0	0	Uncertain
—	—	—	—	S	+(CAD)	0	0	ACHD
500	+	+	0	S	0	0	+	IDC
650	0	0	0	S	0	0	+	HC
450	0	0	0	S	+(Cong)	0	0	L from R
480	0	0	0	S	+(Cong)	0	0	L from R
410	0	0	0	S	0	0	0	Uncertain
—	0	0	0qq	S	0	0	0	Uncertain
—	0	0	0qq	S	0	0	0	Uncertain
410	0	+	(3)	S	+(CAD)	0	0	ACHD
—	+	—	+	S	+(CAD)	0	0	ACHD(AMI)
—	—	+	+	S	+(CAD)	0	0	ACHD
420	—	—	—	S	+(Cong)	0	0	R and L
350	0	+	3	S	+(CAD)	0	0	ACHD
600	—	—	0	S	+(Cong)	0	0	L from R
—	—uu	0	0	S	0	0	+	Myoc
482	0	+	0	S	+(Cong)	0	0	Hypoplastic
—	0	+	0	S	+(Cong)	0	0	L from PT
—	0	+	0	S	+(Cong)	0	0	Single
—	0	0	0	S	+(Cong)	0	0	R from L
—	+	—	0	Svv	+(Cong)	0	0	L from R
—	—	—	—	S	0	0	+	DSAS
—	—	—	—		0	0	0	Ao Dis
—	—	—	—	S	+(Cong)	0	0	Single
—	—	—	—	S	+(Cong)	0	0	L from PT
—	—	—	—	S	+(Cong)	0	0	L from R
—	—	—	—	S	+(Cong)	0	0	L from R
—	—	—	—	S	+(Cong)	0	0	L from R
—	—	—	—	S	+(Cong)	0	0	L from R
—	—	—	—	S	+(Cong)	0	0	L from R
—	—	—	—	S	+(Cong)	0	0	L from R
—	—	—	—	S	+(Cong)	0	0	L from R
—	—	—	—	S	+(Cong)	0	0	L from R
—	—	—	—	S	+(Cong)	0	0	L from R
—	—	—	—	S	+(Cong)	0	0	L from R
—	—	—	—	S	+(Cong)	0	0	L from R
—	—	—	—	S	+(Cong)	0	0	L from R
—	—	—	—	S	+(Cong)	0	0	L from R
—	—	—	—	S	19(CAD)	—4—	—ww	19 ACHD 4 CV

Table 3. Summary of certain clinical and morphologic observations in 158 previously reported

First Author	Year Published	Age (Yrs)	Sex	Type(s) Exercise	Running Hx No. Yrs	Miles Ma	Miles Wkly	FH HD	Hx AP	Hx AMI	Int. from Last Exam	SH	TC	Abn ECG RS	Abn ECG E
Morales (34)	1980	54	M	R	—	—	—	—	0	0	—	—	—	+[yy]	+
		34	M	R	—	—	—	—	0	0	—	—	—	—	—
		17	F	Sw	—	—	—	—	0[xx]	0	—	—	—	—	—
TOTALS: (No. = 158)		11–57 (27)	146M:9F (94%) (6%)		13			22	6	5		160–350 (251)		11	2

Abbreviations: AA = aortic aneurysm; Abn = abnormal, ACHD = atherosclerotic coronary heart disease; AMI = acute myocardial infarction; AP = angina pectoris; Ao Dis = aortic dissection (non-Marfans); Bab = baseball; Bkb = basketball; Box = boxing; CA = epicardial coronary arteries; CAD = coronary artery disease; Cong = congenital coronary anomaly; COR = coronary; CV = cardiovascular abnormality; D = dancing; da = days; DSAS = discrete subaortic stenosis; E = exercise treadmill; ECG = electrocardiogram; F = female; FB = football; FHHD = family history of heart disease; Fi = fibrosis; g = grams; G = gymnastics; H = hiking; HC = hypertrophic cardiomyopathy; HS = heart stroke; HW = heart weight; Hx = history; IDC = idiopathic dilated cardiomyopathy; Int = interval; L from R = left CA arising from right sinus of Valsalva; LV = left ventricular myocardial; M = male; Ma = marathon runner; Mar = marching; mo = months; MV = mitral valve; Myoc = myocarditis; N = necrosis; No. = number; PRIM MYO = primary myocardial abnormality (excludes myocardial damage resulting from ACHD); pt = patient; R = running; R from L = right CA arising from left sinus of Valsalva; Rs = resting; Rug = rugby; S = sudden; SE = subendocardial; SH = systemic hypertension (history of systolic >140 and/or diastolic >90 mmHg); Sk = skipping rope; Ski = skiing; SW = swimming; T = tennis; TC = total serum cholesterol (mg/dl); Tm = transmural; TunCa = tunneled ("bridged") coronary artery; V = variety; W = wrestling; WK = week; WL = weight lifting; XSA = cross-sectional area; Yr = year.

[a]Severe coronary atheromata at necropsy. Details of the 7 individual sportsmen were not provided.

[b]Completed several 32-Km runs

[c]Marked coronary narrowing

[d]Completed several 42-Km races

[e]Resuscitated during race but remained comatose and died 50 days later from infection

[f]Only 1 epicardial coronary artery shown as normal

[g]Completed one 84-Km and one 42-Km race

[h]Normal but no value given

[i]Completed nine 42-Km races, one 56-Km race, one 90-km race, and one 50-km race

[j]Ran several marathons before AMI 28 months before death, and at least 5 marathons and 3624 Km after AMI. Continued to have angina during training after AMI

[k]Hospitalized awaiting bypass surgery and had second fatal AMI

[l]Completed at least 28 marathons over 7 years, including 90-Km and 160-Km track race

[m]Completed four 42-Km races or longer races in 14 months of long distance running

[n]One 42-Km race

[o]13 men with CAD were aged ≥ 42 years. Data reported collectively on 18 pts

[p]14/18 had exercised regularly at least 1 year, 9 for 3 or more years, 2 ≤ 1 month (both with CAD) including 1 for only 9 days. Six ran >160 Km/month and 4 subjects ran >96 Km/month for at least 1 year. One pt over age 40 years ran 23 miles/day and held many running records for the Master's age group.

[q]Three of 6 runners with prodromal symptoms had stomach discomfort, 2 fatigue, and 1 neck discomfort. All 6 had CAD.

[r]AMI 12 years earlier. Another runner was examined 7 years before death for rule out AMI.

[s]Median values of blood pressure and cholesterol. Six of 8 runners had cholesterols >200 mg/dl.

[t]9 of 13 had rest or exercise tests within 2 years of death; 6/9 resting ECGs were nl and 3/9 had LVH, atrial fib, or inferior infarct pattern; four had exercise tests within 1 year of death: 3/4 ml and 1/4 equivocally normal

[u]CHD diagnosis in 13/18 defined as coronary narrowing >50%, severe, marked, or occlusive atherosclerosis.

necropsy subjects dying during or shortly after exercise (*Continued*)

HW (g)	LV Tm N	LV Tm Fi	Major CA ↓ > 75% in XSA (no.)	Mode of Death	Type Cardiac Abnormality			
					Cor	Valve	Prim Myo	Cause of Death
400	0	+	0	S	+(TunCa)	0	0	Uncertain
460	0	+	0	S	+(TunCa)	0	0	Uncertain
260	0	+	0	S	+(TunCa)	0	0	Uncertain
260–650 (435)	14	27			101 (64%)	3 (2%)	22 (14%)	

[v] Only 1 of 13 had a diagnosis of coronary atherosclerotic heart disease but 6 others had histories of CAD risk factors: 4 SH, 1 AMI by Hx, 1 rule out MI. One also had atrial fibrillation on ECG, and 1 had an abnormal myocardial perfusion scan and was advised to stop running.
[w] Value not provided.
[x] Previous history of coronary atherosclerotic heart disease.
[y] History of TIAs
[z] SD while sleeping
[aa] History of prolonged chest pain
[bb] Of the 30 joggers reported by Virmani, 9 had resting ECGs 2 months to 8 years before death: 5/9 normal, 2 LVH, 1 RBBB (× 8 yrs), 1 VPCs
[cc] Coronary thrombi noted in 6 (27%) runners. Of 70 coronary arteries examined, 34 (49%) were narrowed > 75% (in order of decreasing frequency: LAD, R, LC, LM)
[dd] Gradually diminished the number of kilometers/week because of excessive fatigue and dyspnea.
[ee] All highly conditioned competitive athletes.
[ff] Cardiovascular disease suspected or identified during life
[gg] WPW, history of syncope
[hh] LVH, LVOFT gradient = 15 mm Hg at cath. Clinical dx: HC
[ii] Q waves in 3, AVF, V_5, V_6; precordial murmur clinically diagnosed as VSD
[jj] Deep symmetric T-inversion in 2, 3, AVF, V_3-V_6, LVH.
[kk] Deep, symmetric T-inversion in 1, 2, 3, AVF, V_4-V_6, LVH. Resting LVOFT gradient = 0, but cavity obliteration on LV gram with EF = 95%. VT on exercise test.
[ll] LVH + strain, resting LVOFT gradient = 0. History of mild fatigue.
[mm] Completed 23-mile run 1 day before death, had also won the National Amateur Athletics Union Masters 25-Km race.
[nn] Chest pain while playing tennis and jogging 2 years prior to death.
[oo] LVH interpreted as athlete's heart
[pp] History of syncope
[qq] Marked thickening (hyperplasia) of sinus node artery
[rr] 6 weeks before death aching in shoulders and sweating. Hospitalized but pain disappeared the next day
[ss] Two months prior to death collapsed after hard run.
[tt] Two previous episodes of dyspnea after long runs which were atypical for his normal post-marathon experience.
[uu] Subacute myocarditis with interstitial infiltrates of histiocytes and plasma cells
[vv] Died 24 hours after sudden collapse
[ww] Reported collectively. Cause of death listed as acute or chronic ischemia, coronary heart disease in 9 and other cardiovascular disease in 4.
[xx] Chest pain
[yy] Short PR interval

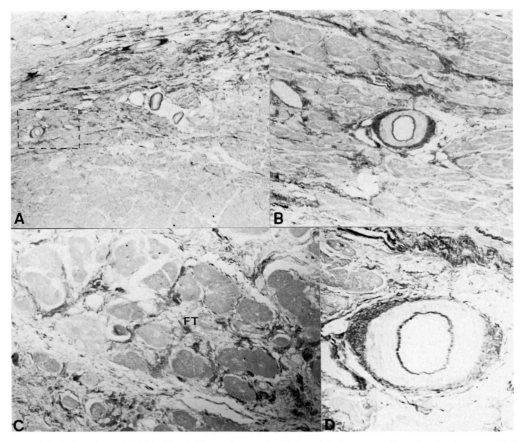

Figure 4. L.G. (number 14), Table 1A. *A*, Photomicrograph of left ventricular myocardium showing hypertrophied myocardial fibers, abnormal intramural coronary arteries, and increased interstitial fibrous tissue (Elastic stain, × 10). *B and D*, Higher magnification of boxed-area in *A*. Abnormally thickened intramural coronary artery (Elastic stains, ×40 and ×80, respectively). *C*, Higher magnification (×80) of left ventricular free wall showing myocardial fiber hypertrophy and extensive interstitial fibrous tissue (FT) (Elastic stain).

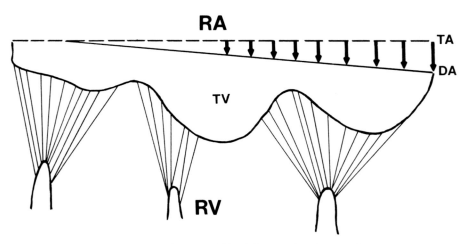

Fibure 5. J.N. (number 15), Table 1A. Diagram of Ebstein's anomaly of tricuspid valve (TV) observed in this athlete. A portion of the annulus (A) is displaced (D) toward right ventricular apex. TA = true annulus; RA = right atrium.

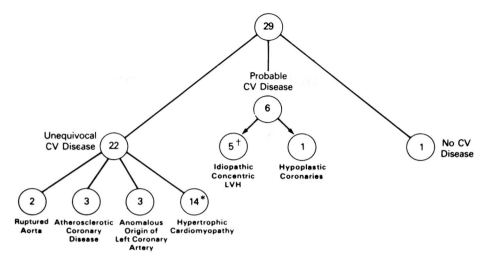

Figure 6. Diagram summarizing the causes of death in 29 competitive athletes. CV = cardiovascular; LVH = left ventricular hypertrophy (From Maron, BJ, Roberts, WC, McAllister, HA, et al,[17] with permission.)

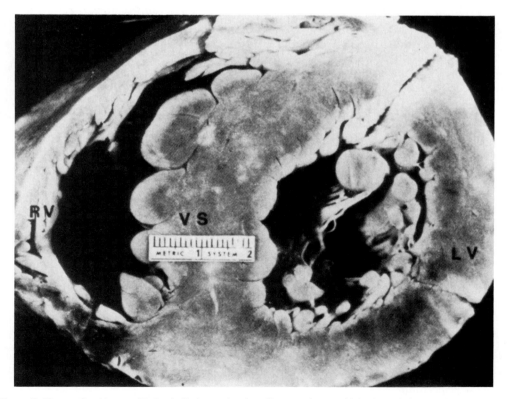

Figure 7. Heart of a 13-year-old football player showing disproportionate thickening of the ventricular septum (VS) with respect to the posterior left ventricular (LV) free wall. RV = right ventricular wall (From Maron, BJ, Roberts, WC, McAllister, HA, et al,[17] with permission.)

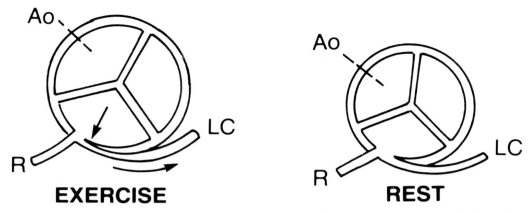

Figure 8. Diagram of anomalous origin of the left coronary (LC) from the right (R) sinus of Valsalva observed in 4 competitive athletes with sudden death studied by Maron et al.[17] During exercise the LC ostium becomes narrowed. Ao = aorta

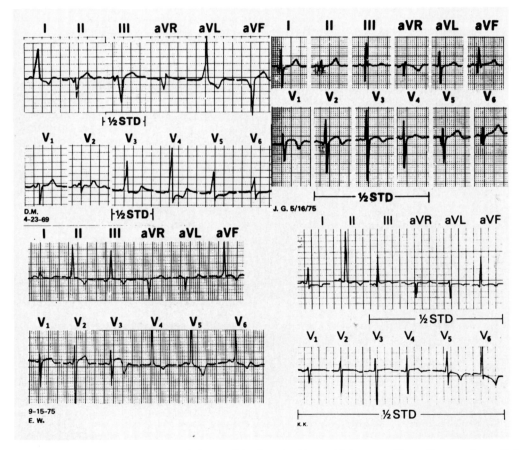

Figure 9. ECGs showing the spectrum of abnormalities from 4 athletes with hypertrophic cardiomyopathy studied at necropsy: *Top left,* From a 14-year-old wrestler showing Wolff-Parkinson-White pattern, diffuse T-wave abnormalities and probable left ventricular hypertrophy (LVH). *Top right,* From a 17-year-old football player with deep Q waves in leads III, aVF, V5, V6, and probable LVH. *Bottom left,* From a 20-year old basketball player showing LVH and T wave abnormalities. *Bottom right,* From a 30-year-old tennis player showing LVH with strain. (From Maron BJ, Roberts, WC, McAllister, HA, et al,[17] with permission.)

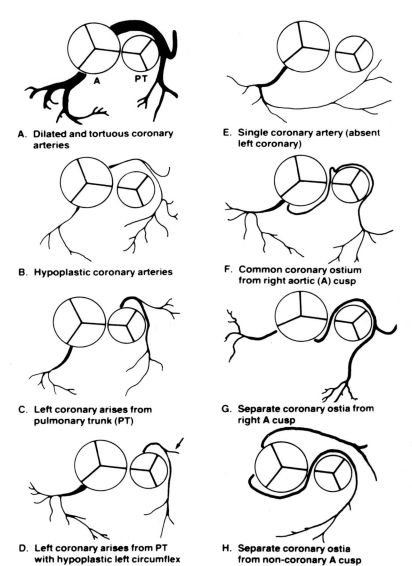

A. Dilated and tortuous coronary arteries

B. Hypoplastic coronary arteries

C. Left coronary arises from pulmonary trunk (PT)

D. Left coronary arises from PT with hypoplastic left circumflex

E. Single coronary artery (absent left coronary)

F. Common coronary ostium from right aortic (A) cusp

G. Separate coronary ostia from right A cusp

H. Separate coronary ostia from non-coronary A cusp

Figure 10. Congenital coronary anomalies associated with sudden death and exercise. (From Jokl, E and McClellan, JT,[25] with permission.)

SUDDEN DEATH IN CONDITIONED SUBJECTS AGED > 30 YEARS

Morphologic observations in exercise-related sudden deaths in conditioned subjects over age 30 years have recently received attention.[12-14,35-39] In this section personal and previously reported necropsy observations in conditioned subjects aged 31 to 65 years will be described.

Personal Series

Of the 12 subjects who constitute this study, 6 have previously been reported.[35,36] All 12 subjects died during or shortly after vigorous exercise. For inclusion in this series, each subject must have been conditioned (defined as exercise performed daily or several times per week) for at least 1 year. Two of the subjects (numbers 5 and 7, Table 1B) were competitive runners having completed 1 or more standard marathons. It was also necessary for inclusion that a complete necropsy examination be performed in each subject.

Demographic Data

The 12 conditioned subjects (Tables 1B and 4 through 6, Figs. 11 through 33) ranged in age from 37 to 65 years (mean 48) and all were males. All of the men were runners, and 1 each participated additionally in tennis and baseball. None of the subjects had symptoms of heart disease *before* starting their conditioning, but 3 subjects (numbers 1, 7, and 9, Table 1B, Figs. 11 and 21 through 24) developed chest pain and/or angina pectoris 2 to 5 years before death. The men had run regularly for 1 to 12 years, covering 4 to 107 miles per week. Runner number 7 (Tables 1B and 4; Figs. 21 through 24) completed six 42-km Boston marathons and 7 JFK 80-km races. Runner number 12 (Table 1B, Figs. 31 and 32) received 4 YMCA awards for the "1000 mile/year club" and had run over 3500 miles during a 4-year period. At least 1 coronary atherosclerotic risk factor was present in 9 of 12 subjects: 4 (33 percent) had systemic hypertension, 7 of 7 with available total serum cholesterol values had levels 240 to 310 mg/dl, and 2 others had ascending aortas morphologically typical of type 2 hyperlipidemia, 6 had other family members with atherosclerotic coronary heart disease, and 5 runners had abnormal resting and/or exercise electrocardiograms (Tables 1B and 4, Figs. 15, 18, 21, 22, and 25).

Necropsy Findings and Causes of Death

The heart weights ranged from 320 to 500 grams (mean 412) (normal adult male heart < 400 grams), with 6 of the 12 hearts weighing greater than 400 grams. Transmural myocardial infarctions were found in 8 of the 12 runners (11 healed, 1 acute), and all 11 healed infarctions were clinically silent. Each of the 12 runners had at least 1 of the 3 major (right, left anterior descending, left circumflex) coronary arteries narrowed 76 to 100 percent in cross-sectional area by atherosclerotic plaques. Seven of the 12 subjects had all 3 arteries so narrowed. No runner had severe left main coronary narrowing. In 8 runners, the entire coronary tree was cut transversely into 5-mm long segments and the degrees of cross-sectional area narrowing graded into 4 categories of percent luminal narrowing: 0 to 25, 26 to 50, 51 to 75, and 76 to 100 percent. The number of segments narrowed 76 to 100 percent in cross-sectional area ranged from 9 to 53 (17 percent) to 31 of 55 segments (56 percent) with an average of 124 of 450 coronary segments (28 percent) so narrowed (Tables 1B and 5, Fig. 33). The cause of sudden death in each of the 12 conditioned subjects over age 30 years was atherosclerotic coronary heart disease. No subject had associated congenital coronary anomalies. One runner (number 5, Table 1B, Figs. 19 and 20) had clinical mitral regurgitation produced by a scarred papillary muscle secondary to a healed inferior myocardial infarction with aneurysm formation. Thus, of 12 conditioned subjects aged 30 years and older, all 12 had fatal atherosclerotic coronary disease.

Previously Reported Subjects

Several previous studies[9,11,12,13,14,16,23,25,33–36,39] have reported causes of death in conditioned subjects over 30 years of age. Few of these studies, however, provide detailed clinical or cardiac morphologic information.

Virmani and colleagues[14] described sudden nontraumatic deaths in 23 men aged 31 to 57 years. Seven of the 23 (30 percent) runners had previous symptoms of coronary heart disease *before* beginning to exercise. Each had run ½ to 28 years and distances from 7 to 105 miles per week. Two runners had completed at least 1 marathon race (Table 3). Of the 23 runners, 21 (91 percent) had severe narrowing by atherosclerotic plaques of at least 1 major coronary artery, and 13 (62 percent) had transmural myocardial infarctions. One runner, a 38-year-old marathoner who had been running 105 miles per week for 23 years, had all 4 major epicardial coronary arteries (including the left main artery) severely narrowed by plaques. In 22 runners the cause of death was CAD, and 1 runner died with a floppy mitral valve.

Thompson and colleagues[13] reported the causes of death in 18 runners and joggers who died during or immediately after jogging (Table 3). Of the 18, 13 were men over 40 years of age who died of atherosclerotic coronary heart disease. Although 6 of the 13 men had clinical histories relevant to the cardiovascular system, only 1 had CAD diagnosed. Two subjects had exercised for less than 1 month, 5 had been exercising regularly for at least 1 year, and 9 had exercised for 3 years or more.

Noakes and associates[11,12] reported sudden death in 5 marathon runners aged 36 to 44 years, 4 of whom had severe coronary atherosclerosis at necropsy, and 1 had hypertrophic cardiomyopathy. One runner with severe CAD died during a 15-mile road race, another died in the hospital awaiting coronary bypass surgery for unstable angina pectoris, and the remaining 2 runners with CAD had traumatic deaths.

Thus, of 48 previously reported conditioned subjects dying suddenly during or shortly after exercise (Table 6), 46 (96 percent) died from atherosclerotic coronary heart disease, 1 (2 percent) had congenitally hypoplastic coronary arteries,[25] and 1 (2 percent) had hypertrophic cardiomyopathy.[11]

COMPARISON OF EXERCISE-RELATED SUDDEN DEATHS IN CONDITIONED SUBJECTS AGES < 30 YEARS AND > 30 YEARS

Combining my personal series with previously reported subjects dying suddenly with exercise, Tables 2, 6, and 7 summarize the causes of death in subjects under and over age 30. Of 87 conditioned subjects ≤ 30 years of age (mean 20), the 3 leading causes of death were: (1) *congenital coronary artery anomalies,* 30 subjects (35 percent); (2) *hypertrophic cardiomyopathy,* 19 (22 percent); and (3) *atherosclerotic coronary heart disease,* 4 (5 percent). Of the 87 subjects, 72 (90 percent) were men. In contrast, of 60 conditioned subjects aged > 30 years (mean 44) studied at necropsy, the 3 causes of death were nearly the opposite of the younger group: 58 (97 percent) had *fatal atherosclerotic coronary heart disease;* 1 (1.5 percent) had *hypertrophic cardiomyopathy,* and 1 (1.5 percent) had a *congenital coronary anomaly.* All of the necropsy subjects over 30 years of age were men.

Thus, in both young (≤ 30 years) and old (> 30 years) conditioned subjects dying suddenly during or shortly after exercise, congenital or acquired disease of the epicardial coronary arteries is the killer.

Table 4. Data for marathon runner (G.B.) at ages 44 and 48

G.B. Age 44 years

Stage	Heart Rate (bts/min)	Blood Pressure (mm Hg)	ST Segment Depression (mm, lead)	Symptoms
Pre-exercise	60	140/94	0	0
Speed (mph)	Grade (%)			
1.7	10 88	140/100	0	0
2.5	12 107	155/100	0	0
3.4	14 125	185/90	0	0
4.2	16 150	180/100	0	0
5.5	18 187	—	3.5(V5)	0
Post-exercise (min)				
2	115	220/100	2(V6)	0
4	96	170/90	1(V6)	0
6	93	—	0	0
8	90	145/94	0	0

G.B. Age 48 years

Stage	Heart Rate (bts/min)	Blood Pressure (mm Hg)	ST Segment Depression (mm, lead)	Symptoms
Pre-exercise	72	135/90	0	0
Speed (mph)	Grade (%)			
3	0 108	150/80	2(2, 3, V5-V6)	0
3	5 112	150/80	2.5(2, 3, V5-V6)	0
3	10 122	150/80	4(2, 3VF, V5-6)	0
Post-exercise				
0	122	184/96	2 (diffuse)	0
2	85	170/90	2 (diffuse)	0
5	85	160/90	2 (diffuse)	0
10	75	150/90	0	0

Table 5. Number and percent of 5-mm segments of 21 major epicardial coronary arteries and the grade of cross-sectional area luminal narrowing by atherosclerotic plaque in 7 conditioned runners dying suddenly

Major Coronary Artery	Percent Cross-sectional Area Luminal Narrowing (No. [%])				
	0–25	26–50	51–75	76–100	Totals
LAD	22 (16)	38 (26)	35 (24)	49 (34)	144 (100)
LC	23 (21)	37 (33)	26 (24)	24 (22)	110 (100)
R	19 (17)	34 (30)	25 (22)	36 (31)	114 (100)
	64 (17)	109 (30)	86 (23)	109 (30)	368 (100)

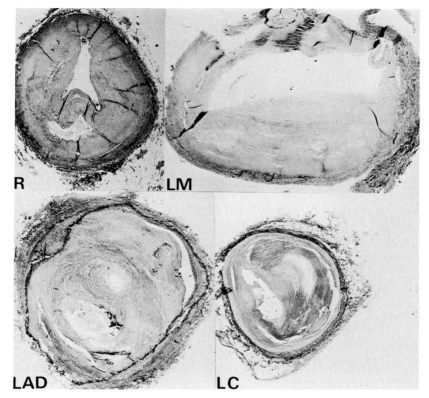

Figure 11. J.H. (number 1), Table 1B. Cross-sections at sites of maximal narrowing of the right (R), left main (LM), left anterior descending (LAD), and left circumflex (LC) coronary arteries. (Elastic stain, ×12)

Table 6. Causes of sudden death in 60 necropsy athletes age >30 years dying during or shortly after exercise

Condition	Present study ages 37–65 (48) 12 M (100%)	Previous studies ages 31–57 (42) 48 M (100%)	Totals ages 31–65 (44) 60 M (100%)
A. Congenital Coronary Anomaly	0	1(2%)	1(1.5%)
1. Hypoplastic coronary arteries		(1)	(1)
B. Atherosclerotic Coronary Heart Disease	12(100%)	46(96%)	58(97%)
C. Hypertrophic Cardiomyopathy	0	1(2%)	1(1.5%)
TOTALS:	12(100%)	48(100%)	60(100%)

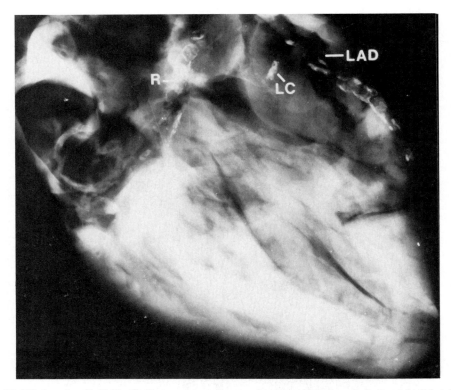

Figure 12. P.S. (number 2), Table 1B. Postmortem radiogram showing calcific deposits in the right (R), left anterior descending (LAD), and left circumflex (LC) coronary arteries. (From Waller, BF and Roberts, WC[35], with permission.)

Table 7. Cardiovascular causes of sudden death in conditioned athletes

Abnormal Structure	Age at Death (Years)		
	≤30	>30	Total
1. Coronary Artery	34 (47%)[a]	59[c] (98%)	93 (71%)
2. Myocardium	31 (43%)[b]	1 (2%)	32 (24%)
3. Valve	4 (6%)	0	4 (3%)
4. Aorta	3 (4%)	0	3 (2%)
TOTALS:	72 (100%)	60 (100%)	132 (100%)

[a]Includes 30 congenital anomalies and 4 atherosclerotic coronary heart disease subjects
[b]Includes hypertrophic cardiomyopathy, discrete subaortic stenosis, idiopathic dilated cardiomyopathy, myocarditis and 10 subjects with idiopathic left ventricular hypertrophy
[c]Includes 1 congenital anomaly

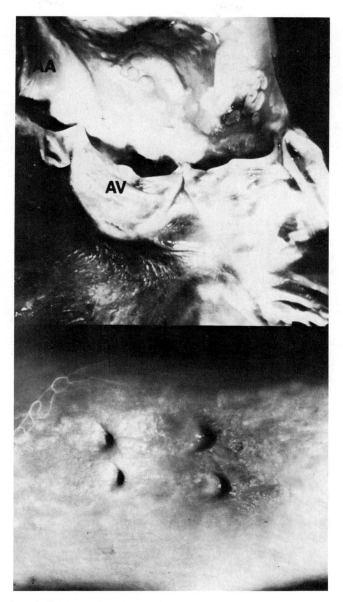

Figure 13. P.S. (number 2), Table 1B. Postmortem views of intimal surface of ascending aorta (AA) *(upper)* showing heavy atherosclerotic plaques and intimal surface of descending aorta *(lower)* showing minimal atherosclerotic plaques. (From Waller, BF and Roberts, WC,[35] with permission.)

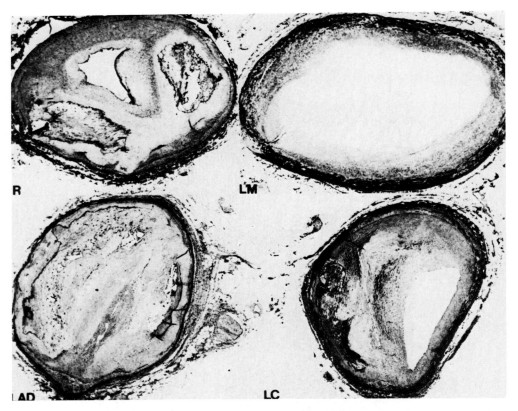

Figure 14. P.S. (number 2), Table 1B. Cross-sections at sites of maximal narrowing of the right (R), left main (LM), left anterior descending (LAD), and left circumflex (LC) coronary arteries. (From Waller, BF and Roberts, WC,[35] with permission.)

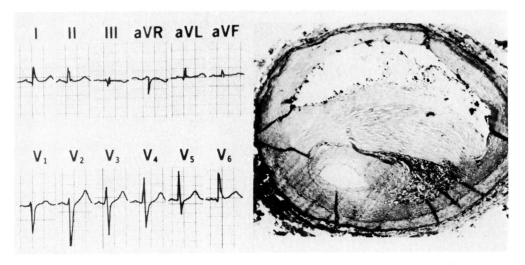

Figure 15. L.W. (number 3), Table 1B. Normal resting ECG obtained 90 days before death *(left)* and a cross-section of the severely narrowed left anterior descending coronary artery *(right)* (From Waller, BF and Roberts, WC,[35] with permission.)

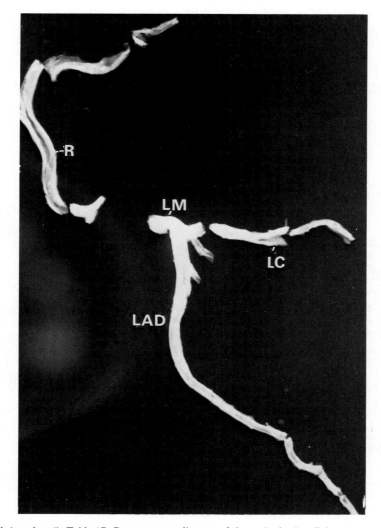

Figure 16. T.V. (number 4), Table 1B. Postmortem radiogram of the excised epicardial coronary arteries showing mild calcific deposits in the right (R), left anterior descending (LAD), and left circumflex (LC) coronary arteries. LM = left main

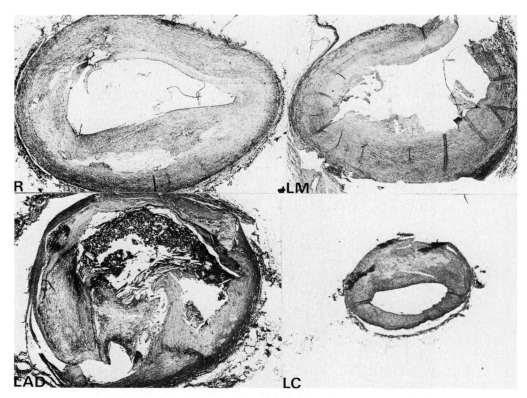

Figure 17. T.V. (number 4), Table 1B. Cross-sections at sites of maximal narrowing of the right (R), left main (LM), left anterior descending (LAD), and left circumflex (LC) coronary arteries. (Elastic stain, ×14)

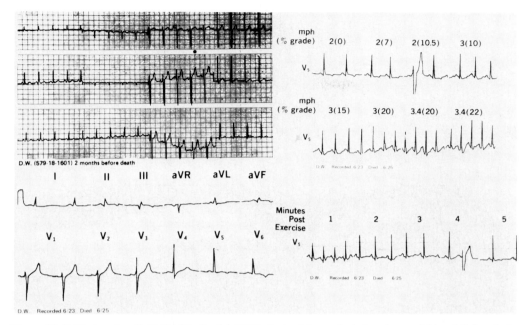

Figure 18. D.W. (number 5) Table 1B. Resting ECG obtained 2 months before *(upper left)* and 2 days before *(lower left)* showing nonspecific ST-segment and T wave abnormalities in leads 11,111, and aVF. Exercise treadmill test *(right)* obtained 2 days before death showing a normal ST-segment and T wave response during exercise up to 3.4 miles per hour (mph) at 22 percent grade *(upper right)* and up to 5 minutes after exercise *(lower right)*. A single ventricular premature beat is seen in the fourth minute postexercise.

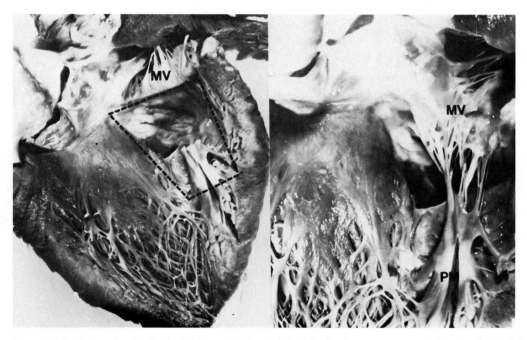

Figure 19. D.W. (number 5), Table 1B. Opened left ventricle *(left)* showing an aneurysm at the site of a healed left ventricular basal myocardial infarct (dashes). Close-up view *(right)* of dashed area showing a scarred and atrophied papillary muscle (PM). MV = mitral valve (From Waller, BF and Roberts, WC,[35] with permission.)

37

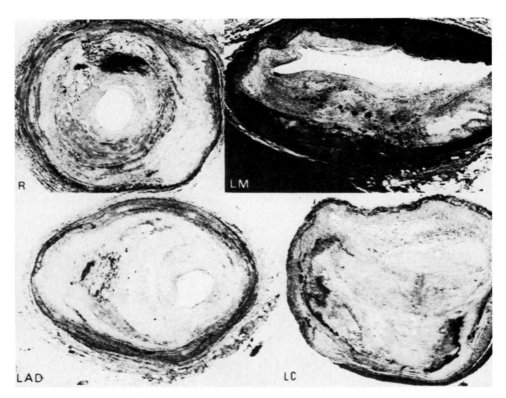

Figure 20. D.W. (number 5), Table 1B. Sites of maximal cross-sectional area narrowing of the right (R), left main (LM), left anterior descending (LAD), and left circumflex (LC) coronary arteries. (From Waller, BF and Roberts, WC,[35] with permission.)

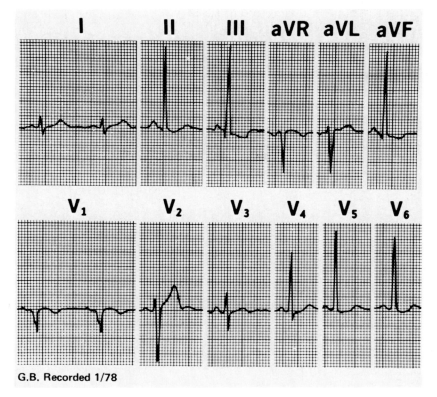

Figure 21. G.B. (number 7), Table 1B. Resting ECG obtained 10 months before death showing left ventricular hypertrophy and ST-segment and T wave abnormalities.

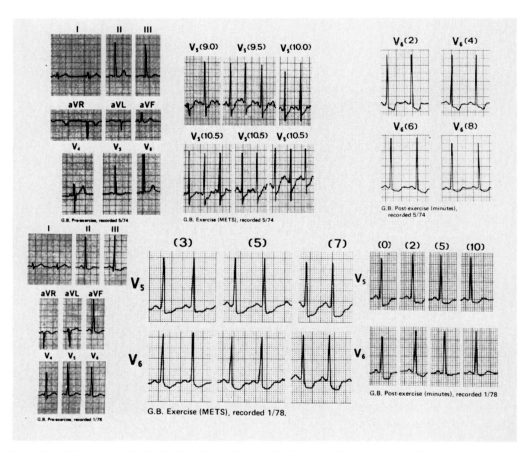

Figure 22. G.B. (number 7), Table 1B. *Upper,* Exercise ECG before *(left),* during *(middle),* and after *(right)* treadmill test performed 4 years before death showing severe ST-segment depression at a maximal speed of 5.5 mph at 18 percent grade. *Lower,* Another exercise test performed 10 months before death at 3.0 mph at 10 percent grade. Both tests are strongly positive for myocardial ischemia. METS = metabolic equivalents (From Waller, BF and Roberts, WC,[35] with permission.)

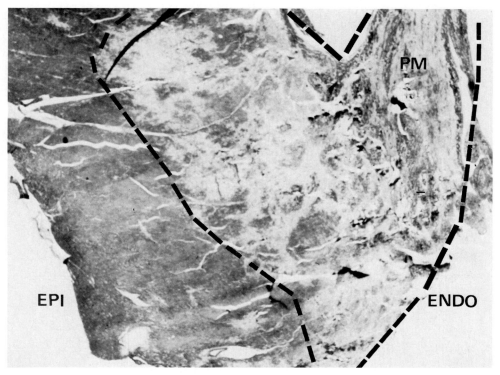

Figure 23. G.B. (number 7), Table 1B. Photograph of a portion of left ventricular free wall showing extensive scarring (dashed area). ENDO = endocardial surface; EPI = epicardial surface; PM = papillary muscle (From McManus, BM, Waller, BF, Graboys, TB, et al,[37] with permission.)

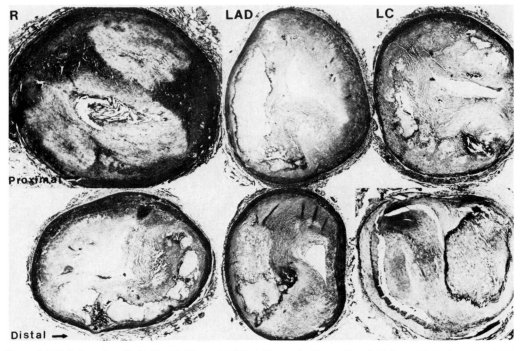

Figure 24. G.B. (number 7), Table 1B. The right (R), left anterior descending (LAD), and left circumflex (LC) arteries at sites of maximal narrowing in the proximal *(upper panel)* and distal *(lower panel)* halves of the respective arteries. (From Waller, BF and Roberts, WC,[35] with permission.)

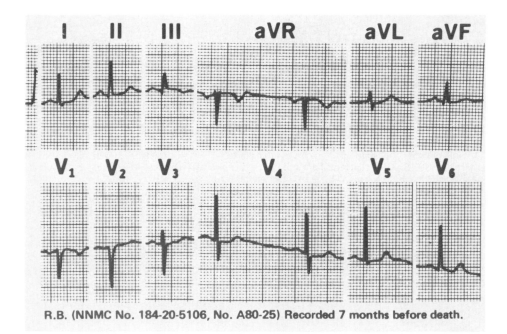

R.B. (NNMC No. 184-20-5106, No. A80-25) Recorded 7 months before death.

Figure 25. R.B. (number 8), Table 1B. ECG recorded 4 months before death showing absence of R wave in V2 and nonspecific ST-segment and T-wave changes. (From Waller BF, Csere, RS, Baker, WP, et al,[36] with permission.)

42

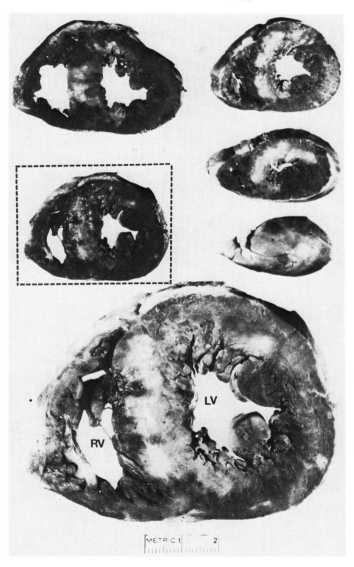

Figure 26. R.B. (number 8), Table 1B. Transverse ventricular myocardial sections. *Upper,* Healed transmural infarct extending from base to apex and involving primarily ventricular septum. *Lower,* Close-up of bracketed section. LV and RV = left and right ventricular cavities, respectively. Compare infarct location at necropsy with the loss of R wave on ECG (Fig. 25) (From Waller, BF, Csere, RS, Baker, WP, et al,[36] with permission.)

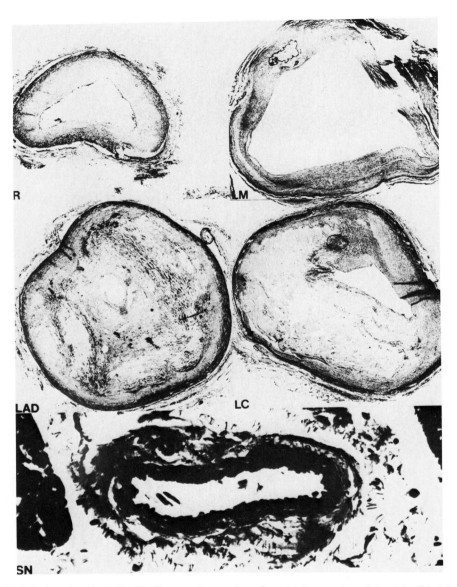

Figure 27. R.B. (number 8), Table 1B. Cross-sections at sites of maximal narrowing of the right (R), left main (LM), left anterior descending (LAD), left circumflex (LC), and sinus node (SN) arteries. (From Waller, BF, Csere, RS, Baker, WP, et al,[36] with permission.)

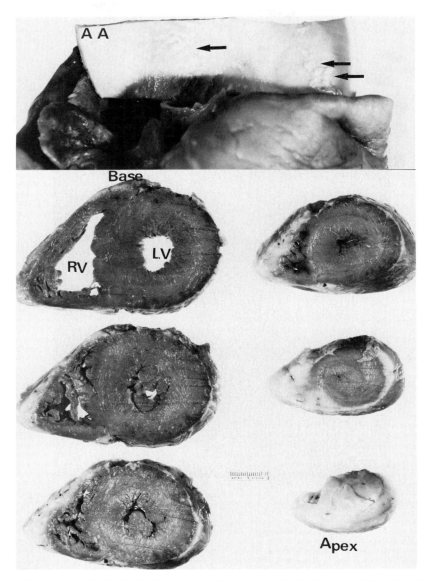

Figure 28. D.C. (number 11), Table 1B, *Upper,* Ascending aorta (AA) showing intimal lipid deposits (arrows) characteristic of hyperlipidemia type 2. *Lower,* Transverse ventricular myocardial sections from base to apex are normal. RV and LV = right and left ventricular cavities, respectively. (from McManus, BM, Waller, BF, Graboys, TB,[37] et al, with permission.)

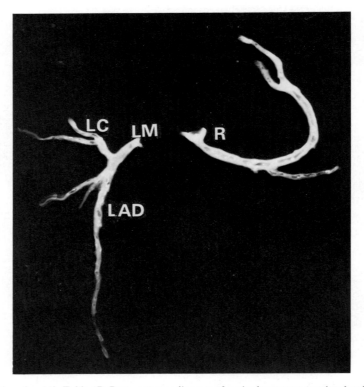

Figure 29. D.C. (number 11), Table 1B. Postmortem radiogram of excised coronary arteries showing heavy calcific deposits in the left anterior descending (LAD), left circumflex (LC), and right (R) coronary arteries. LM = left main.

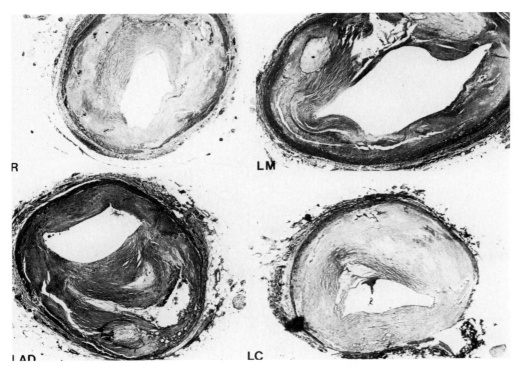

Figure 30. D.C. (number 11), Table 1B. Sites of maximal cross-sectional area narrowing of the right (R), left anterior descending (LAD), left main (LM), and left circumflex (LC) coronary arteries. (From Waller, BF and Roberts, WC,[35] with permission.)

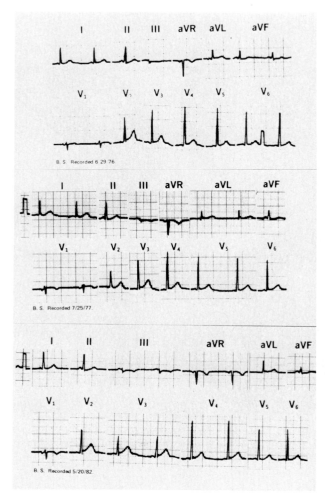

Figure 31. B.S. (number 12), Table 1B. Resting ECGs obtained 6 years *(upper)*, 5 years *(middle)*, and 1 month *(lower)* before sudden death show minor ST-segment and T-wave changes.

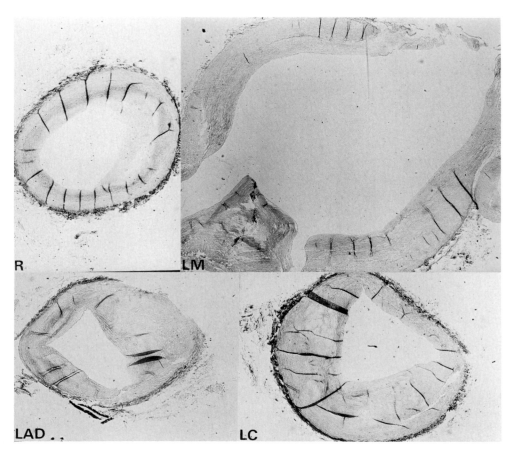

Figure 32. B.S. (number 12), Table 1B. Sites of maximal cross-sectional area narrowing of the right (R), left main (LM), left anterior descending (LAD), and left circumflex (LC) coronary arteries. (Elastic stain, ×16)

PERCENT OF 5-mm SEGMENTS OF THE MAJOR EPICARDIAL CORONARY ARTERIES NARROWED TO
VARIOUS DEGREES BY ATHEROSCLEROTIC PLAQUES IN 7 CONDITIONED RUNNERS

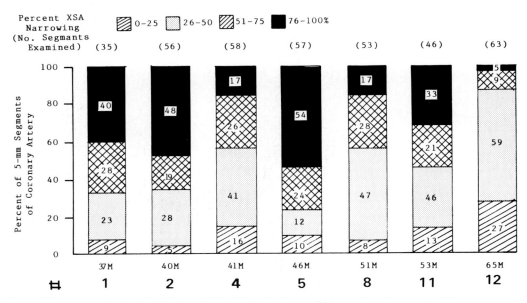

Figure 33. (numbers 1, 2, 4, 5, 8, 11, and 12), Table 1B. Bar graph comparing the percent of 5-mm coronary segments of the major epicardial coronary arteries narrowed to various degrees in cross-sectional (XSA) by atherosclerotic plaques in 7 runners with sudden death.

CARDIOVASCULAR STRUCTURAL ABNORMALITIES IN EXERCISE-RELATED SUDDEN DEATHS

Cardiovascular morphologic abnormalities associated with sudden death during exercise can be grouped into 4 categories: (1) *coronary arterial* factors; (2) *myocardial* factors; (3) *valvular* factors; and (4) *aortic* factors. Of 183 conditioned subjects dying suddenly (Tables 1 A and B and 3), 132 (72 percent) had an identifiable cardiovascular structural abnormality (Table 7): 93 (71 percent) subjects had abnormal coronary arteries, 32 (24 percent) had abnormalities of the myocardium, 4 (3 percent) had abnormal valves, and 3 (2 percent) subjects had abnormalities of the aorta.

Coronary Arterial Factors

Sudden death from coronary abnormalities is the most frequent cause of all sudden *cardiac* deaths with or without associated exercise or physical exertion. These coronary arterial abnormalities may be subgrouped as: (1) coronary *atherosclerosis;* (2) *congenital* coronary *anomalies;* (3) *tunneled epicardial* coronary arteries; (4) *high take-off* coronary *ostia;* (5) coronary *trauma;* and (6) coronary *spasm.*

Coronary Atherosclerosis

Coronary atherosclerosis is the most frequent cause of exercise-related sudden death, accounting for 83 (45 percent) of 183 instances of sudden death (Tables 1A and B and 3), and 58 (97 percent) of 60 sudden deaths in conditioned subjects over 30 years of age (Table 6). The amount of coronary narrowing by atherosclerotic plaques in runners and nonrunners with sudden coronary death is compared in Figure 34. By assigning arbitrary numbers for each category of cross-sectional area narrowing (Table 5; Fig. 33), a total coronary score can be calculated.[37] Dividing the total coronary score by the total number of coronary segments examined results in a number representing the average amount of luminal narrowing per coronary segment. Of 7 conditioned male runners aged 37 to 65 dying suddenly, the average amount of coronary luminal narrowing was 51 percent (Fig. 34). Of 15 necropsy patients (nonrunners) with sudden coronary death aged 40 to 60 years,[36] the average amount of cross-sectional area narrowing was similar at 56 percent. Furthermore, of 24 necropsy patients (nonrunners) aged 40 to 60 with fatal coronary events other than sudden death, the average luminal reduction was more severe at 67 percent (Fig. 34).

Of historic interest are the coronary necropsy findings in Clarence DeMar ("Mr. Marathon").[41] In 1909 at the age of 21, he placed in a long-distance cross-country run. His last race was in 1957, when at the age of 69, he completed a 9-mile race. The intervening 49 years is a saga unequaled in the annals of marathon running: over 1000 long-distance races including 100 true marathons of 26 miles or more. His blood pressure was 14/8 cm H_2O, his resting pulse 60 beats per minute, and his precordial examination was normal. He never had symptoms of myocardial ischemia, and he died from metastatic carcinoma. At necropsy, his heart weighed 340 grams and the myocardium was free of necrosis and fibrosis. The sites of maximal luminal cross-sectional area narrowing by atherosclerotic plaques of the left main, "left" and right coronary arteries are shown in Figure 35. A striking necropsy observation was the large caliber of the coronary arteries, estimated to be 2 or 3 times the normal diameter for a heart of this weight.

Anomalous Origin of a Major Coronary Artery

Anomalous origin of a major coronary artery from the sinuses of Valsalva is the second most frequent morphologic coronary abnormality observed in exercise-related sudden death, accounting for 31 (17 percent) of 183 instances of sudden death (Tables 1 and 3), and 30 (35

51

percent) of 87 sudden deaths in conditioned subjects aged $\leq$ 30 years (Table 2). Until the study of Cheitlin and colleagues[31] in 1974, single coronary arteries and the origin of both left and right coronary arteries from the same sinus of Valsalva were regarded as having little clinical significance. In the study by Cheitlin,[31] 51 necropsy patients with anomalous coronary origins were examined: 33 (61 percent) with origin of the left main and right coronary arteries from the *right* sinus of Valsalva (Fig. 36) and 18 with origin of the right and left coronary arteries from the *left* sinus of Valsalva (Fig. 36). Of the 51 patients, 7 (14 percent) had sudden death with exercise (Table 3), all of whom had origin of the left main from the *right* sinus (Fig. 36). None of the 18 patients with origin of the right from the left sinus had exercise-related sudden death. Liberthson and colleagues[32] also reported sudden death with exercise in 2 (10 percent) of 21 necropsy patients with anomalous origin of major coronary arteries. The 2 patients with exercise-related sudden death had the left main artery arising as the first branch of the right coronary artery (Fig. 37), with leftward passage between the walls of the aorta and pulmonary trunk. Four patients with origin of the left main artery from the right sinus but with passage around the anterior surface of the pulmonary trunk did not have sudden death.

Of 10 necropsy patients studied by Roberts and colleagues,[15] in whom the right coronary artery arose from the *left* coronary sinus and then passed to the right atrioventricular sulcus by coursing between the aorta and pulmonary trunk, 3 died suddenly, 1 of whom had exercise-related sudden death. Thus, origin of the right coronary artery from the left sinus may produce cardiac dysfunction that can be fatal.

The mechanism(s) of sudden death with exercise in subjects with origin of *both* coronary arteries from a *single* coronary sinus and passage of 1 artery between the walls of aorta and pulmonary trunk is depicted in Figures 38 through 40. The acute angle take-off of the anomalous coronary artery appears to be an important factor in producing myocardial ischemia.[15,31]

At least 8 additional subjects with various types of congenital coronary anomalies associated with sudden death during exercise have been reported[17,25-27] (Table 3) and are diagrammed in Figures 10 and 37.

Tunneled Epicardial Coronary Arteries

Tunneled epicardial coronary arteries (myocardial bridges) have received renewed attention in a recent report by Morales and colleagues[34] (Table 3), who reported sudden death during strenuous exercise in 3 patients in whom a tunneled portion of the left anterior descending coronary artery was present at necropsy (Fig. 41). Two patients had sudden death during running and 1 while swimming. Morales and associates[34] concluded that this morphologic finding represented a potentially lethal anatomic variant. Tunneled coronary arteries were observed in 2 (7 percent) of the 27 subjects in my series (Table 1A and B), and in 5 (3 percent) of 158 previously reported subjects with sudden death and exercise (Table 3). In view of the wide range (5 to 85 percent)[34] of tunneled coronary arteries found at autopsy, the linking of tunneled coronary arteries to sudden death is questioned. However, a potential mechanism for sudden death in subjects with tachycardia (including exercise-induced) is postulated in Figures 42 and 43. However, the significance of the intramural portions of epicardial coronary arteries in relation to myocardial ischemia and sudden death remains unsettled.

High Take-off of Coronary Ostia

High take-off of coronary ostia is defined as origin of coronary ostia 5 mm or more above the aortic sinotubular junction (Fig. 2). It has been suggested that high take-off of a coronary artery may precipitate sudden death.[43] One of my subjects, a 17-year-old basketball player (number 4, Table 1A) with sudden death, had the left coronary artery ostium arising about 5 mm above the sinotubular junction as well as anomalous origin of the right coronary artery from the left sinus of Valsalva. This combination appears to be the first such observation in an athlete dying suddenly with exercise.

Coronary Arterial Trauma

Coronary arterial trauma is an infrequently reported cause of sudden death associated with physical exertion. Recently, Roberts and Maron[22] reported sudden death in a professional football player while walking back to the huddle after having run a pass pattern in a professional football game (Fig. 44). Although this subject had severe coronary atherosclerosis, the unusual feature was extensive atherosclerotic plaque hemmorrhage. Roberts and Maron postulated that tackling and blocking caused trauma to the severely narrowed left anterior descending coronary artery producing atherosclerotic cracks with subsequent bleeding into them.

Exercise-induced Coronary Spasm

Exercise-induced coronary spasm has recently been proposed[37] as a mechanism for sudden death in athletes. Circadian variation in exercised-induced coronary spasm has also been reported. Yasue and colleagues[42] noted that of 13 subjects with exercise-induced coronary spasm, all 13 had ST segment elevation with exercise in the morning, but only 2 of the 13 had ST segment elevation in the afternoon with similar amounts of exercise. Thus, although coronary spasm as a real factor in *exercise-related* sudden death has not been reported, its potential seems logical. It would seem logical, therefore, that if patients with evidence of coronary spasm desire to participate in regular exercise, exercise testing should be performed to detect the small subgroup of patients with exercise-induced spasm, and these patients should be advised to exercise in the afternoon hours.

Myocardial Factors

Structural abnormalities of ventricular myocardium are the second most frequently observed morphologic cardiac alteration in conditioned subjects dying suddenly. Of 132 conditioned subjects with exercise-related sudden death (Table 7), 32 (24 percent) had abnormalities of ventricular muscle, including 10 subjects with idiopathic LVH. Of the myocardial abnormalities, hypertrophic cardiomyopathy was most frequent, occurring in 20 (63 percent) subjects. Of the 20 subjects, 19 (95 percent) were aged 30 years and under (Table 2). The second most frequent myocardial abnormality was idiopathic LVH, occurring in 10 (31 percent) of 32 conditioned subjects, all of whom were young ($\leq$ 30 years) individuals. The remaining myocardial abnormalities associated with exercise-related sudden death include idiopathic dilated cardiomyopathy (familial), 1 (3 percent);[19] and myocarditis in a 25-year-old gymnast.[25]

Recently, 2 joggers who each ran 12 to 14 miles per week were studied at necropsy (Table 3).[16] Their initial symptom had been dyspnea on exertion that became progressive and ultimately prevented each runner from exercising. Both died within 1 year of discontinuing running, and at necropsy, both had cardiac amyloidosis. The mode of death in these 2 runners was not provided.

Valvular Factors

Structural abnormalities of cardiac valves in conditioned subjects dying suddenly with exercise are the third most frequent cardiac abnormality observed at necropsy, occurring in 4 (3 percent) of 132 conditioned subjects (numbers 7 and 12, Table 1A; Virmani,[14] Maron,[17] Table 3). All 4 subjects had floppy mitral valves and the floppy valve was the only cardiac abnormality in 2 of the 4 subjects. The remaining 2 subjects had associated idiopathic LVH. A fifth subject (number 15, Table 1A), a 29-year-old runner, had Ebstein's anomaly of the tricuspid valve (Fig. 5), but in view of absence of a history of cardiac arrhythmias the abnormality could not be definitely related to sudden death. Thus, floppy mitral valves appear to be the major valvular abnormality observed at necropsy in conditioned subjects dying suddenly with exercise.

Aortic Factors

Diseases affecting the aorta accounted for sudden death in 3 (2 percent) of 132 subjects (Table 7). Two of the 3 athletes[17] were basketball players and at least 1 had typical physical stigmata of the Marfan syndrome. Both men, ages 18 and 21, had rupture of a markedly dilated ascending aorta. Histologic examination of the aortic wall in each disclosed a diminished number of medial elastic fibers (cystic medial necrosis). The third subject was a 15-year-old weight lifter and wrestler[25] who had aortic dissection unassociated with Marfan syndrome.

EXERCISE UNMASKING NONFATAL CARDIOVASCULAR DISEASE

Exercise may bring out symptoms or abnormal physical findings that are not present at rest. Exercise, such as jogging or running, may serve as a built-in exercise stress test that might uncover an underlying illness sooner than would have been apparent without the strenuous exercise (Fig. 45).[16] I have studied 3 patients since September 1982, in whom exercise unmasked aortic valve stenosis (Table 8, Figs. 46 through 48). Two of the 3 men (aged 55 and 60) had just started to jog (< 2 months) when each developed symptoms (syncope, chest pain) during exercise not previously present at rest. Medical evaluation disclosed aortic valve stenosis in both men, who subsequently had aortic valve replacement and have resumed mild exercise activities. The third man, a 35-year-old tennis player (Fig. 46), had been exercising for 4 to 5 years before beginning to feel fatigued, lightheaded, and dizzy while running short distances. He also experienced near-syncope while running on a hot day. Medical evaluation in this patient also disclosed aortic valve stenosis, and he underwent aortic valve replacement and has resumed mild exercise.

At least 6 previously reported runners also had cardiac disease *unmasked* during vigorous exercise (Table 8).[44-47] Four of these 6 runners were competitive, well-conditioned long-distance runners.[44-45,47] Five of the 6 runners had severe coronary narrowing by coronary angiography treated by percutaneous coronary angioplasty in 2 runners. The remaining 20-year-old female[6] had sudden death during jogging but was successfully resuscitated. At cardiac catheterization, the left ventricular end-diastolic pressure rose to 55 mm Hg with exercise. The left ventricular dysfunction was interpreted as that of an idiopathic cardiomyopathy.

It is interesting to speculate that running may unmask CAD or cardiomyopathies at an early stage, when perhaps the disease, particularly CAD, is more amenable to therapy.

SUDDEN DEATH WITH EXERCISE IN CONDITIONED PATIENTS WITH *KNOWN* CARDIAC DISEASE

Although it is known that patients with clinically apparent coronary heart disease may begin supervised exercise programs and ultimately become marathon runners,[48] only 2 reports[7,38] are available that describe cardiac findings at necropsy in subjects dying suddenly during exercise who have had previously recognized cardiac disease. Three conditioned subjects (Table 9, Figs. 49 and 50) with previously recognized valvular or coronary heart disease died suddenly during exercise. A 30-year-old male with mitral valve replacement 10 years earlier had exercised over 2 years and suddenly collapsed while roller skating. At necropsy

(Fig. 49), the prosthetic valve had extensive fibrous overgrowth around the base and struts of the caged-ball prosthesis, preventing complete opening and closing of the poppet. With exercise, an increased cardiac output was associated with increased flow across the abnormally functioning prosthesis, creating severe and fatal mitral stenosis. The left atrium also contained thrombus, but emboli were not observed in the lungs, brain, or coronary arteries.

Two runners aged 49 and 52 years (Fig. 50) misused exercise to *treat* chest pain in unsupervised settings. Both men had documented acute myocardial infarction with subsequent recurrent angina pectoris. Both men ran regularly (10 to 40 miles per week) for at least 2 years before sudden death, and both ran intentionally when they developed angina at rest. Both men had been very athletic before their infarction and had strong beliefs regarding exercise and health and well being. These men are similar to a jogger, described by Opie,[7] who fought his heart disease by running 7 miles per day.

Thus, patients with known cardiac disease require educational programs, supervision, and close medical followup if vigorous exercise is to be undertaken.

ACKNOWLEDGMENTS

The invaluable secretarial assistance of Janet Chastain and talents of artist Lynn Waller are gratefully acknowledged.

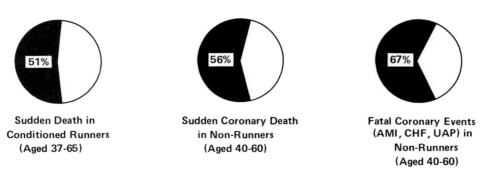

51%	56%	67%
Sudden Death in Conditioned Runners (Aged 37-65)	Sudden Coronary Death in Non-Runners (Aged 40-60)	Fatal Coronary Events (AMI, CHF, UAP) in Non-Runners (Aged 40-60)

Figure 34. Comparison of average amounts of luminal cross-sectional area narrowing by atherosclerotic plaques in 3 groups of necropsy patients of similar age and sex. (From McManus, BM, Waller, BF, Graboys, TB,[37] et al, with permission.)

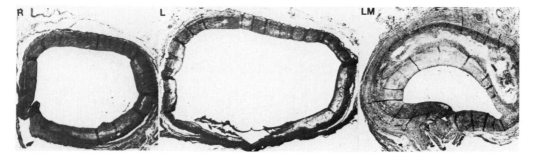

Figure 35. Cross-sections of the right (R), left (L), and left main (LM) coronary arteries at sites of maximal narrowing from "Mr. Marathon." (From Currens, JH and White, PD,[41] with permission.)

Table 8. Nonfatal heart disease unmasked by exercise

Item	Present Study			Asay[44]	Handler[45]	Fletcher		Noakes[47]	
	No. 1	No. 2	No. 3	1981	1982	1981[6]	1969[46]	1977	1977
Age (yr)	35	55	60	54	48	20	48	50	46
Sex/Race	MW	MW	MW	M/-	M/-	F/-	MW	MW	MW
Type of E	R, T	R	R	R	R[m]	R	R	R	R,Sw, O
Running Hx:									
Miles	<1½/da	<1/da	1½/da	2-4[i]/da	50-70/wk	—	80-90/wk[r]	40/wk[u]	—
Duration	<5 yr	<2 mo	<2 wk	20 yr	>8 yrs	—	10 yrs	10 yrs	14 yrs
Sx During E	D[a]	S	CP	CP	CP	SD[p]	AMI	CP	CP
FH HD	0	0	0	+[j]	0	0	+	+[v]	+
Angina pectoris	0	0	0	0	+[n]	0	0	0	+
Hx AMI	0	0	0	0	0	0	0	0	0
SAP (mmHg)	105/75	135/70	170/80	130/78	—	—	130/90	110/80	130/90
TC (mg/dl)	160	—	—	212	185	—	268	216	—
Abn ECG									
Rest	+[b]	+[b]	+[b]	0	0	—	+	+	+
E	—	—	—	+[k]	+[k]	—	—	—	+[y]
LV-Ao (mm Hg)	112[c]	55[e]	70[g]	—	—	—	—	—	—
Abn Ca by Angio	0	0	0	+[l]	+[o]	0[q]	+[s]	+[w]	+[z]
Treatment	AVR[d]	AVR[f]	AVR[h]	PTCA	PTCA	D	0	0	0
Resumed E	+	0	+	+	—	+	+[t]	+[t]	+[t]
Type C Abn									
Cor	0	0	0	+	+	0	+	+	+
Valve	+	+	+	0	0	0	0	0	0
Myo	0	0	0	0	0	+	0	0	0

Abbreviations: Abn = abnormal/abnormality; AMI = acute myocardial infarction; Angio = angiogram; Ao = aorta; AVR = aortic valve replacement; C = cardiac; CA = coronary artery; Cor = coronary; CP = chest pain; D = digoxin; da = day; E = exercise; ECG = electrocardiogram; F = female; FH HD = family history of heart disease; Hx = history; LV = left ventricle; M = male; Mo = month; Myo = primary myocardial; O = oarsman; PTCA = percutaneous coronary angioplasty; R = running; S = syncope; SD = sudden death; Sw = swimming; Sx = symptoms; T = tennis; Tc = total serum cholesterol; W = white; wk = week; yr = year.

[a] Onset of lightheadedness, dizziness, and fatigue while running. Near syncope while running on hot day.

[b] Left ventricular hypertrophy with strain

[c] Ao = 106/26; LV = 218/14; LV-PCW = 0; 1+/4 + AR

[d] Unicuspid aortic valve

[e] Ao = 135/70; LV = 190/8; LV-PCW = 0; 1+/4 + AR

[f] Congenitally bicuspid AV

[g] Ao = 170/80; LV = 240/22; LV-PCW = 0; 2+/4 + AR

[h] Three-cuspid AV

[i] 3 to 6 runs/week

[j] Onset 20 years after beginning running. Onset of pain after running 2¼ miles.

[k] Developed angina with 1 mm ST segment depression

[l] LAD reduced 90%, LOM reduced 50%

[m] Completed 7 marathons and other races ranging from 6.2 miles to 52 mile ultramarathon.

[n] Angina onset after 8 years of conditioned running

[o] LAD reduced 99%

[p] Sudden death while running but successfully resuscitated from ventricular fibrillation

[q] LV end-diastolic pressure after exercise = 55 mm Hg. Interpretation of LV dysfunction was that of an idiopathic cardiomyopathy.

[r] Completed over 7 Comrades marathons and over 20,000 miles in training.

[s] Ten months after AMI: LAD reduced 50–75% and LM, LC, and R normal. LV angiogram disclosed dilated cavity with anterior akinesis.

[t] Continues to run marathons

[u] Completed 18 marathons

[v] Onset during a marathon. Five years before had episode of CP while running. AMI 48 hours after completion of marathon.

[w] One month after AMI, significant distal R narrowing, normal left coronary system and dyskinetic apex on LV angiogram

[x] Onset of chest pain while running. Five days later ECG showed AMI.

[y] Ventricular bigeminy

[z] Two years after AMI: PD reduced 70%, LAD 80%, and mild but diffuse LC disease. LV angiogram disclosed an anterior akinetic area.

57

Table 9. Sudden death during exercise in conditioned men with *known* cardiac disease

Item	Patient		
	No. 1 (RB)	No. 2 (DB)[37]	No. 3 (PH)[37]
Age (years)	30	49	52
Sex/Race	MW	MW	MW
History of:			
AMI	0	+	+
AP	0	+	+
CHF	+[a]	0	0
SH	0	+	0
CS	0	+	+
Exercise Hx:			
Type	RS	R	R
Duration (mo)	>24	4	>24
Miles Run/Wk	—	10	40
Abn ECG:			
Rest	+	+	—
Exercise	—	+	+
TC (mg/dl)	—	291	—
HW (g)	600	370	470
LV damage:			
Tm Necrosis	0	+	0
Scar	0	+	+
CAD	0	+(3)[c]	+[d]
Valve abn	MVR[b]	0	0

Abbreviations: Abn = abnormal/abnormality; AMI = acute myocardial infarction; AP = angina pectoris; CAD = coronary atherosclerotic disease; CHF = congestive heart failure; CS = cigarette smoker; ECG = electrocardiogram; g = grams; HW = heart weight; Hx = history; LV = left ventricular; R = running; RS = roller skating; SH = systemic hypertension; TC = total serum cholesterol; Tm = transmural; wk = week.

[a]Mitral regurgitation requiring MV replacement 10 years before death (Starr-Edwards)

[b]Thrombus in left atrium despite anticoagulation

[c]LAD, LC, and R coronary arteries narrowed >75% in cross-sectional area by plaques

[d]Two arteries narrowed 51–75% in cross-sectional area by plaques

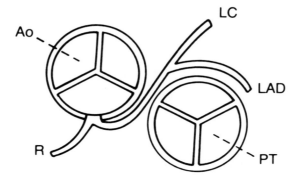

33 Necropsy Patients (31 M, 2 F) Aged 13-87 Years (mean 36)
(7/33 [21%] had sudden death with exercise)

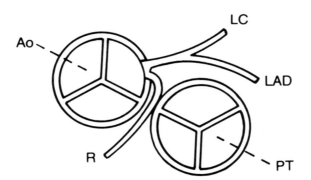

18 Necropsy Patients (14 M, 4 F) Aged 28-80 Years (mean 59)
(0/18 had sudden death with exercise)

Figure 36. Anomalous origin of the left main and right (R) coronary arteries in 51 necropsy patients. Of 33 patients with anomalous origin of the LM, 7 had sudden death with exercise *(upper),* but none of 18 patients with anomalous origin of the R from the left sinus of Valsalva had sudden death with exercise. Ao = aorta; LAD = left anterior descending; LC = left circumflex; PT = pulmonary trunk (From Cheitlin, MD, DeCastro, CM, and McAllister, HA,[31] with permission.)

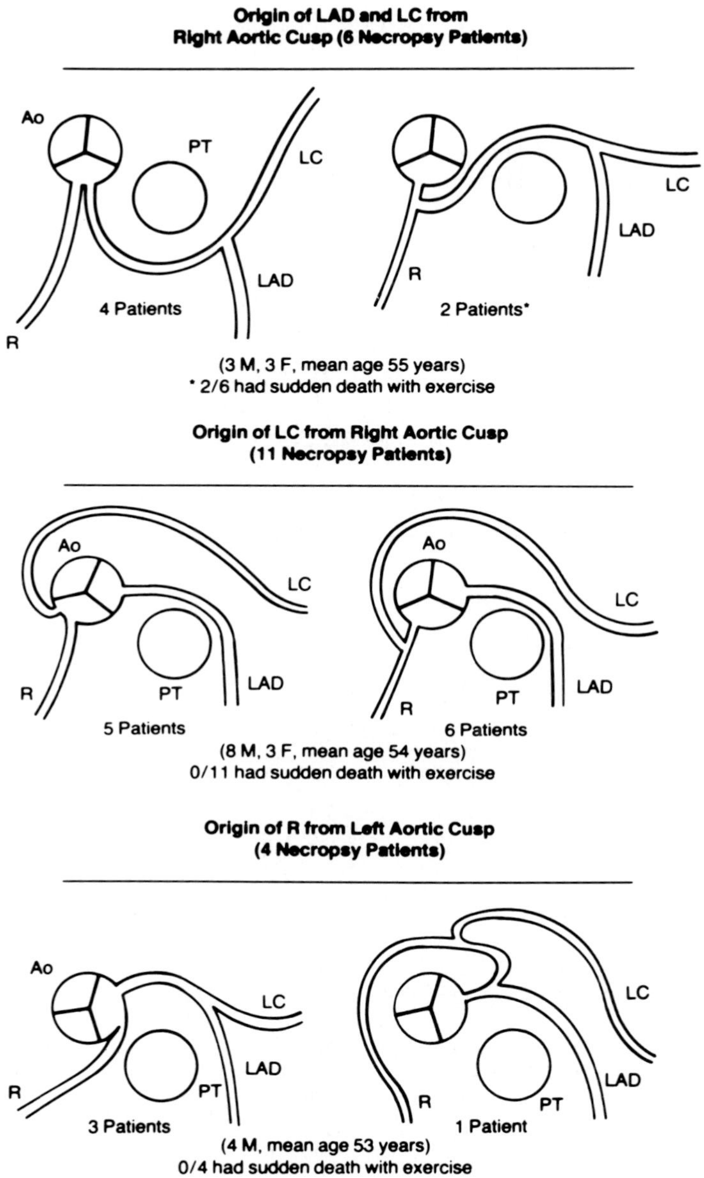

**Origin of LAD and LC from
Right Aortic Cusp (6 Necropsy Patients)**

4 Patients

2 Patients*

(3 M, 3 F, mean age 55 years)
* 2/6 had sudden death with exercise

**Origin of LC from Right Aortic Cusp
(11 Necropsy Patients)**

5 Patients

6 Patients

(8 M, 3 F, mean age 54 years)
0/11 had sudden death with exercise

**Origin of R from Left Aortic Cusp
(4 Necropsy Patients)**

3 Patients

1 Patient

(4 M, mean age 53 years)
0/4 had sudden death with exercise

Figure 37. Frequency of anomalous origin of coronary arteries associated with sudden death and exercise. Same abbreviations as Figure 36. (From Liberthson, RR, Dinsmore, RE, Bharati, S, et al[32], with permission.)

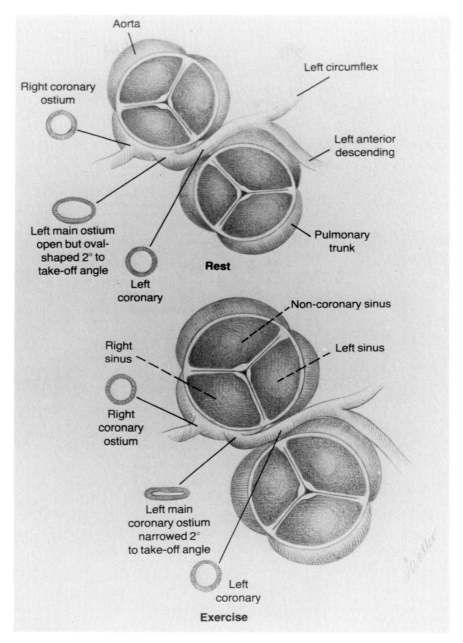

Figure 38. Diagram illustrating a proposed mechanism of sudden death with exercise associated with anomalous origin of the *left main* coronary artery from the *right* sinus of Valsalva. At rest, the acute angle take-off of the left main ostium is oval in shape, but with exercise, the ostium becomes slitlike and severely narrowed, presumably producing myocardial ischemia. Compression of the left main artery during exercise by the walls of the aorta and pulmonary trunk probably cause no reduction in the coronary lumen. (Modified from Roberts, WC, Siegel, RJ, and Zipes, DP[15])

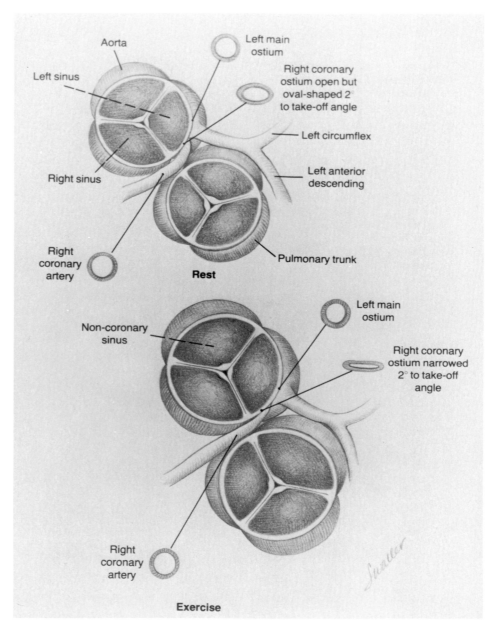

Figure 39. Diagram illustrating a proposed mechanism of sudden death with exercise associated with anomalous origin of the *right* coronary artery from the *left* sinus of Valsalva. At rest, the acute angle take-off of the right coronary ostium is oval in shape, but with exercise, the ostium becomes slitlike and severely narrowed, presumably producing myocardial ischemia. Compression of the right artery during exercise by the walls of aorta and pulmonary trunk probably causes no reduction in the coronary lumen. (Modified from Roberts, WC, Siegel, RJ, and Zipes, DP[15])

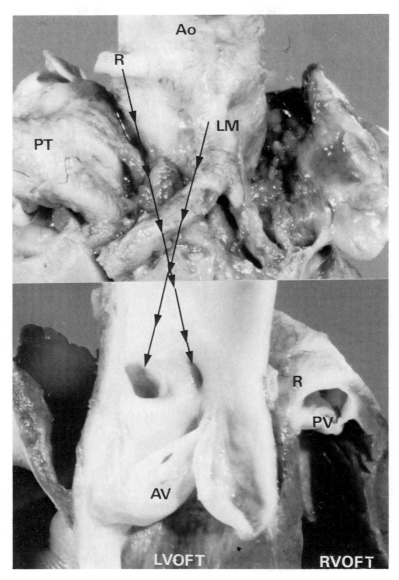

Figure 40. Photograph showing anomalous origin of the right (R) coronary artery from the left sinus of Valsalva with passage of the artery between the walls of aorta (Ao) and pulmonary trunk (PT) (arrow). *Upper,* Posterior view of ascending aorta showing the acute angle take-off of the R coronary artery. *Lower,* Opened aorta showing the oval or slitlike shape of the R coronary ostium compared with the normal round shape of the left main (LM) coronary ostium. LVOFT and RVOFT = left and right ventricular outflow tract, respectively.

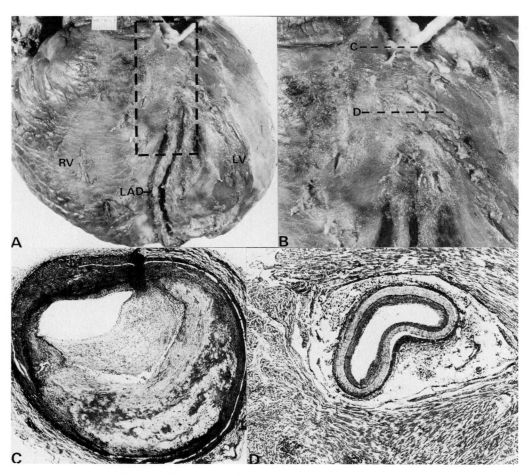

Figure 41. *A,* Postmortem view of a tunneled left anterior descending (LAD) coronary artery. LV and RV = left and right ventricles. *B,* Close-up of tunneled segment of LAD with sites of cross-sections shown in *C* and *D. C,* Severe cross-sectional area narrowing by atherosclerotic plaques. *D,* Intramural (tunneled) segment of LAD with mild atherosclerotic plaque. (From McManus, BM, Waller, BF, Graboys, TB,[37] et al, with permission.)

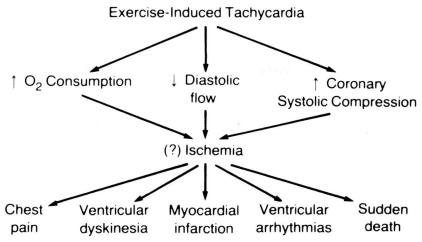

Exercise-Induced Tachycardia

↑ O$_2$ Consumption   ↓ Diastolic flow   ↑ Coronary Systolic Compression

(?) Ischemia

Chest pain   Ventricular dyskinesia   Myocardial infarction   Ventricular arrhythmias   Sudden death

Figure 42. Proposed mechanism(s) of myocardial ischemia from tunneled epicardial coronary arteries.

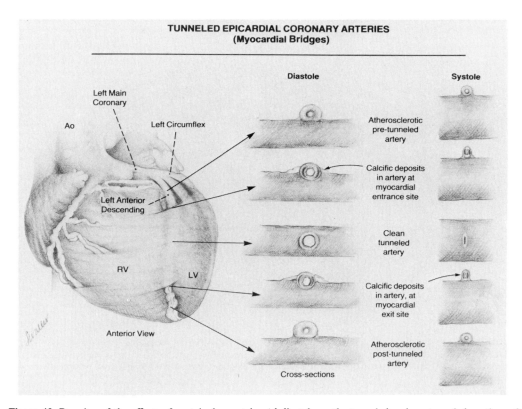

TUNNELED EPICARDIAL CORONARY ARTERIES
(Myocardial Bridges)

Diastole   Systole

Left Main Coronary

Ao   Left Circumflex

Atherosclerotic pre-tunneled artery

Calcific deposits in artery at myocardial entrance site

Left Anterior Descending

Clean tunneled artery

RV   LV

Calcific deposits in artery, at myocardial exit site

Anterior View

Atherosclerotic post-tunneled artery

Cross-sections

Figure 43. Drawing of the effects of ventricular systole and diastole on the tunneled and nontunneled portions of the left anterior descending coronary artery. During ventricular systole the intramyocardial segment of epicardial coronary artery becomes severely narrowed by surrounding contracting left ventricular myocardium. Ao = aorta; LV = left ventricle; RV = right ventricle.

65

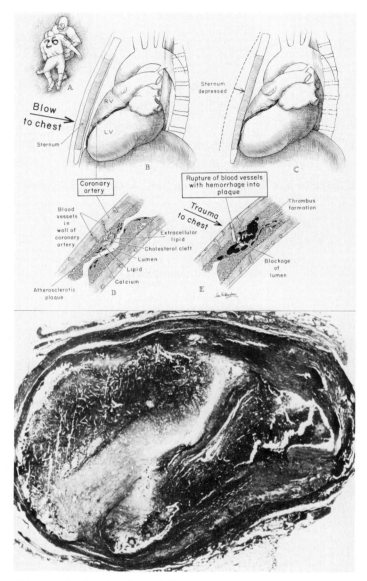

Figure 44. *Upper,* Diagram showing the effects of chest wall blows during football to a severely narrowed and calcified left anterior descending coronary artery. *Lower,* Cross-section of the left anterior descending coronary artery showing extensive hemorrhage into atherosclerotic plaque. (From Roberts, WC and Maron, BJ,[22] with permission.)

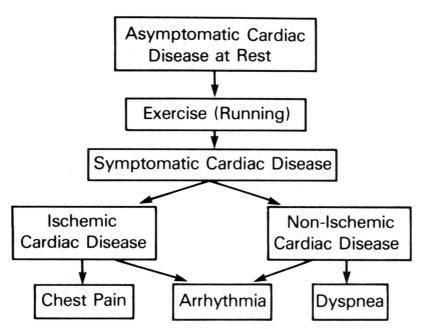

Figure 45. Exercise may unmask asymptomatic cardiac disease. (From Siegel, RJ, French, WJ, and Roberts, WC,[16] with permission.)

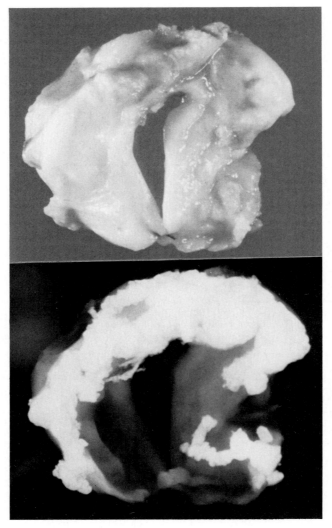

Figure 46. Patient number 1, Table 8. Operatively excised stenotic unicommissural (unicuspid) aortic valve showing heavy calcific deposits on a postexcision radiogram *(lower)*.

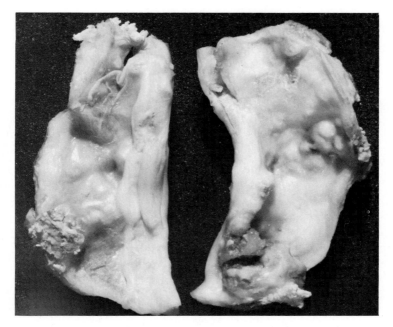

Figure 47. Patient number 2, Table 8. Operatively excised stenotic congenitally bicuspic aortic valve.

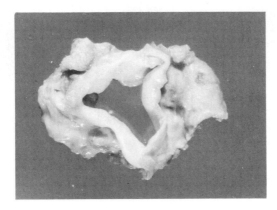

Figure 48. Patient number 3, Table 8. Operatively excised stenotic 3-cuspid aortic valve.

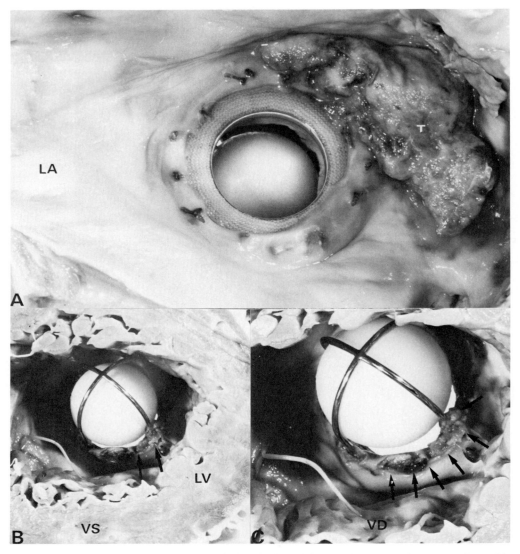

Figure 49. Patient number 1, Table 9. Photograph of a mitral caged-ball prosthesis inserted 10 years before sudden death during exercise. *A*, View of mitral prosthesis from opened left atrium (LA) showing mural thrombus (T). *B* and *C*, Views of prosthesis from left ventricle (LV) during simulated ventricular systole (VS) and diastole (VD) showing impaired movement of the poppet from fibrous tissue overgrowth (arrows).

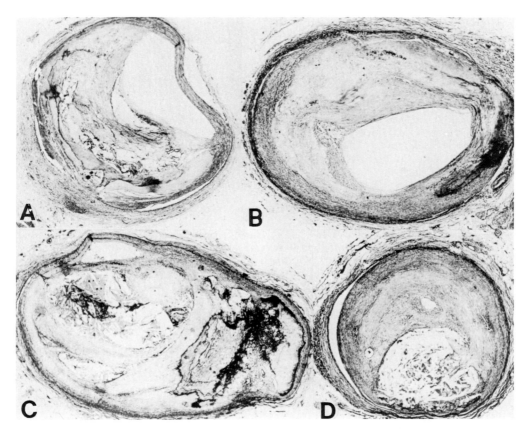

Figure 50. Patient number 3, Table 9. Sites of maximal cross-sectional area narrowing of the right (*A*), left main (*B*), left anterior descending (*C*), and left circumflex (*D*) coronary arteries. (From McManus, BM, Waller, BF, Graboys, TB, et al,[38] with permission.)

REFERENCES

1. The President's Council on Physical Fitness and Sports: *Adult Physical Fitness Survey.* Opinion Research Corporation, 1972, 1975.

2. *American Exercise Survey,* The Gallup Poll, 1978.

3. *Perrier Survey of Fitness in America,* Study No. S2813, Louis Harris and Associates, Inc., 1978.

4. *Healthy People: The Surgeon General's Report on Health Promotion and Disease Prevention,* 1979. Department of Health, Education, and Welfare, PHS Publication No. 79-55071, 1979.

5. *Exercise and Participation in Sports Among Persons 20 Years of Age and Over: United States, 1975.* National Center for Health Statistics, Department of Health, Education, and Welfare PHS Publication No. 78-1250, 1978.

6. FLETCHER, GF: *The dangers of exercise.* In *The Heart. Update V.* McGraw-Hill, New York, 1981, pp 161–174.

7. OPIE, LH: *Sudden death and sport.* Lancet 1:263, 1975.

8. OPIE, LH: *Long distance running and sudden death.* N Engl J Med 293:941, 1975.

9. GREEN, LH, COHEN, SI, AND KURLAND, G: *Fatal myocardial infarction in marathon racing.* Ann Intern Med 84:704, 1976.

10. CANTWELL, JD AND FLETCHER, GF: *Sudden death and jogging.* Phys Sports Med 3:94, 1978.

11. NOAKES, TD, ROSE, AG, AND OPIE, LH: *Hypertrophic cardiomyopathy associated with sudden death during marathon racing.* Br Heart J 41:624, 1979.

12. NOAKES, TD, OPIE, LH, ROSE, AG, ET AL: *Autopsy-proved coronary atherosclerosis in marathon runners.* N Engl J Med 301:86, 1979.

13. THOMPSON, PD, STERN, MP, WILLIAMS, P, ET AL: *Death during jogging or running. A study of 18 cases.* JAMA 242:1265, 1979.

14. VIRMANI, R, ROBINOWITZ, M, AND MCALLISTER, HA, JR: *Nontraumatic death in joggers. A series of 30 patients at autopsy.* Am J Med 72:874, 1982.

15. ROBERTS, WC, SIEGEL RJ, AND ZIPES, DP: *Origin of the right coronary artery from the left sinus of Valsalva and its functional consequences: Analysis of 10 necropsy patients.* Am J Cardiol 49:863, 1982.

16. SIEGEL, RJ, FRENCH, WJ, AND ROBERTS, WC: *Spontaneous exercise testing. Running as an early unmasker of underlying cardiac amyloidosis.* Arch Intern Med 142:345, 1982.

17. MARON, BJ, ROBERTS, WC, MCALLISTER, HA, JR, ET AL: *Sudden death in young athletes.* Circulation 62:218, 1980.

18. ULLYOT, J: *The Medical Report.* Runners World. II Sept. 16, 1976.

19. WARREN, SE, BOICE, JB, BLOOR, C, ET AL: *The athletic heart revisited. Sudden death of a 28-year-old athlete.* West J Med 131:441, 1979.

20. TSUNG, SH, HUANG, TY, AND CHANG, HH: *Sudden death in young athletes.* Arch Pathol Lab Med 106:168, 1982.

21. JAMES, TN, FROGGATT, P, AND MARSHALL, TK: *Sudden death in young athletes.* Ann Intern Med 67:1013, 1967.

22. ROBERTS, WC AND MARON, BJ: *Sudden death while playing professional football.* Am Heart J 102:1061, 1981.

23. COLT, E: *Coronary-artery disease in marathon runners.* N Engl J Med 302:57, 1980.

24. HANZLICK, R AND STIVERS, RR: *Sudden death in a marathon runner with origin of the right coronary artery from the left sinus of Valsalva.* Am J Cardiol 51:1467, 1983.

25. JOKL, E AND MCCLELLAN, JT: *Exercise and cardiac death.* Med and Sport Vol. 5: 1, 1971.

26. ROBERTS, TJ AND LOUBE, SD: *Congenital single coronary artery in man.* Am Heart J 34:188, 1947.

27. ROTTER, W: *Uber den abnormen Abgang der linken Herzkranzarterie aus der Lungenschlagader.* Zentralbl Allg Path Anat 89:160, 1952.

28. NIEOD, JL: *Anomalie coronaire et mort subite.* Cardiologia 20:172, 1952.

29. COHEN, LS AND SHAW, LD: *Fatal myocardial infarction in an 11-year-old boy associated with a unique coronary artery anomaly.* Am J Cardiol 19:420, 1967.

30. BENSON, PA AND LACK, AR: *Anomalous aortic origin of left coronary artery.* Arch Pathol 86:214, 1968.

31. CHEITLIN, MD, DECASTRO, CM, AND MCALLISTER, HA: *Sudden death as a complication of anomalous left coronary origin from the anterior sinus of Valsalva. A not-so-minor congenital anomaly.* Circulation 50:780, 1974.

32. LIBERTHSON, RR, DINSMORE, RE, BHARATI, S, ET AL: *Aberrant coronary artery origin from the aorta.* Circulation 50:774, 1974.

33. VUORI, I, MAKARAINEN, M, AND JAASKELAINEN, A: *Sudden death and physical activity.* Cardiology 63:287, 1978.

34. MORALES, AR, ROMANELLI, R, AND BOUCEK, RJ: *The mural left anterior descending coronary artery, strenuous exercise and sudden death.* Circulation 62:230, 1980.

35. WALLER, BF AND ROBERTS, WC: *Sudden death while running in conditioned runners aged 40 years or over.* Am J Cardiol 45:1292, 1980.

36. WALLER, BF, CSERE, RS, BAKER, WP, ET AL: *Running to death.* Chest 79:346, 1981.

37. MCMANUS, BM, WALLER, BF, GRABOYS, TB, ET AL: *Exercise and sudden death—Part 1.* Cur Prob Cardiol 9:1, 1981.

38. MCMANUS, BM, WALLER, BF, GRABOYS, TB, ET AL: *Exercise and sudden death—Part 2.* Cur Prob Cardiol 10:1, 1982.

39. THOMPSON, PD, FUNK, EJ, CARLETON, RA, ET AL: *Incidence of death during jogging in Rhode Island from 1975 through 1980.* JAMA 247:2535, 1982.

40. KOPLAN, JP: *Cardiovascular deaths while running.* JAMA 242:2578, 1979.

41. CURRENS, JH AND WHITE, PD: *Half a century of running. Clinical, physiologic and autopsy findings in the case of Clarence DeMar ("Mr. Marathon").* N Engl J Med 265:988, 1961.

42. YASUE, H, OMOTE, S, TAKIZAUA, A, ET AL: *Circadian variation of exercise capacity in patients with Prinzmetal's variant angina: Role of exercise-induced coronary arterial spasm.* Circulation 59:938, 1979.

43. VLODAVER, Z, AMPLATZ, K, BURCHELL, H, ET AL: *Coronary Heart Disease. Clinical, Angiographic and Pathologic Profiles.* Springer-Verlag, New York, 1976.

44. ASAY, RW AND VREWEG, WVR: *Severe coronary atherosclerosis in a runner: An exception to the rule?* J Cardiac Rehab 1:413, 1981.

45. HANDLER, JB, ASAY, RW, WARREN, SE, ET AL: *Symptomatic coronary artery disease in a marathon runner.* JAMA 248:717, 1982.

46. CANTWELL, JD AND FLETCHER, GF: *Cardiac complications while jogging.* JAMA 210:13, 1969.

47. NOAKES, T, OPIE, L, BECK, W, ET AL: *Coronary heart disease in marathon runners.* Proc NY Acad Sci 301:593, 1977.

48. KAVANAGH, T, SHEPHARD, RH, AND PANDIT, V: *Marathon running after myocardial infarction.* JAMA 229:1602, 1974.

Distance Running in the 1980s:
Cardiovascular Benefits and Risks

Herman K. Hellerstein, M.D.* and T. William Moir, M.D.*

Major changes have transpired in the past four decades in the management of patients with coronary heart disease. For example, changes during and after acute myocardial infarction include reduction of the period at bed rest, early mobilization, exercise testing before discharge from the hospital, return to work in a variety of occupations (many with significant physical and emotional demands), and subsequent high-level exercise testing and training in exercise programs. Some cardiologists have advocated extreme caution, with exercise training restricted to supervised and monitored programs, whereas others recommend vigorous participation in sports training, including marathon and long-distance running.[1]

In part, these changes in attitude have paralleled the dramatic increase in the United States in recent years in the popularity of jogging and of marathon running (26.2 miles, 42.2 km). A recent Gallup Poll showed that over 45 percent of Americans engage in some type of regular exercise activity.[2] This percentage is more than twice that found in a similar poll in the 1960s and includes 12 percent of people who report that they jog regularly. There has been a 300 percent increase in the number of marathon competitions in the United States during the 9-year period from 1968 to 1976.[3] Not only has the number of marathons increased but so has the number of runners capable of completing the race in under 3 hours.

The enthusiasm for running has extended to marathon running for cardiac patients and has led to the revival of the ultramarathon.[3] The latter consists of two classes of longer races: those requiring repetitive days of running long distances (generally at speeds slower than a marathon pace) and continuous runs of up to 100 miles. In the 1928 transcontinental foot race from Los Angeles to New York City (3484 miles), the contestants averaged approximately 41 miles a day for 84 consecutive days. Limited medical studies performed on the contestants 3 to 10 days after the race revealed no major adverse effects, although "The Race (1928) was characterized by almost every violation of the accepted principles of diet, hygiene and disregard for injuries, infection and human endurance."[3] In the long-distance race from Aomori to Tokyo in 1931, the total distance of 464.9 miles was divided into 12 unequal sections ranging from 22.2 to 52.8 miles, with one section to be run each day of the race. Motivated by concern for the runners' health, more sophisticated studies were performed in the South African 54-mile Comrades Marathon. The studies in 1970 stimulated further investigations of renal function and fluid and electrolyte balance.

---

*Supported in part by grants from Mr. and Mrs. Leo Demsey, Mr. and Mrs. Harry Figgie, Messrs. Neil, David, and Arthur Genshaft, Mr. and Mrs. Donald Krush, William L. Luntz, and Mr. and Mrs. Harry Mann.

The capacities and goals of the people running long distances, marathons, and ultramarathons are diverse:[3] some are competitors intending to win the race; a large number of runners of lesser training and/or ability have goals to improve their personal times and to compete against runners of similar capabilities or limitations; some intend just to complete the distance (a stimulating challenge); others hope to enhance self-esteem and to solve deep-seated emotional problems, especially depression; and many have the impression or hope that meeting this challenge will either preclude their developing coronary heart disease or, if already so identified clinically, will prevent or delay recurrence of myocardial infarction and prolong life.

A remarkable change in attitude toward long-distance running has transpired. Early investigators were concerned about the possible adverse repercussions of marathon running on the cardiovascular system; more recently the question being asked is whether the training required for a marathon in some way protects the individual against cardiovascular disease.

The change in emphasis stemmed in large part from the demonstration in the 1960s that a large majority (75 to 85 percent) of patients with myocardial infarction have responded favorably in a multitude of fashions to carefully supervised, comprehensive exercise reconditioning programs.[4,5] The exercise prescription is designed to exercise each subject at approximatley 60 to 80 percent of his or her aerobic capacity, during three one-hour training periods each week. At this relative load, many physiologic and biochemical changes transpire: the respiratory exchange ratio approaches unity and there are increases in blood lactate, fibrinolytic activity, urinary catecholamine excretion, capacity to oxidize fatty acids, release of fatty acids from adipose tissue, capacity to regenerate ATP by oxidative phosphorylation, and so on—desirable changes that are associated with favorable adaptation and health benefits.[6] The exercise sessions generally include run-walk and then jogging sequences to increase endurance, as well as calisthenics and recreational exercise. In the past, participants usually were not encouraged to run longer distances, that is, more than 6 to 10 miles each week.

The health benefits associated with such programs for cardiac patients include marked improvement of work capacity; reduction of exercise-induced blood pressure elevations; decrease of peripheral vascular resistance during exercise; diminution of the heart rate at rest, during sleep, and during exercise at submaximal effort; lowering of triglycerides and low-density lipoprotein cholesterol (LDL-C) and elevation of high-density lipoprotein cholesterol (HDL-C); enhanced extraction of the oxygen by the peripheral tissues; lessening of electrocardiographic ST segment displacement; increased fibrinolytic activity; and improvement of subjective well-being, with lowering of the depression, hypochondriasis, hysteria, and psychasthenia scales of the Minnesota Multiphasic Personality Inventory test.[5,7] The low mortality of participants in the early studies was not considered to be persuasive, because these studies were not randomized.[4] The inability of the early exercise trials to alter convincingly the natural history of coronary disease was attributed to the view that proper study of the effects of physical exercise on the cardiac patient must involve exercise levels above the "protective threshold of 6+ mile units to a total dose of 10,000 miles, a dose that is predicted to be able to promote regression of arteriosclerosis and to improve angiograms."[1]

Four prospective randomized studies were organized and conducted in the 1970s, employing a relatively moderate level of intensity of exercise training for patients following myocardial infarction.[5] In 1983, Dr. Roy J. Shephard (a prominent, enthusiastic proponent of marathon running for post-myocardial infarction patients) analyzed the combined data from 1318 subjects enrolled in several large controlled studies (U.S. National Exercise and Heart Disease Project, Finland, and Sweden) and found similar beneficial effects. Subjects allocated to exercise programs had a 25 to 35 percent survival advantage over control subjects and also had fewer recurrent events and fewer fatal outcomes for recurrences throughout a four-year period.[5,8]

In the midst of the aforementioned studies, in the early 1970s, the question was raised as to whether more vigorous training and marathon running programs were desirable and valuable in the rehabilitation of patients with coronary heart disease. Our personal enthusiasm for marathon running by such patients was dampened by the experience of one of our patients who completed the Boston Marathon on April 9, 1970, in 4 hours and 15 minutes.[6] His performance was remarkable. He completed the run within the time achieved by the first 35 percent of the participants who finished the 1970 Boston Marathon. However, his subsequent history was noteworthy. He continued to maintain his exercise training program. In February and March 1971, he experienced five episodes of Stokes-Adams syndrome and ventricular tachycardia and required emergency resuscitative treatment. Coronary arteriography revealed involvement of three coronary arteries; that is, complete occlusion of the proximal third of the right coronary artery, 90 percent stenosis of the proximal third of the left anterior descending coronary artery, and 30 percent stenosis of the left circumflex coronary artery. This experience highlighted the potential hazard of serious arrhythmias occurring during a marathon run, at which time immediate resuscitative efforts might not be available. For this reason, and because of the lack of substantial proof of the medical value of such athletic virtuosity, one of us (HKH) subsequently discouraged other similarly trained coronary subjects from marathon running.[6]

In 1973, Shephard and associates[9] reported their first experience with postcoronary marathon runners at an international scientific meeting in Magglinger. Substantial numbers of their patients had participated in various events from 1973 onward.[9]

Considerable fuel was added to the fires of enthusiasm for marathon running when Bassler claimed that marathon running conferred immunity to coronary disease, that is, "Marathon runners are immune to fatal atherosclerosis."[10] Although Shephard later (1983) disavowed "any particular enthusiasm for Bassler's immunity hypothesis . . . ," he and his associates have continued to promote marathon running for patients following myocardial infarction.[9] Although a majority of post-infarction patients were considered to have the *necessary potential* to undertake marathon training, to date "the total number of individuals referred to the Toronto program who chose to prepare themselves for running 42 km remained relatively small (1.1 percent 50 of 4,522 patients)."[1,9]

The Toronto Rehabilitation Center population was remarkable. They averaged 42 years of age. Only 2 percent had severe left ventricular dysfunction, and 34 percent of 610 patients had mild to moderate angina.[9] In other communities, long-distance or marathon running is considered to have a more limited applicability to patients discharged from the hospital after an acute myocardial infarction. They are usually older, the average ages of the men and women being 60 and 65 years, respectively, and only 5 percent are less than 45 years of age.[6] In our experience, only 5 to 7 of 1000 subjects discharged from a coronary care unit have the potential capacity to attain a $\dot{V}O_2$ max sufficient to complete a marathon run in 5 hours or less;[6] the limitations are motivation, age, presence of previous myocardial infarctions (in over one third), angina pectoris (in over one half), left ventricular dysfunction (in 20 to 30 percent), and the need for implanted pacemakers (especially in the elderly subjects with complete A-V block).

Because controversy continues to surround the effects of vigorous exercise on the morbidity and mortality of patients after myocardial infarction, as well as of coronary-prone subjects, and because conclusive proof is lacking that long distance or marathon running has any better effect on prognosis than does less vigorous physical or recreational activity, one can question the desirability of long-distance or marathon running in primary or secondary prevention programs.

This discussion reviews the cardiovascular adaptations, possible benefits, and risks of long-distance and marathon running. The psychologic benefits will not be presented inasmuch as they are similar to those that occur in participants of less intensive programs.[5,7]

CARDIOVASCULAR ADAPTATIONS AND BENEFITS

Long-distance or marathon running typically involves many months of careful preparation[11] and considerable time, with a minimum of running 10 miles a week usually required for long-distance (more than 500 miles per year) running, and more prolonged training before a marathon.[11] The success in distance running is related to the frequency, intensity, and duration of the training program prior to the competitive event.[12] World class distance runners usually run twice a day and between 110 and 240 km per week for 45 to 52 weeks per year. Less talented runners train below these levels. Marathoners usually train for more than 3 months at progressive weekly distances up to an average of 60 km per week for cardiac patients and 80 km per week for healthy persons.[12] This training requires at least 5 to 6 hours per week, exclusive of the additional time to stretch, warm up, and cool down, plus more time and energy allotted in usual rehabilitation exercise programs. The devotion to a training regimen often involves other beneficial changes. It requires a comprehension of and adherence to a prudent, hygienic life style including optimal nutrition, careful dietary modification (with reduction of fats and calories), weight control, abstinence from tobacco, avoidance of drug abuse, and adequate rest and sleep; in addition there is usually acquisition of considerable insight into the principles and practices of exercise training, stretching, warm up, dynamic activity, pacing of the intensity of effort, awareness of signs and symptoms of excessive activity, and cool down. Recently Bassler revised his concept that marathon running confers immunity to coronary disease and champions the view that marathon running involves a lifestyle conducive to freedom from coronary disease.

EFFECTS OF LONG-DISTANCE AND MARATHON RUNNING ON CARDIAC ARRHYTHMIAS DURING USUAL ACTIVITIES, OTHER THAN RUNNING, AND DURING MAXIMAL TREADMILL AND DISTANCE RUNNING. The recent interest in running as a means of enhancing physical fitness has focused interest on the mode of exercise-induced or exercise-related sudden cardiac death.[13] Although the majority of individuals who die suddenly during strenuous physical activity have coronary artery disease, some, especially those who are young, have no demonstrable heart disease.[14-17] Physicians are often asked to determine whether it is safe for an individual to enter or to continue in strenuous exercise training. The appearance of ventricular ectopy in high-level exercise tests has been used to give advice either to not run in order to avoid exposure to similar or worse arrhythmias, or to continue a jogging or running program to "obviate" the arrhythmia.[13]

To determine whether the latter approach is correct, Talan and associates[18] recently studied 20 21-year-old men who were experienced long-distance runners (running an average of 63 miles per week, training an average of 328 days per year for 6 years) and 50 healthy and untrained men. The two groups did not differ with respect to the prevalence of ventricular premature beats, R on T phenomenon, ventricular couplets, or ventricular tachycardia during 24 hours of ambulatory electrocardiographic monitoring during normal activities other than running. The long-distance runners consistently had slower sinus heart rates and a greater prevalence of marked sinus bradycardia than the untrained men. Average waking and sleeping rates in the long-distance runners were slower than in the untrained men, by 7 and 9 beats per minute, respectively. Considering the extreme cardiovascular functional differences between the long-distance runners and the untrained men, the difference in heart rates between the trained and the untrained men was not very striking.[13] Few significant differences in the various arrhythmias were noted between long-distance runners and untrained males. Atrial dysrhythmias were more common among the athletes. Runners had a significantly greater prevalence of isolated premature atrial beats (100 percent vs 56 percent) and of atrial couplets (25 percent vs 0 percent). There were no significant differences in the prevalence of isolated or complex ventricular ectopy (70 percent and 20 percent, respectively). Runners had a significantly greater prevalence of first degree A-V block (45 percent vs 8 percent) and of type 1 second degree A-V block (40 percent vs 6 percent) over a 24-hour recording period.[18]

Pantano and Oriel[13] used Holter monitoring to evaluate young (33-year-old) well-conditioned runners for arrhythmias during both a distance run and a maximal treadmill test. Sixty percent had some ventricular arrhythmias during a monitored run; 35 percent had occasional ventricular premature beats (VPBs), 10 percent ventricular bigeminy, 10 percent ventricular couplets or salvos, and 5 percent multiform VPBs. Treadmill testing significantly underestimated the frequency and grade of both atrial and ventricular arrhythmias. Although the grade of ventricular ectopy was higher during a distance run than in similar subjects during usual activities other than running, a high level of physical fitness did not "obviate" these potentially fatal arrhythmias.

These findings indicate that healthy, well-trained endurance runners commonly have variations in heart rhythm that could be ominous, possibly explaining sudden cardiac deaths in cardiac patients, and in the 10 percent of noncardiac subjects during cross-country ski touring, jogging, and marathon running.[13] The observed frequency of high-grade dysrhythmias in healthy subjects suggests that this is a statistically "normal" finding during prolonged strenuous exercises, and only long-term prospective studies will determine whether runners with these dysrhythmias are at increased risk of sudden death. As yet, there is no proof that enhanced physical fitness resulting from endurance running protects healthy persons or cardiac patients with coronary artery disease from exercise-induced dysrhythmias and sudden cardiac death.

ADAPTIVE CARDIOVASCULAR CHANGES PRODUCED BY REGULAR INTENSIVE TRAINING (ENDURANCE RUNNING). Noninvasive evaluation by echocardiographic techniques has shown consistent differences between endurance runners and control subjects (Table 1), both at rest and after effort.[19-23] Increased left ventricular mass, diastolic volume, stroke volume, and ejection fraction have been confirmed by many studies. However, the left ventricular peak velocity of circumferential fiber shortening of the runners relative to that of the control subjects was significantly reduced, both at rest and during submaximal supine exercise at a similar absolute workload. Since peak Vcf is a more sensitive index of fiber shortening than mean Vcf and may be able to detect small changes in fiber shortening rates that do not affect mean Vcf of the runners, the reduced peak Vcf may indicate a reduction of intrinsic myocardial contractility.[22] An increase in parasympathetic and a decrease in sympathetic activity have been postulated to account for the reduced heart rate in athletes. Paulsen and associates[22] suggest that these influences could also exert a negative inotropic effect on the myocardium and reduce contractility, and hence Vcf, in parallel with the reduction in heart rate. However, reduction in Vcf was directly related to the lower pressure-rate product of the runners; and this finding suggested that endurance training did not produce a change in the contractile proteins of the myocardial cell.[22] Moreover, the reduction in Vcf was no different in runners than in normal control subjects, indicating that running neither increased nor decreased intrinsic myocardial contractility.

Intense and prolonged exercise training of eight patients with coronary heart disease produced echocardiographic changes similar to those found in normal, healthy younger runners,

Table 1. Characteristics of marathon and long-distance runners compared with untrained sedentary controls

Left Ventricle	Other
+ Muscle mass	+ Left atrial diameter
+ Wall thickness	− Heart rate at rest, submaximal effort
+ End-diastolic volume	+ QRS (ECG) amplitude
+ Stroke volume	+ Third and fourth heart sounds
− Systolic volume	
+ Ejection fraction	
+ Cardiac output	
+ Diastolic thickness of interventricular septum	
− Peak velocity of circumferential fiber shortening; at rest, submaximal effort	

+ = Increased
− = Decreased

including increased left ventricular end-diastolic volume and, surprisingly, a higher mean velocity of circumferential shortening during static exercise after training.[24] These changes occurred in addition to the increased maximal oxygen uptake, increased oxygen pulse, lower heart rate at rest and at submaximal exercise, and lower systolic blood pressure at a given workload after training. Systolic blood pressure at maximal exercise increased after training; this increase may reflect improvement in the overall left ventricular performance, inasmuch as myocardial ischemia results in a lower peak systolic pressure during exercise.[24] The cardiac enlargement and the significant increases in end-diastolic diameter and posterior wall thickness are similar responses to those observed in young and middle-aged long-distance runners. The results of this preliminary study of coronary patients indicate that in addition to the well-known peripheral adaptations, prolonged and intense exercise training may have resulted in favorable cardiac adaptations.

The question as to whether training produces significant central adaptations in addition to the well-established peripheral adaptations has still not been resolved. In the special case of patients with impaired left ventricular function, improvement of left ventricular ejection fraction at rest and after effort occurred more frequently in trained than in control groups.[25] However, training produced no significant change in the ejection fraction at rest and during exercise in a large group (99 patients) who trained on an average of 6.5 weeks following myocardial infarction.[25]

As yet there has been no evidence that marathon or long-distance running has reversed or halted the rate of progression of coronary atherosclerosis or has increased intercoronary collateral circulation. The effects of physical training in patients with coronary artery disease has been studied by angiography and isotope techniques. Although an increase in coronary collaterals has been documented in some patients, similar changes have also been found in other patients with coronary artery disease who have not participated in a physical training program.[26] In this regard, it appears that myocardial ischemia (progression of atherosclerosis) has a greater effect than physical training. The evidence that physical training enhances intercoronary collateral formation in humans with coronary artery disease is equivocal. The reason may be the insensitivity of angiography. Because present day angiography does not visualize vessels smaller than 100 micra, changes in lesser size vessels cannot be excluded.[27] Future technologic advances using computer processing may permit detection of changes in smaller coronary vessels similar to those currently being demonstrated in the aorta and iliac arteries.[28] Radionuclide testing is now being used to evaluate this possibility. Froelicher and associates[29] reported that 6 of 16 patients with coronary artery disease participating in a physical training program for at least 3 months showed some improvement in myocardial perfusion during exercise testing with thallium-201. However, several larger studies found no evidence that collateral vessel development was different in a group of exercise-trained patients when compared with control subjects with coronary heart disease. Although physical training improved exercise performance, there was no difference between the resting or exercise myocardial perfusion index as studied by thallium-201 scintigraphy before and after a 12-week treadmill training program.[30]

LIPOPROTEIN LEVELS IN DISTANCE AND MARATHON RUNNERS. Population studies suggest that there is an inverse relationship between the amount of physical activity and the incidence of coronary heart disease[11] but do not necessarily prove a causal relationship. A prospective long-term study of 50 distance runners and 43 control subjects showed that the runners had significantly lower pulse rates and relative weights, higher levels of high-density lipoprotein (HDL) cholesterol, and lower levels of low-density lipoprotein (LDL) cholesterol. Multiple factors have been cited to account for the elevation of HDL-cholesterol, namely, the distance run, relative body weight, diet, and body fatness. The hypothesis that exercise elevates HDL-cholesterol and results in protection from coronary heart disease is an attractive, well-publicized theory. Undoubtedly, this possibility motivates some of the millions of healthy Americans and a growing number of cardiac patients who have taken up distance and marathon running. This hypothesis remains unproved. Many years of observation of comparable numbers of long-distance runners and control subjects will be required to clarify this issue.[11] Meanwhile, long-distance running cannot be rcommended for coronary patients solely on the basis of the possibility that distance running will prevent, reverse, or retard the development of coronary atherosclerosis.

CARDIOVASCULAR RISKS

The enthusiasm for jogging has caused large numbers of participants to move into long-distance, endurance running. Included in this group are an increasing number of patients with known coronary heart disease, and their participation has included training for and completing full marathons.[3,9] For both normal individuals and patients known to have coronary disease, these levels of exercise seem far beyond those required to attain a cardiovascular training effect and the other direct and indirect cardiovascular benefits ascribed to such efforts.[11] In all of this enthusiasm, however, consideration must be given to the cardiovascular risks involved, particularly for presumably normal individuals in whom the need for restraint is not as easily accepted as it is more likely to be in the case of patients with known coronary heart disease.

Among normal individuals with widely patent coronary arteries, there is an extremely small but definite prevalence of sudden cardiac death associated with long-distance training and running, as documented by postmortem studies.[14–16] Additionally, a limited number of incidence studies confirm an association between distance running and sudden cardiac death, although this occurrence may be chance or, at the most, constitutes an extremely low risk.[31–33] In the majority of cases, sudden cardiac death is associated with coronary artery disease, which was previously undiagnosed in most of these cases. This association is particularly apt to occur in men over the age of 40, in contrast to a variety of other cardiovascular causes (for example, hypertrophic cardiomyopathy) that are more likely to be encountered in younger individuals.[34] An important epidemiologic feature of the sudden cardiac deaths associated with coronary heart disease is that, in the majority of cases, the presence of the disease was either known or could have been suspected by accompanying signs or symptoms. In other words, the death was not entirely unheralded. Of additional importance, data from these studies indicate a high prevalence of coronary risk factors among these individuals and suggest that potential candidates for sudden cardiac death might be identified by appropriate medical screening.

Although the risk of exercise-induced ventricular fibrillation has been estimated to be low (between one in 116,000 and one in 300,000 person-hours)[9] for cardiac patients, and even lower for normal subjects, defibrillators, trained medical personnel, and appropriate emergency transportation should be available throughout a marathon course. Ledingham and associates[35] have reported effective defibrillation and resuscitation of a 47-year-old man who collapsed within 30 meters of the finishing line during the Glasgow Marathon. The success of the resuscitation under field conditions may be attributable to the ready availability of a ventricular defibrillator and of trained personnel in a mobile intensive care unit.[35] Other subjects have not been so fortunate.

Education is of primary importance in identifying possible candidates for sudden cardiac death related to subclinical coronary heart disease, among individuals already participating in endurance running or those who wish to begin such a program. The education should include the meaning of symptoms such as exercise-related chest discomfort, arrhythmias, sudden changes in levels of fatigue, and so on. For established distance runners, this recognition is a difficult problem because of the high level of denial of discomfort that accompanies endurance training. For individuals who wish to begin an exercise program and who visit their physicians for advice in this regard, such education can be included in the medical screening.

MYOCARDIAL DAMAGE. It has been suspected that distance running produces myocardial damage. Creatine kinase MB isoenzyme levels become elevated in most (65 percent) marathon runners after a race.[36] Although infarct scintigraphy (technetium Tc 99^m pyrophosphate) may be normal, this study does not exclude the presence of small transmural myocardial infarctions or nontransmural infarctions.[37] Another cardiac source such as myocytolysis[38] or a combination of cardiac and skeletal muscle sources may account for the observed increases in serum CK-MB.

Firm guidelines do not exist for the pre-exercise assessment of coronary risk for subjects who wish to begin an endurance training program. However, based on available epidemiologic and clinical pathologic data the following algorithm is suggested for use by clinicians. First, individuals younger than 40 years of age, without known cardiopulmonary disease (implying that they have had some type of physical examination in the past) should be able to begin a rigorous training program without further evaluation. For people over age 40, or for younger people with coronary risk factors, a history and physical examination and a resting electrocardiogram is advisable prior to beginning training. If this examination discloses information that is suggestive of coronary heart disease or identifies major coronary risk factors (hypercholesterolemia, untreated hypertension, cigarette smoking, diabetes mellitus, family history of premature coronary artery disease, or an abnormal resting electrocardiogram), a multistage exercise test is advisable. However, the clinician must recognize that there are limitations to this test because of the occurrence of both false-positive and false-negative responses, the latter being the more important with respect to screening for subclinical coronary heart disease. Thus, the exercise test should not be used for general screening despite the recommendation of the American College of Sports Medicine that people over age 35 should have an exercise test prior to beginning a vigorous exercise program.[39] The efficacy of this recommendation as a practical screening device is not supported by available data nor by present clinical usage.[40] Rather, the predictive value of exercise testing for the detection of coronary heart disease in presumably normal people is directly related to the prevalence of the disease in the population of interest, as manifested by the presence of coronary risk factors. Using the latter indication for exercise testing, an abnormal response might appropriately call for exclusion of coronary disease by arteriography in individuals over 40 who wish to pursue an endurance training program for long-distance running. However, there is the residual problem of false-negative responses to exercise in individuals with coronary risk factors. In this circumstance, consideration should be given to the use of an exercise test with myocardial imaging, which if normal in conjunction with a normal electrocardiographic response to exercise, absence of coronary disease can be assumed to be accurate with a high level of certainty.[41] Again, these technical applications would be appropriate only for those individuals with prominent coronary risk factors who wish to begin an endurance training program.

The issue of safety in endurance training and running in patients with known coronary heart disease seems more straightforward than the unknown risks in presumably normal individuals. Data from rehabilitation exercise programs for patients after myocardial infarction indicate that levels of exercise training that produce a cardiovascular training effect can be safely used by appropriately screened patients. However, these training programs are usually less rigorous than those required for endurance exercise.[4,6] This being the case, it appears reasonable to advise coronary arteriography in all patients with known coronary heart disease, in addition to the usual maximal exercise test for assessment of safe levels of intensive physical activity.[42] This anatomic evaluation, together with exercise testing, will provide the clinician with information regarding the degree of risks and the advisability of such patients beginning endurance training programs, particularly if unsupervised.

Although coronary heart disease is the major cardiovascular risk associated with long-distance and marathon running, one must also consider the presence of other cardiovascular abnormalities as possible impediments to such physical activities. Among these disorders are valvular heart disease, cardiomyopathies, cardiac arrhythmias without associated heart disease, and uncontrolled essential hypertension.

In almost all circumstances, cardiomyopathy is incompatible with endurance training. With congestive cardiomyopathies the inherent abnormality of left ventricular function will severely limit cardiovascular adaptations to distance training. Although in the hypertrophic cardiomyopathies, left ventricular function may be perfectly normal and patients may be able to attain high levels of training, the risk of sudden cardiac death has been clearly documented and competition should be prohibited.[34,43]

Similarly, significant valvular heart disease is incompatible with endurance training and long-distance running. In particular, syncope is a clear cardiovascular risk in patients with hemodynamically significant aortic valvular stenosis because of the failure of cardiac output to compensate for peripheral vasodilation. In patients with mitral stenosis, the rise in left atrial pressure that occurs because of a decreased diastolic filling time incident to an increased heart rate could lead to acute pulmonary edema. Although the left ventricular volume overload associated with aortic and mitral regurgitation might be compatible, in the early stages, with endurance training and running, the inherent limitation of cardiac reserve and the possibility of accelerating left ventricular dysfunction contraindicates endurance type physical activity for patients with these conditions.

A special case for consideration with regard to distance running and valvular heart disease is the presence of mitral valve prolapse. Because of the high prevalence of this abnormality, it is of practical significance to assess the cardiovascular risk associated with endurance exercise. Fortunately, sudden cardiac death is rare in this syndrome despite a relatively high prevalence of arrhythmias. However, if individuals with mitral valve prolapse have symptomatic cardiac arrhythmias, it would be prudent to perform an exercise test prior to beginning an endurance training program. Interestingly, there are data suggesting that exercise training in patients with mitral valve prolapse can decrease the frequency of arrhythmia events.[44]

The cardiovascular risk associated with the presence of premature ventricular beats in individuals without evidence of cardiac disease is not known but is probably extremely small. With respect to the pre-exercise training assessment of such individuals, the presence of premature ventricular beats at rest probably requires an electrocardiogram both to identify the morphology of the beats and to screen for possible electrocardiographic manifestations of underlying heart disease. However, because ventricular premature beats per se are not a coronary risk factor, an exercise test is not required unless the patient gives a history of awareness of this arrhythmia during exercise. In that case, the exercise test would serve to establish whether complex forms of premature ventricular beats were present which possibly entail an increased risk of fatal arrhythmia during strenuous exertion. As mentioned earlier, recent studies indicate that a maximal treadmill exercise test is not very sensitive with respect to the induction of premature ventricular beats, in comparison with similar arrhythmias discovered by Holter monitoring during a distance run.[13] The latter data also demonstrate that ventricular arrhythmias (and atrial arrhythmias), including some complex forms, are present in over half of well-trained runners who were monitored during training. Thus, premature ventricular beats are of importance with respect to cardiovascular risk in distance running only when they are associated with overt heart disease or when they are the sole manifestation of some underlying disease. As with most patients with premature ventricular beats and no evidence of heart disease, treatment should be directed at control of symptoms rather than prevention of a fatal cardiac arrhythmia, and these individuals should not be excluded from endurance training and long-distance running.

Although there is increasing evidence that exercise training may be beneficial as part of a treatment program for patients with mild to moderate hypertension,[45–47] there are no data with respect to hypertension as a specific risk factor for endurance training and long-distance running. Exercise testing has shown that systolic and diastolic pressures in young patients with sustained essential hypertension are significantly higher during exercise than in normal individuals or in those with labile high blood pressure.[48] Although these young people had no deleterious cardiac effects of the blood pressure elevations, the response of older individuals with respect to induction of abnormalities of cardiac function is not known and, therefore, untreated hypertensive patients should be advised to avoid strenuous endurance training. Patients with labile hypertension and those with fixed hypertension under treatment should have an exercise test prior to beginning an endurance training program, in order to identify excessive elevations in blood pressure that would require appropriate modification of treatment. It should be recognized that antihypertensive drug therapy may limit participation in endurance training because of modification of the cardiovascular responses, especially those associated with the use of beta-blocking agents, and the possible deleterious electrolyte and metabolic effects of diuretics.

Heat injury, which is a general risk in long-distance running, may have a specific deleterious cardiac effect: myocardial infarctions have been documented as a consequence of hyperthermia.[49] However, the cardiac risk is small in comparison with the fatal central nervous system and metabolic consequences of heat injury.

The final cardiovascular risk associated with endurance training and running is failure of clinicians to recognize that highly trained athletes may show cardiovascular "abnormalities" incident to an extreme training effect. These changes include sinus and junctional bradycardias, first and second degree heart blocks (Wenckebach), electrocardiographic signs of advanced left ventricular hypertrophy, systolic heart murmurs, third heart sounds, and increased heart size on x-ray examinations.[50,51] Clinicians must be aware of the possibility of such changes in endurance athletes in order to avoid a misdiagnosis of cardiovascular disease.

SUMMARY

Although within the capacity of perhaps one to two percent of highly motivated patients after myocardial infarction, long-distance and marathon running do not confer on normal subjects immunity from coronary atherosclerosis or freedom from high grades of ventricular ectopy during running and nonrunning activities. The presence of significant coronary heart disease does not preclude participation in long-distance and marathon running, provided appropriate safety precautions are taken.[5,6,52] There is no conclusive proof that the long-term prognosis is improved by long-distance or marathon running or by increasing the intensity of training above the generally accepted level of 60 to 80 percent of $\dot{V}O_2$ max. Marathon running for coronary patients and for coronary-prone persons remains experimental and awaits further scientific evaulation employing a prospective randomized study of subjects with angiographic proof of significant coronary artery disease.[1]

REFERENCES

1. Hellerstein, HK: *Marathon jogging in post-MI patients*. J Cardiac Rehab 3:441, 1983.

2. The Gallup Poll. Princeton, N.J., 1980, p 109.

3. Maron, MB and Horvath, SM: *The marathon: A history and review of the literature*. Med Sci Sports 10:137, 1978.

4. Hellerstein, HK: *Exercise therapy in coronary disease*. Bull NY Acad Med 44:1028, 1968.

5. Shephard, RJ: *The value of exercise in ischemic heart disease: A cumulative analysis*. J Cardiac Rehab 3:294, 1983.

6. Hellerstein, HK: *Limitations of marathon running in the rehabilitation of coronary patients: Anatomic and physiologic determinants*. Ann NY Acad Sci 301:484, 1977.

7. Hellerstein, HK and Franklin, BA: *Exercise testing and prescription*. In Wenger, NK and Hellerstein, HK (eds): *Rehabilitation of the Coronary Patient*, ed 2. John Wiley & Sons, New York, 1983.

8. Shaw, LW: *Effects of a prescribed supervised exercise program on mortality and cardiovascular morbidity in patients after a myocardial infarction. The National Exercise and Heart Disease Project*. Am J Cardiol 48:39, 1981.

9. Shephard, RJ, Kavanagh, RT, Tuck, J, et al: *Marathon jogging in post-myocardial infarction patients*. J Cardiac Rehab 3:321, 1983.

10. BASSLER, TJ: *Marathon running and immunity to atherosclerosis.* Ann NY Acad Sci 301:579, 1977.

11. ADNER, MM AND CASTELLI, WP: *Elevated high-density lipoprotein levels in marathon runners.* JAMA 243:534, 1980.

12. HAGAN, RD, SMITH, MG, AND GETTMAN, LR: *Marathon performance in relation to maximal aerobic power and training indices.* Med Sci Sports and Exercise 13:185, 1981.

13. PANTANO, JA AND ORIEL, RJ: *Prevalence and nature of cardiac arrhythmias in apparently normal well-trained runners.* Am Heart J 104:762, 1982.

14. VIRMANI, R, ROBINOWITZ, M, AND MCALLISTER, HA: *Nontraumatic death in joggers. A series of 30 patients at autopsy.* Am J Med 72:874, 1982.

15. THOMPSON, P, STERN, M, WILLIAMS, P, ET AL: *Death during jogging or running: A study of 18 cases.* JAMA 242:1265, 1979.

16. WALLER, B AND ROBERTS, W: *Sudden death while running in conditioned runners aged 40 years or over.* Am J Cardiol 45:1292, 1980.

17. HAYASHI, KD AND LEWIS, ER: *Sudden death in a marathon runner with widely patent coronary arteries.* Clin Cardiol 3:288, 1980.

18. TALAN, DA, BAUERNFEIND, RA, ASHLEY, WW, ET AL: *Twenty-four hour continuous ECG recordings in long-distance runners.* Chest 82:19, 1982.

19. PARKER, BM, LONDEREE, RR, GUPP, GV, ET AL: *The non-invasive cardiac evaluation of long-distance runners.* Chest 73:376, 1978.

20. IKAHEIMO, MJ, PALATSI, IJ, AND TAKKUNEN, JT: *Non-invasive evaluation of the athletic heart: Sprinters versus endurance runners.* Am J Cardiol 44:24, 1979.

21. LONGHURST, JC, KELLY, AR, GONYEA WJ, ET AL: *Echocardiographic left ventricular masses in distance runners and weight lifters.* J Appl Physiol 48:154, 1980.

22. PAULSEN, W, BOUGHNER, RR, KO, P, ET AL: *Left ventricular function in marathon runners: Echocardiographic assessment.* J Appl Physiol 51:881, 1981.

23. MUMFORD, M AND PRAKASH, R: *Electrocardiographic and echocardiographic characteristics of long distance runners. Comparison of left ventricular function with age- and sex-matched controls.* Am J Sports Med 9:23, 1981.

24. EHSANI, AA, MARIN, WH, HEATH, GW, ET AL: *Cardiac effects of prolonged and intense exercise training in patients with coronary artery disease.* Am J Cardiol 50:246, 1982.

25. GRODZINSKI, E, KREUTZ, E, BLUMCHEN, G, ET AL: *The behavior of the ejection fraction (EF) at rest and exercise in cardiac infarct patients before and after a 4-week training period. Comparison to a control group.* Z. Kardiol 72:105, 1983.

26. SCHEUER, J: *Effects of physical training on myocardial vascularity and perfusion.* Circulation 66:491, 1982.

27. HELLERSTEIN, HK: *Panel V: Acceleration of collaterals due to physical activity—Dogma or fact. A misguided goal or unrealized objective?* In KELLERMANN, JJ AND DENOLIN, H (EDS): *Critical Evaluation of Cardiac Rehabilitation.* S. Karger, Basel, Switzerland, 1977, p 125.

28. MALINOW, MR AND BLATON, V (EDS): *Regression of Atherosclerosis in Humans.* Plenum Press, New York (in Press).

29. FROELICHER, V, HENSEN, D, ATWOOD, JE, ET AL: *Cardiac rehabilitation evidence for improvement in myocardial perfusion and function.* Arch Phys Med Rehab 61:517, 1980.

30. VERANI, MS, HARTUNG, GH, HOEPFEL-HARRIS, J, ET AL: *Effects of exercise training on left ventricular performance and myocardial perfusion in patients with coronary artery disease.* Am J Cardiol 47:797, 1981.

31. KOPLAN, J: *Cardiovascular deaths while running.* JAMA 242:2578, 1979.

32. GIBBONS, L, COOPER, K, MEYER, B, ET AL: *The acute cardiac risk of strenuous exercise.* JAMA 244:1799, 1980.

33. THOMPSON, P, FUNK, E, CARLETON, R, ET AL: *Incidence of death during jogging in Rhode Island from 1975 through 1980.* JAMA 247:2535, 1982.

34. MARON, B, ROBERTS, W, AND MCALLISTER, H: *Sudden death in young athletes.* Circulation 62:218, 1980.

35. LEDINGHAM, IM, MACVICAR, S, WATT, I, ET AL: *Early resuscitation after marathon collapse.* Lancet 2:1096, 1982.

36. KIELBLOCK, AJ, MANJOO, M, BOOYENS, J, ET AL: *Creatine phosphokinase and lactate dehydrogenase levels after ultra long-distance running.* S Afr Med J 55:1061, 1979.

37. KASTE, M AND SHERMAN, DG: *Creatine kinase isoenzyme activities in marathon runners.* Lancet 2:327, 1982.

38. ALI, M: *Elevated CK-MB levels in marathon runners.* JAMA 247:2368, 1982.

39. AMERICAN COLLEGE OF SPORTS MEDICINE: *Guidelines for Graded Exercise Testing and Exercise Prescription,* ed 2. Philadelphia, Lea & Febiger, 1980.

40. RYNEARSON, R, ROBERTS, J, AND STEWART, W: *Occasional notes: Do physician athletes believe in pre-exercise examinations and stress tests?* N Engl J Med 301:792, 1979.

41. PATTERSON, R, HOROWITZ, S, ENG, C, ET AL: *Can exercise electrocardiography and thallium-201 myocardial imaging exclude the diagnosis of coronary artery disease?* Am J Cardiol 49:1127, 1982.

42. HELLERSTEIN, HK: *Anatomic factors influencing effects of exercise therapy of ASHD subjects.* In ROSKAMM, H AND REINDELL, H (EDS); *Das Chronisch Kranke Herz.* FK Schattauer Verlag-Stuttgard, New York, 1973, p 513.

43. NOAKES, T, ROSE, A, AND OPIE, LH: *Hypertrophic cardiomyopathy associated with sudden death during marathon racing.* Br Heart J 41:624, 1979.

44. ALEXANDER, L AND SCHAAL, S: *Effects of exercise on mitral valve prolapse syndrome patients.* Med Sci Sports Exerc 14:165, 1982.

45. KRATKIEWSKI, M, MANDROUKOS, K, SJOSTROM, L, ET AL: *Effects of long-term physical training on body fat, metabolism, and blood pressure in obesity.* Metabolism 28:650, 1979.

46. ROMAN, O, CAMUZZI, A, VILLALON, E, ET AL: *Physical training program in arterial hypertension.* Cardiology 67:230, 1981.

47. WILCOX, R, BENNETT, T, BROWN, A, ET AL: *Is exercise good for high blood pressure?* Br Med J 285:767, 1982.

48. NUDEL, D, GOOTMAN, N, AND BRUNSON, S: *Exercise performance of hypertensive adolescents.* Pediatrics 65:1073, 1980.

49. KNOCHEL, JP: *The marathon: Physiological, medical, epidemiological, and psychological studies. Part II. Body temperature and fluid balance discussion.* Ann NY Acad Sci 301:185, 1977.

50. OAKLEY, D, AND OAKLEY, C: *Significance of abnormal electrocardiograms in highly trained athletes.* Am. J Cardiol 50:985, 1982.

51. VIITASALO, M, KALA, R, AND EISALO, A: *Ambulatory electrocardiographic recordings in endurance athletes.* Br Heart J 47:213, 1982.

52. HANDLER, JB, ASSAY, RW, WARREN, SE, ET AL: *Symptomatic coronary artery disease in a marathon runner.* JAMA 248:717, 1982.

Effects of Exercise on the Myocardium: Echocardiographic Studies

Ezra A. Amsterdam, M.D., and Lawrence J. Laslett, M.D.

Echocardiography provides a unique approach to the investigation of the effects of exercise training on the myocardium and may help to clarify important aspects of a number of changes.[1] This noninvasive method affords accurate serial analysis of cardiac structure and function with no known risk and at reasonable cost. These advantages have recently stimulated a number of studies using echocardiography to determine the cardiac effects of habitual exercise in both normal individuals and cardiac patients.

Previous reports concerning a cardiac component in the response to exercise training have been restricted to the demonstration of augmented cardiac pump performance[2] and assessment of heart volume and mass from chest roentgenography[3,4] and electrocardiography.[5] These methods are inadequate to evaluate this problem because alterations in cardiac pump function may be related to extracardiac factors as well as to intrinsic contractility.[6] Furthermore, radiography and electrocardiography are imprecise for assessing cardiac volume and mass. Cardiac ultrasound studies, using M-mode echocardiography, have assessed the anatomic and functional response to exercise by measurement of myocardial wall thickness and ventricular dimensions and by calculation of derived indexes such as left ventricular mass, shortening fraction and circumferential fiber shortening rate (V_{CF}). These data have been obtained almost entirely in the resting state following a training program, inasmuch as echocardiography poses substantial technical problems during exercise.[7]

METHODOLOGIC CONSIDERATIONS

Although echocardiography is superior to previous methods used to assess the response of the myocardium to exercise training, this technique has certain inherent limitations, particularly in relation to anatomic alterations that are small (measured im millimeters) and that develop over extended periods. Such changes are illustrated by the echocardiographic recordings shown in Figure 1 from one study depicting the magnitude of changes in morphology and function following exercise training.[8] Echocardiographic analysis entails subjective interpretation that may present problems with regard to quantitative data. It should be appreciated that endocardial surface recognition is not always precise and reproducible, thereby resulting in a potential source of error involving this factor. It is therefore essential that more than one observer be involved in the analysis. The observers should function independently and should be blinded as to the origin of each echocardiogram. To minimize sources of error related to transducer angulation in a longitudinal study, echocardiographic measurements should be made at the same intracardiac site, for example, the level of the chordae tendineae. Calculations of cardiac mass from data obtained at a specific site assume uniformity of myo-

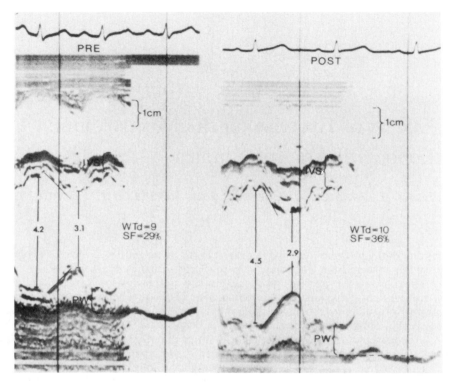

Figure 1. Pre- and post-exercise training echocardiograms. Illustrated are the echograms obtained prior to (PRE) and following (POST) training in a representative subject from this study. The solid lines depict the course of interventricular septal and posterobasal endocardial motion during systole. PW = left ventricular posterior wall; WTd = left ventricular wall thickness; SF = left ventricular shortening fraction.[8] (Reproduced with permission from the American Heart Association.)

cardial thickness, which may not apply because of normal variability in this factor or abnormal asymmetry. However, despite any error in absolute values, directional changes in measurements that occur over time are meaningful. Nonetheless, it is important that caution be exercised in the interpretation of changes noted at echocardiography. For example, an increase in end-diastolic dimension following training may reflect an intrinsic cardiac structural adaptation or may be related to augmented diastolic filling associated with the bradycardia of training.

There is more than one convention for performing echocardiographic measurements such as thickness of the interventricular septum, posterior wall, and diameter of the left ventricle. Several such standards have been presented,[9] differing in the point in the cardiac cycle and the precise sites on the myocardial wall used for measurements. Despite these technical limitations, however, echocardiographic determination of cardiac chamber dimensions, wall thickness, and ventricular mass correlate well with data obtained from ventriculographic and anatomic measurements.[10,11]

INDIVIDUALS IN THE TRAINED STATE

Studies in Man

Several echocardiographic studies have been performed in athletes at a time when they were already in the trained state.[5,12,13] Although these evaluations did not assess these subjects longitudinally, prior to and after a program of exercise training, they did include control groups for comparison. Of note is the superior level of aerobic capacity of those athletes for whom these data were available, reflected by group mean maximal oxygen consumptions of 70.9[12] and 62.0[13] ml/kg/min for distance runners and 57.0 ml/kg/min for cycle racers.[13] The findings in these reports were consistent in demonstrating that, in association with this very high aerobic capacity, echocardiographically measurable alterations were consistent with increased left ventricular volume and mass. Thus, as a group, professional basketball players,[5] distance runners,[12,13] and cyclists[13] had, compared with less active matched control subjects, increased left ventricular end-diastolic dimension,[5,13] end-diastolic volume,[12] end-diastolic volume index,[12] posterior wall thickness,[5,12,13] and interventricular septal thickness[13] and mass.[12,13] In addition, there were also increases in right ventricular end-diastolic dimensions.[5,12] In the two studies that reported left ventricular ejection fraction and V_{CF}, there was either no change[5] or a slight decrease in the athletes,[12] the latter believed to be an appropriate conservation of contractile function in the trained, enlarged, bradycardic heart, which thereby required less mechanical effort to maintain resting cardiac output. These studies provide evidence that the heart adapts to intense aerobic training with an increase in both mass and volume, in addition to the well-recognized bradycardia, and that there is little alteration in indices of function at rest.

The cardiac adaptations to exercise appear to be related somewhat to the mode of training. It has thus been reported that isometric exercise, such as weight lifting or wrestling, is primarily associated with increases in left ventricular wall thickness and thereby mass,[14] whereas isotonic activity, such as running and swimming, increases cardiac mass mainly through dilatation.[14] Other reports are less clear in this regard in that increased left ventricular wall thickness has been found in individuals who engage in isotonic (running), combined isotonic-isometric (cycling), and isometric (weight lifting) activities.[13] Moreover, the increments in wall thickness were greater with isotonic than with isometric exercise.[13] In weight lifters, the only increase was in left ventricular wall thickness, whereas in runners and cyclists wall thickness and end-diastolic dimensions were both elevated. Thus, the reports[13,14] are consistent in suggesting that increased wall thickness is the major cardiac adaptation to isometric exercise. Discrepancies between the studies concerning the cardiac response to isotonic training may reflect differences in training state as well as the ages of the subjects.

Animal Data

Rippe and colleagues[15] recently combined cardiac catheterization studies with echocardiography to assess the anatomy, hemodynamics, systolic mechanics, and diastolic properties of the heart in relation to the level of physical activity in dogs. Their experimental animals included highly trained racing greyhounds, greyhounds that had been detrained for six months or more, and mongrel dogs of comparable weight. Both left ventricular wall thickness and mass were greater in the greyhounds than in the mongrel dogs, although there were no differences between the two groups of greyhounds. However, the diastolic properties of the left ventricle (peak negative dp/dt, peak negative V_{CF}, and stiffness) were similar in racing greyhounds and mongrels. These findings are of considerable interest in their implication that cardiac hypertrophy induced by physiologic stimuli such as aerobic training is not associated with the abnormal diastolic properties (for example, reduced compliance) characteristic of hypertrophy related to abnormal or disease conditions such as chronic pressure overload.

LONGITUDINAL STUDIES IN NORMAL SUBJECTS

Most but not all investigations using pre- and post-training echocardiography in healthy individuals show some evidence of cardiac structural changes in association with physiologic evidence of a trained state (for example, increased functional capacity, increased maximal oxygen consumption, and attenuation of heart rate response to submaximal exercise). Echocardiographic evidence of alteration in cardiac performance is more variable.

Alterations in Cardiac Structure and Function

In an early study, DeMaria and coworkers demonstrated that aerobic training was accompanied by significant echocardiographic changes in ventricular mass and performance.[8] Twenty-six normal individuals (15 men, 11 women) ranging in age from 20 to 34 years engaged in a walk-jog-run program at 70 percent of maximal heart rate for one hour four days per week for 11 weeks. The estimated peak oxygen consumption rose from 35.5 ml/kg/min before training to 40.6 ml/kg/min after training. Compared with pre-training, echocardiography following training (Figures 1 through 4) revealed an increase in left ventricular end-diastolic dimension, wall thickness, and mass; decrease in left ventricular end-systolic dimension; and increases in stroke volume, shortening fraction, and V_{CF}. There was also electrocardiographic evidence of left ventricular hypertrophy. The changes noted in this study were small but consistent, and limitation of the investigation to young, healthy individuals in whom high quality echocardiograms could be obtained and who served as their own controls further supported the validity of the results.

A combination of dynamic and static exercise training during seven months in the form of competitive rowing by members of a Dutch college crew resulted in cardiac alterations that were related to the initial training state and cardiac dimensions.[16] Thus, in freshman oarsmen

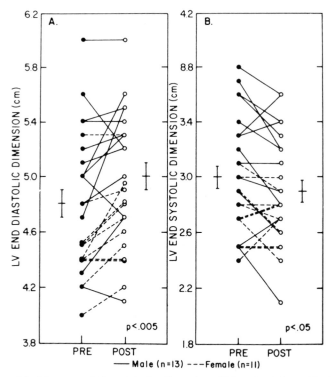

Figure 2. Influence of training upon left ventricular dimensions. Values for left ventricular (LV) end-diastolic (panel A) and end-systolic (panel B) dimensions are exhibited for the pre- and post-training periods.[8] (Reproduced with permission from the American Heart Association.)

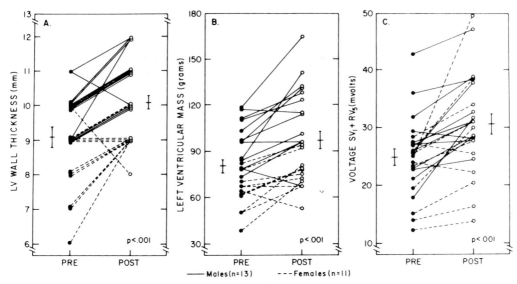

Figure 3. Effects of exercise upon left ventricular mass. Displayed are the values of left ventricular wall thickness (panel A), mass (panel B), and the sum of the electrocardiographic voltage of the S wave in lead V_1 and R wave in lead V_5 ($SV_1 + RV_5$) (panel C) before and after the training program.[8] (Reproduced with permission from the American Heart Association.)

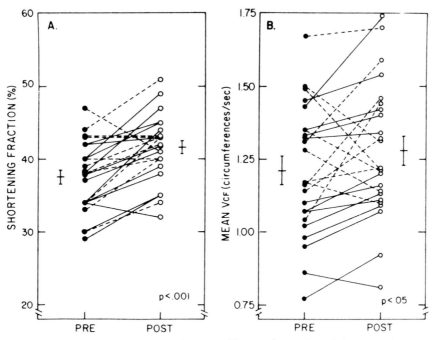

Figure 4. Effect of training upon ventricular performance. Illustrated are values of shortening fraction (panel A) and mean velocity of circumferential fiber shortening (V_{CF}) (panel B) before and after exercise training.[8] (Reproduced with permission from the American Heart Association.)

an increase in maximal oxygen consumption from 58.0 to 65.4 ml/kg/min was associated with increases in left ventricular end-diastolic dimension and interventricular septal and posterior wall thickness. In senior rowers, however, who had augmented left ventricular end-diastolic dimension and wall thickness at the beginning of the training season, echocardiography showed a further increase only in left ventricular end-diastolic dimension during training in which maximal oxygen consumption rose from 62.1 to 71.7 ml/kg/min. There was no alteration in left ventricular shortening fraction in either group. The investigators interpreted these results as indicating that chronic heavy exercise had induced physiologic cardiac hypertrophy and dilatation in the seniors that was altered only slightly by further training, whereas in the freshmen, more extensive exercise-induced cardiac changes occurred in relation to their initial, less altered cardiac morphology.

Augmentation of cardiac anatomy after training and regression of enlargement with detraining have been reported by Ehsani and coworkers.[17] Evaluating eight competitive swimmers in whom maximal oxygen uptake increased from 52 to 60 ml/kg/min, they demonstrated increases in left ventricular end-diastolic dimension, posterior wall thickness, and the derived indices of left ventricular end-diastolic volume, mass, and stroke volume. Conversely, in six competitive runners who were assessed during detraining over three weeks in which maximal oxygen consumption fell from 62 to 57 ml/kg/min, there were significant reductions in left ventricular end-diastolic dimension, posterior wall thickness, and the derived indices.

Augmentation in cardiac dimensions and performance not only at rest but also during exercise was demonstrated after training by Stein and associates.[18] In their study of 14 healthy students who underwent 14 weeks of vigorous interval bicycle training that resulted in a 31 percent increase in maximal oxygen consumption (28.7 to 37.6 ml/kg/min), training was associated with an increase at rest in left ventricular end-diastolic dimension, stroke dimension, and dimensional shortening. Measurements of ventricular wall thickness were not reported. A unique aspect of this investigation was the performance of echocardiographic measurements *during* exercise before and after training. Exercise after training, compared with the pre-trained state, was associated with an increase in stroke dimension related to a decrease in end-systolic dimension, whereas end-diastolic dimension during exercise remained unaltered compared with pre-training values. The authors interpreted these findings as being indicative of a training-induced enhancement of contractile state during exercise, inasmuch as a Starling effect was not apparent in this state.

Enlarged cardiac dimensions without an accompanying increase in wall thickness after training have been reported by Adams and colleagues.[19] A program of aerobic exercise (jogging) for 11 weeks in 25 male students 18 to 25 years old that resulted in enhanced physiologic status (maximal oxygen consumption: 48.6 to 56.2 ml/kg/min) also induced an increase in measured left ventricular end-diastolic dimension and calculated end-diastolic volume and stroke volume—changes that did not occur in the control group. The trained subjects, however, had no alterations in left ventricular posterior and septal wall thickness or in ejection fraction.

Minimal Cardiac Changes

Several studies have shown little or no echocardiographically detectable changes in cardiac structure and function in association with development of a trained state.[20-22] Aerobic exercise (running) produced significant improvement in predicted[20] and measured[21] maximal oxygen consumption (42.4 to 50.0 and 58.4 to 64.2 ml/kg/min, respectively), without alterations in left ventricular wall thickness or its dimensions.[20,21] However, in one of these studies[20] derived stroke volume increased slightly but significantly, and in the other,[21] the small increase in calculated left ventricular mass was significant. Similarly, only calculated left ventricular mass at rest during autonomic blockade increased significantly in a study of arm or leg endurance training that produced a significant training effect.[22] Of interest was a group of subjects who underwent strength training[21] with significant improvement in upper body strength and similar echocardiographic results as in the runners in the same study, that is, slight but significant increase in left ventricular mass without significant changes in wall thickness or dimension.

In all three of the foregoing investigations, minimal but significant changes occurred in derived indices calculated from measured data that were not significantly altered. The interpretations of the investigators in each instance were that the changes observed probably related more to the training bradycardia and small secondary increase in end-diastolic dimension than to an intrinsic modification of cardiac structure. It was further asserted that the trained state could be attained without echocardiographic evidence of cardiac adaptations. In this regard, in one of the studies an enhanced contractile state during exercise was suggested on the basis of systolic time interval data.[22]

LONGITUDINAL STUDIES IN PATIENTS WITH CORONARY HEART DISEASE

Limited longitudinal studies using echocardiography to assess the cardiac effects of training in coronary patients have yielded variable findings. Ehsani and coworkers[23] demonstrated significant increases in left ventricular end-diastolic and end-systolic diameters and in posterior wall thickness in association with a 12-month aerobic training program that increased maximal oxygen uptake from 26 to 37 ml/kg/min. Additionally, left ventricular fractional shortening and V_{CF} decreased in response to isometric handgrip exercise before but not after training. By contrast, Ditchey and associates[9] found that the attainment of a training effect (rise in peak exercise capacity from 8.8 to 10.7 METs) from an aerobic exercise program over a seven-month interval was unaccompanied by echocardiographic evidence of cardiac adaptations. There were no changes in left ventricular end-diastolic diameter, posterior wall or interventricular septal thickness, or cross-sectional area. They concluded that the improved functional capacity after exercise training in patients with coronary heart disease is not due to exercise-induced left ventricular hypertrophy. The disparate echocardiographic findings in these two studies cannot be related to differences in the pre-and post-training levels of aerobic capacity, the duration of training, or the ages of the subjects, all of which were similar in the two groups.

CONCLUSIONS

Echocardiographic studies indicate that cardiac enlargement is a frequent finding after exercise training. This structural alteration most commonly consists of an increase in left ventricular end-diastolic dimension consistent with volume overload hypertrophy. However, the change in this factor is small, the increase in end-diastolic dimension in the studies reviewed here averaging 1.9 mm. Increases in left ventricular wall thickness and functional alterations are less common than dimensional changes but do occur. Again, they are usually of modest magnitude. Cardiac structural adaptation that accompanies isometric, strength-building exercise, when it does occur, is primarily an increase in left ventricular wall thickness, but this has not been a consistent finding. Factors that may account for some inconsistencies in current echocardiographic studies of the effects of exercise on the myocardium include the mode, intensity, and duration of training; the age of the subjects, inasmuch as cardiac responsiveness to training may be inversely related to age;[20] and the differing echocardiographic techniques employed.

Whether an increase in end-diastolic dimension in the presence of a training effect represents an intrinsic cardiac change or is secondary to augmented diastolic filling is a recurring question in these echocardiographic studies. An accompanying increase in wall thickness is evidence for a primary cardiac alteration. An increase of as much as 34 beats per minute produces a reduction of end-diastolic dimension of only 2 mm.[23] Therefore, similar enlargement in end-diastolic dimension in association with training-induced decrements in heart rate of 5 to 10 beats per minute is unlikely to be related to changes in heart rate alone.

Echocardiography has provided a previously unavailable means of directly assessing the effects of physical training on the heart. This application of cardiac ultrasound is still in its early stages; it is anticipated that its full potential in this setting is yet to be realized.

REFERENCES

1. AMSTERDAM, EA, LASLETT, LJ, DRESSENDORFER, RH, ET AL: *Exercise training in coronary heart disease: Is there a cardiac effect?* Am Heart J 101:870, 1981.

2. CLAUSEN, J: *Circulatory adjustments to dynamic exercise and effect of physical training in normal subjects and in patients with coronary artery disease.* Progr Cardiovasc Dis 18:459, 1976.

3. FRICK, NH, KONITTINEN, A, AND SARAJAS, HSS: *Effects of physical training on circulation at rest and during exercise.* Am J Cardiol 12:142, 1963.

4. EKBLOM, B, ASTRAND, PO, SALTIN, B, ET AL: *Effect of training on circulatory response to exercise.* J Appl Physiol 24:518, 1968.

5. ROESKE, WR, O'ROURKE, RA, KLEIN, A, ET AL: *Noninvasive evaluation of ventricular hypertrophy in professional athletes.* Circulation 53:287, 1976.

6. MASON, DT, SPANN, JF, ZELIS, R, ET AL: *Comparison of the contractile state of the normal, hypertrophied and failing heart in man.* In ALPERT, N (ED): *Cardiac Hypertrophy.* Academic Press, New York, 1971, p 433.

7. FEIGENBAUM, H (ED): *Echocardiography.* Lea & Febiger, Philadelphia, 1981.

8. DEMARIA, AN, NEUMANN, A, LEE, G, ET AL: *Alterations in ventricular mass and performance induced by exercise training in man evaluated by echocardiography.* Circulation 57:237, 1978.

9. DITCHEY, RV, WATKINS, J, McKIRNAN, MD, ET AL: *Effects of exercise training on left ventricular mass in patients with ischemic heart disease.* Am Heart J 101:701, 1981.

10. TROY, BL, POMBO, J, AND RACKLEY, CE: *Measurement of left ventricular wall thickness and mass by echocardiography.* Circulation 45:602, 1972.

11. SAHN, DJ, DEMARIA, A, KISSLO, J, ET AL: *Recommendations regarding quantitation in M-mode echocardiography. Results of a survey of echocardiographic measurements.* Circulation 58:1072, 1978.

12. GILBERT, CA, NUTTER, DO, FELNER, JM, ET AL: *Echocardiographic study of cardiac dimensions and function in the endurance-trained athlete.* Am J Cardiol 40:528, 1977.

13. SNOECKX, LHEH, ABELING, HFM, LAMBREGTS, JAC, ET AL: *Echocardiographic dimensions in athletes in relation to their training programs.* Med Sci Sports Exer 14:428, 1982.

14. MORGANROTH, J, MARON, BJ, HENRY, WL, ET AL: *Comparative left ventricular dimensions in trained athletes.* Ann Intern Med 82:521, 1975.

15. RIPPE, JM, PAPE, LA, ALPERT, JS, ET AL: *Studies of systolic mechanics and diastolic behavior of the left ventricle in the trained racing greyhound.* Basic Res Cardiol 77:619, 1982.

16. WIELING, W, BORGHOLS, EA, HOLLANDER, AP, ET AL: *Echocardiographic dimensions and maximal oxygen uptake in oarsmen during training.* Br Heart J 46:190, 1981.

17. EHSANI, AA, HAGBERG, JM, AND HICKSON, RC: *Rapid changes in left ventricular dimensions and mass in response to physical conditioning and deconditioning.* Am J Cardiol 42:52, 1978.

18. STEIN, RA, MICHIELLI, D, DIAMOND, J, ET AL: *The cardiac response to exercise training: Echocardiographic analysis at rest and during exercise.* Am J Cardiol 46:219, 1980.

19. ADAMS, TD, YANOWITZ, FG, FISHER, AG, ET AL: *Noninvasive evaluation of exercise training in college-age men.* Circulation 64:958, 1981.

20. WOLFE, LA, CUNNINGHAM, DA, RECHNITZER, PA, ET AL: *Effects of endurance training on left ventricular dimensions in healthy men.* J Appl Physiol: Respirat Environ Exer Physiol 47:207, 1979.

21. RICCI, G, LAJOIE, D, PETITCLERC, R, ET AL: *Left ventricular size following endurance, sprint, and strength training.* Med Sci Sports Exer 14:344, 1982.

22. THOMPSON, PD, LEWIS, S, VARADY, A, ET AL: *Cardiac dimensions and performance after either arm or leg endurance training.* Med Sci Sports Exer 13:303, 1981.

23. EHSANI, AA, MARTIN, WH, III, HEATH, GW, ET AL: *Cardiac effects of prolonged and intense exercise training in patients with coronary artery disease.* Am J Cardiol 50:246, 1982.

Predischarge Exercise Testing After Myocardial Infarction: Prognostic and Therapeutic Features

Donald A. Weiner, M.D.

The exercise test has been the standard noninvasive procedure to help confirm or exclude the diagnosis of coronary artery disease. Recently, exercise testing using a modified, low-level protocol has been applied to patients early after myocardial infarction.[1-3] These so-called postinfarction or predischarge exercise tests have been shown to be safe and feasible even when performed as early as 10 to 21 days after an uncomplicated myocardial infarction.[4-8] The widespread use of standard exercise tests was documented in a survey of physician practices in the management of patients with uncomplicated myocardial infarction in the year 1979.[9] Eighty-three percent of the cardiologists and 59 percent of the internists surveyed stated they used exercise testing. Both percentages represented substantial increases from a similar survey in 1970. Thus, the use of exercise testing early after an infarction has now become an accepted procedure not only to assess a patient's functional capacity in preparation for an exercise rehabilitation program, but also as a diagnostic, prognostic, and therapeutic guide (Table 1).

RATIONALE FOR EARLY EXERCISE TESTING

Risk stratification of patients soon after myocardial infarction can serve two purposes. Those patients ascertained to be at high risk for a future coronary event could be treated with more intensive medical or surgical therapy. On the other hand, those patients who are identified as being at low risk would not need more complicated noninvasive or invasive studies and could have an accelerated rehabilitation and return to normal daily activities.

Many studies have identified subgroups of patients with complicated myocardial infarctions who are at higher risk for subsequent cardiac events. The presence of a large infarction, diagnosed by clinical, electrocardiographic, laboratory, or scintigraphic studies at rest, identifies patients who have severe mechanical damage.[10,11] Complex ventricular arrhythmias before hospital discharge have been shown to have important prognostic value.[12-14] These arrhythmias may, however, simply reflect poor left ventricular function, which in turn determines the patient's poorer prognosis.[15] Finally, patients with persistent or recurrent angina early after infarction have a higher mortality.[16,17] Timely cardiac catheterization appears indicated in these patients to define the coronary anatomy and determine surgical feasibility.

Approximately 75 percent of patients do not have ventricular dysfunction, complex arrhythmias, or angina after myocardial infarction and are initially considered to be at low risk. Some of these patients may still develop complications including severe angina pectoris, recurrent myocardial infarction, or even sudden death during the first year after hospital discharge. In these initially uncomplicated patients, exercise testing prior to hospital discharge may identify subgroups of patients with considerably worse prognoses.

Table 1. Objectives of predischarge exercise testing

I. Functional Capacity
   A. Assess capacity for performing tasks at home
   B. Clearance for return to work
   C. Prescription for cardiac rehabilitation
II. Diagnostic
   A. Detection of multivessel coronary disease and jeopardized myocardium
   B. Assess overall ventricular function and segmental wall abnormalities
   C. Provocation of ventricular arrhythmias
III. Prognostic
   A. Prediction of future coronary events and cardiac death

METHODS

Patient Selection

In order to ensure the safety of testing, it is important to identify patients after myocardial infarction who would not be appropriate for predischarge exercise testing. Patients with rest angina, angina at low activity levels, congestive heart failure at rest, complex ventricular arrhythmias, rest or postural hypotension, or untreated hypertension should be excluded. Severe pulmonary, orthopedic, or neurologic problems may limit a patient's ability to perform even low-level exercise. A stable resting electrocardiogram should be established before starting the exercise test. Using these guidelines for excluding patients, many studies have shown that predischarge exercise testing is remarkably safe.[4-7] Only one study reported any major complications—two nonfatal reinfarctions (representing less than 1 percent of the population undergoing testing) within 24 hours of the exercise test.[8]

Protocol

All patients should be fully ambulatory before testing. The exercise test is usually performed on a treadmill, which uses a familiar form of exercise-walking. Alternatively, a bicycle ergometer may occasionally be more feasible in selected patients. Whichever mode of effort is used, the exercise tests should be performed in a fashion modified in two important ways: the tests should begin with a low initial level of effort and proceed with smaller workload increments than the usual diagnostic protocols. The two most commonly used protocols for predischarge exercise testing are the modified Bruce[18] and Naughton[19] protocols (Table 2).

Table 2. Representative post-myocardial-infarction treadmill test protocols

Stage	Speed (mph)	Grade (%)	METS*
A. Modified Bruce			
0	1.7	0	1.7
½	1.7	5	2.9
1	1.7	10	4.0
B. Modified Naughton			
1	2.0	0	2
2	2.0	3.5	3
3	2.0	7	4
4	2.0	10.5	5

*METS = Multiples of resting energy expenditure

End Points

The predischarge exercise test is always performed with physician supervision. After each stage of exercise, a clinical assessment and electrocardiographic and blood pressure measurements should be made before advancing the patient. The end points of exercise should be predetermined with three general guidelines:

(1) Cardiac signs—the development of 1 to 2 mm of ischemic ST segment depression or complex ventricular arrhythmias on the monitoring electrocardiogram, a fall in the systolic blood pressure, or an unsteady gait.

(2) Symptoms—the occurrence of mild anginal chest pain, dyspnea, or dizziness.

(3) Attainment of a target heart rate (usually 60 to 70 percent of the age-predicted maximal heart rate) or workload (usually 4 to 5 METs).

Whether the predischarge exercise test should be symptom limited or heart rate limited is still controversial. A symptom-limited exercise test appears to yield a higher frequency of abnormal exercise responses in terms of the development of ischemic ST segment depression or angina without increasing the risk of the test.[20,21]

DIAGNOSTIC VALUE OF PREDISCHARGE EXERCISE TESTING

Three studies have correlated the results of early exercise testing with subsequent cardiac catheterization findings in 145 patients[22-24] (Figure 1). Eighty percent of the 77 patients with exercise-induced ischemic ST segment depression or angina had multivessel coronary artery disease; 59 percent had three-vessel disease. In contrast, 40 percent of the 68 patients without evidence of ischemia on exercise testing had multivessel coronary disease, and three-vessel disease was found in 19 percent. Thus, inducible myocardial ischemia on a predischarge exercise test correlates very highly with the presence of multivessel disease, but a classically negative exercise test is not necessarily a reliable indicator of single vessel disease.

Patterson and coworkers[25] analyzed multiple exercise variables in 40 patients who underwent exercise testing 3 to 24 months after myocardial infarction in an attempt to identify

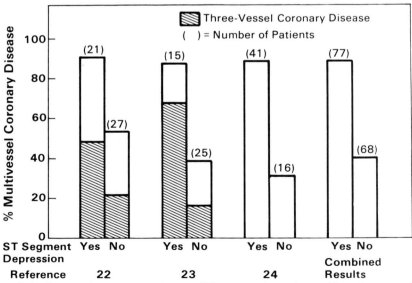

Figure 1. Correlation between the presence or absence of ST segment depression, multivessel coronary disease (top of bars), and three-vessel coronary disease (shaded areas). The data presented are from three separate studies and the combined results.

patients with left main or three-vessel coronary artery disease. If ischemic ST segment depression occurred at a heart rate less than 70 percent of the age-predicted maximal heart rate, there was an 86 percent probability of left main or three-vessel disease. Other useful non ST segment parameters included the failure to achieve 85 percent of the age-predicted maximal heart rate (in the absence of propranolol) and a decrease in the systolic blood pressure during exercise.

The presence of ST segment elevation during exercise testing in the electrocardiographic leads overlying the area of infarction is believed to reflect severe segmental ventricular abnormality rather than myocardial ischemia.[26,27] Thus, it has not been predictive of the extent of coronary artery disease.[26] However, it is generally found in those patients with anterior myocardial infarctions and is associated with a greater degree of impairment of left ventricular contraction and a lower ejection fraction.[22]

PROGNOSTIC SIGNIFICANCE OF EXERCISE TESTING

The results of five independent studies that employed predischarge exercise testing two weeks after infarction to stratify the risk of patients with uncomplicated myocardial infarction are shown in Table 3.[4-8] A total of 838 patients underwent a low-level exercise test using the modified Bruce or Naughton protocol and were followed for a mean of 15 months after the initial infarction to determine the risk of recurrent coronary events (severe angina, a second myocardial infarction, or cardiac death).

ST Segment Depression

The most powerful exercise predictor of recurrent coronary events and cardiac deaths was the occurrence of ischemic ST segment depression. This abnormality occurred in 30 percent of patients and conferred a 36 percent risk of a coronary event and a 16 percent probability of cardiac death (Figure 2). For patients without ischemic ST segment depression, the risk of recurrent coronary events and cardiac death was 16 and 4 percent, respectively. These results indicate that inducible ischemia by exercise testing is a powerful prognostic abnormality, indicating that areas of myocardium away from the infarction are supplied by stenosed coronary vessels and are still in jeopardy.

Table 3. Representative studies evaluating exercise testing postinfarction

	Patients (n)	Mean Age (years)	Type of Protocol	End Point of Exercise	Mean Days Post-MI (n)	Follow-up (months)
Smith et al, 1979[4] (University of Arizona)	62	60	Modified Naughton	60 % HR max	18	21
Theroux et al, 1979[5] (Montreal Heart Institute)	210	53	Modified Naughton	70 % HR max	11	12
Sami et al, 1979[6] (Stanford)	200	53	Modified Naughton	Symptoms	21	19
Starling et al, 1980[7] (University of Texas, San Antonio)	130	54	Modified Naughton	130 beats/min	15	11
Weld et al, 1981[8] (Columbia)	236	57	Modified Bruce	4 mets	16	12

n = number; HR max = maximal age-predicted heart rate

98

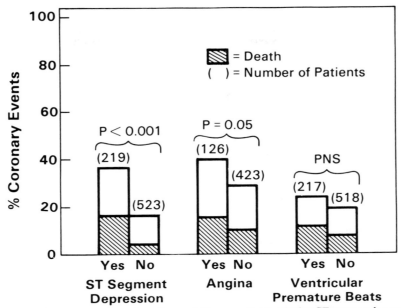

Figure 2. Frequency of coronary events and cardiac mortality according to whether ST segment depression, angina, or ventricular premature beats were present or not. The data are from references 4 through 8.

The effects of medications such as digitalis or beta-adrenergic blocking agents on the ST segment response during exercise testing have uncertain prognostic implications. It may be that beta-adrenergic blocking agents help prevent cardiac mortality after an infarction by inhibiting the ischemic potential.

Further analysis of the ST segment response, such as the amount, configuration, time of onset, and duration of ST segment depression, may further define risk. In one study, the risk of a coronary event was two times greater for patients with ≥0.2 mv of ST segment depression compared with patients with 0.1 to 0.19 mv ST segment depression.[6]

Angina

Angina during exercise testing occurred in 23 percent of patients undergoing predischarge exercise testing. This finding alone conferred an 11 percent additional risk of recurrent coronary events (Figure 2). Anginal pain that occurs concomitantly with ST segment depression probably does not add additional predictive power above that of ST segment abnormalities alone. However, the presence of angina during exercise testing does correlate with the recurrence of angina after hospital discharge and may indicate the need for a more intensive antianginal drug regimen.[28]

Ventricular Arrhythmias

The occurrence of any ventricular arrhythmias during predischarge exercise testing did not add significant prognostic information (Figure 2); the incremental risk averaged only 5 percent. These results are at variance with the clear-cut relationship of ventricular arrhythmias with prognosis postinfarction when ambulatory electrocardiographic monitoring was employed.[12-14] The greater duration of ambulatory monitoring compared with the exercise period may explain this discrepancy. Moreover, the presence of ventricular arrhythmias during exercise testing may have greater implications for patients with either baseline ventricular dysfunction, inducible ischemia, or complex ventricular arrhythmias.[15] Because therapy may be different if either inducible ischemia or left ventricular dysfunction is present, it is best to evaluate the arrhythmic status of a patient with both exercise testing and ambulatory ECG monitoring.

Abnormal Blood Pressure Response

Although an abnormal systolic blood pressure response to exercise occurs infrequently, its presence may have important prognostic implications.[29] Two independent studies found that either a fall in the systolic blood pressure[7] or a maximal systolic blood pressure less than 130 mm Hg[8] was associated with increased risk of recurrent coronary events. The risk was even greater when the abnormal blood pressure response was associated with other exercise test abnormalities such as inducible ischemia.[7] It should be emphasized that the effects of certain medications such as beta-adrenergic blocking agents may blunt the systolic blood pressure rise with exercise but rarely lead to an actual fall in blood pressure during exercise.

Exercise Duration

The functional status of the left ventricle during exercise is reflected by the total exercise duration.[30] Two independent studies have confirmed the importance of total treadmill time as a prognostic indicator.[8,31] A low-risk population (<1 percent mortality) included those patients able to complete 9 minutes on a modified Bruce protocol during a predischarge exercise test[8] or 10 minutes on a regular Bruce protocol when exercise testing was performed 6 to 8 weeks after infarction.[31]

REPRODUCIBILITY OF EXERCISE ABNORMALITIES

When exercise testing at 7 weeks after infarction was compared with the predischarge test, it appeared that the presence of inducible ST segment depression was highly reproducible, but the occurrence of angina pectoris and ventricular arrhythmias was not as reproducible.[32,33] Exercise capacity generally increases over the 3 to 6 weeks after discharge, especially if the patient is enrolled in a cardiac rehabilitation program.[34] The heart rate response to a given workload also declines in the first 3 months after infarction, probably related to a conditioning effect.

TIMING OF A POSTINFARCTION EXERCISE TEST

As many as 10 percent of patients who undergo predischarge exercise testing do not return for repeat testing 3 months later because of a recurrent myocardial infarction or cardiac death.[20,33] Therefore, because the safety of early exercise testing has been confirmed in many studies, it is reasonable to assess the ischemic response and risk of a patient with uncomplicated myocardial infarction during a predischarge low-level exercise test. The exercise test may be repeated with a more standard protocol 6 to 12 weeks after infarction to plan for cardiac rehabilitation, evaluate the work potential, and further assess cardiac risk.

EXERCISE RADIONUCLIDE STUDIES

Thallium-201 Scintigraphy

Diagnosis

Several studies have demonstrated that exercise thallium-201 scintigraphy early after myocardial infarction is useful in predicting the extent of coronary artery disease.[35,36] The presence of reversible ischemia, especially in areas of the myocardium distant from the infarction, identified more than 70 percent of patients with multivessel coronary disease in two separate investigations.[35,36] This abnormality on thallium testing had a sensitivity of 65 percent and a specificity of 96 percent in identifying postinfarction patients with left main or three-vessel coronary disease.[25]

Prognosis

Thallium testing was also found to have prognostic significance in a study by Gibson and colleagues.[37] In a study of 140 consecutive patients postinfarction undergoing early exercise thallium testing postinfarction, the investigators found that an abnormal thallium uptake or washout in 2 or 3 different vascular regions or increased lung uptake of thallium identified 86 percent of patients who had late cardiac events, including 89 percent of patients who died.[37]

Exercise Radionuclide Ventriculography

The determination of the left ventricular ejection fraction at rest and during exercise has been extremely helpful in noninvasively assessing the extent of left ventricular damage, which in turn determines the postinfarction risk. Wasserman and coauthors investigated the diagnostic value of exercise radionuclide ventriculography in predicting multivessel coronary disease.[38] Using the criteria of either a new wall motion abnormality or a fall in the ejection fraction during exercise, the investigators found that the sensitivity and specificity was 80 and 92 percent, respectively, for patients with inferior myocardial infarctions but only 69 and 40 percent, respectively, for patients with anterior myocardial infarctions.[38]

Two other studies have investigated the prognostic value of exercise radionuclide ventriculography, with divergent results.[39,40] Borer and coworkers found that the resting but not the exercise left ventricular ejection fraction was helpful in identifying patients with subsequent cardiac deaths,[39] whereas Corbett and coinvestigators concluded that the change in the ejection fraction with exercise rather than the resting ejection fraction was the most important variable in predicting future cardiac events during a three month followup.[40]

THERAPEUTIC IMPLICATIONS OF PREDISCHARGE EXERCISE TESTING

Patients who sustain complicated myocardial infarctions are not candidates for early exercise testing. Those patients who develop severe angina after infarction should have prompt cardiac catheterization and timely coronary bypass surgery if feasible. Patients with large infarctions who develop congestive heart failure or have severely depressed left ventricular ejection fractions constitute the majority of individuals with postinfarction deaths and are the most difficult to treat. These patients should have optimal inotropic and vasodilator therapy aimed at treating congestive heart failure and the frequently concomitant ventricular arrhythmias. They would not be candidates for cardiac catheterization unless they were found to have inducible ischemia or a discrete ventricular aneurysm by noninvasive testing. Those patients who develop complex ventricular arrhythmias but have preserved left ventricular function should be controlled by antiarrhythmic therapy, perhaps guided by electrophysiologic testing, and then would be candidates for exercise testing.

The remaining patients with initially uncomplicated myocardial infarctions should undergo modified exercise testing if feasible (Figure 3). Based on current data, patients who manifest either ischemic ST segment depression (especially greater than 0.2 mv), angina, or a fall in the systolic blood pressure at low levels of exercise would be classified as high risk with an expected 15 to 20 percent one-year mortality. Inasmuch as this subgroup of patients still has residual jeopardized myocardium, they should be treated with intensive medical therapy and

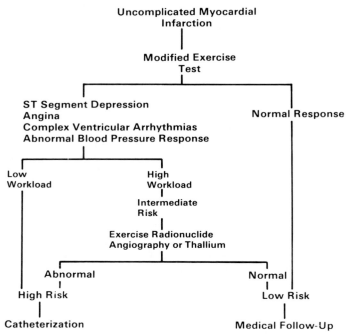

Figure 3. Therapeutic implications of predischarge exercise testing, with suggested guidelines.

probably should undergo cardiac catheterization to more precisely determine the extent of their coronary disease and the feasibility of revascularization procedures.[41]

If the exercise abnormalities occur only at a higher workload or if medications such as digitalis interfere with the interpretation of the ECG results, an exercise radionuclide study such as thallium-201 scintigraphy or radionuclide ventriculography might be helpful in further clarifying the risk.

Patients without exercise abnormalities who maintain preserved exercise capacity on a predischarge exercise test are in a low-risk prognostic subgroup with an expected one-year mortality of less than 2 percent. These patients would not be candidates for immediate cardiac catheterization and could have a more accelerated cardiac rehabilitation program with a less restricted lifestyle.

REFERENCES

1. FEIN, SA, KLEIN, NA, AND FRISHMAN, WH: *Exercise testing soon after uncomplicated myocardial infarction. Prognostic value and safety.* JAMA 245:1863, 1981.

2. DeBusk, RF: *Should exercise testing be standard practice after acute MI?* J Cardiovasc Med 7:261, 1982.

3. WEINER, DA: *Prognostic value of exercise testing early after myocardial infarction.* J Cardiac Rehab 3:114, 1983.

4. SMITH, JW, DENNIS, CA, GASSMANN, A, ET AL: *Exercise testing three weeks after myocardial infarction.* Chest 75:12, 1979.

5. THEROUX, P, WATERS, DD, HALPHEN, C, ET AL: *Prognostic value of exercise testing soon after myocardial infarction.* N Engl J Med 301:341, 1979.

6. SAMI, M, KRAEMER, H, AND DeBUSK, RF: *The prognostic significance of serial exercise testing after myocardial infarction.* Circulation 60:1238, 1979.

7. STARLING, MR, CRAWFORD, MH, KENNEDY, GT, ET AL: *Exercise testing early after myocardial infarction: Predictive value for subsequent unstable angina and death.* Am J Cardiol 46:909, 1980.

8. WELD, FM, CHU, KL, BIGGER, JT, JR, ET AL: *Risk stratification with low-level exercise testing 2 weeks after acute myocardial infarction.* Circulation 64:306, 1981.

9. WENGER, NK, HELLERSTEIN, HK, BLACKBURN, H, ET AL: *Physician practice in the management of patients with uncomplicated myocardial infarction: Changes in the past decade.* Circulation 65:421,1982.

10. SOBEL, BE, BRESNAHAN, GE, SHELL, WE, ET AL: *Estimation of infarct size in man and its relation to prognosis.* Circulation 46:640, 1972.

11. NORRIS, RM, CAUGHEY, DE, MERCER, CJ, ET AL: *Prognosis after myocardial infarction—Six year follow-up.* Br Heart J 36:786, 1974.

12. KOTLER, MH, TABATZNIK, B, MOWER, MM, ET AL: *Prognostic significance of ventricular ectopic beats with respect to sudden death in the late post-infarction period.* Circulation 47:969, 1973.

13. VISMARA, L, AMSTERDAM, EA, AND MASON, DT: *Relation of ventricular arrhythmias in the late hospital phase of acute myocardial infarction to sudden death after hospital discharge.* Am J Med 59:6, 1975.

14. BIGGER, JT, HELLER, CA, WENGER, TL, ET AL: *Risk stratification after acute myocardial infarction.* Am J Cardiol 42:202, 1978.

15. SCHULZE, RA, JR, STRAUSS, HW, AND PITT, B: *Sudden death in the year following myocardial infarction. Relation to ventricular premature contractions in the late hospital phase and left ventricular ejection fraction.* Am J Med 62:192, 1977.

16. CHATURVEDI, NC, WALSH, MJ, EVANS, A, ET AL: *Selection of patients for early discharge after acute myocardial infarction.* Br Heart J 36:533, 1974.

17. SCHUSTER, EH AND BULKLEY, BH: *Early postinfarction angina: Ischemia at a distance and ischemia in the infarct zone.* N Engl J Med 305:1101, 1981.

18. BRUCE, RA AND HORNSTEN, TR: *Exercise stress testing in evaluation of patients with ischemic heart disease.* Prog Cardiovasc Dis 11:371, 1969.

19. NAUGHTON, J, SEVELIUS, G, AND BALKE, B: *Physiological responses of normal and pathological subjects to a modified work capacity test.* J Sports Med 3:201, 1963.

20. DeBUSK, RF AND HASKELL, W: *Symptom-limited vs. heart-rate-limited exercise testing soon after myocardial infarction.* Circulation 61:738, 1980.

21. STARLING, MR, CRAWFORD, MH, AND O'ROURKE RA: *Superiority of selected treadmill exercise protocols predischarge and six weeks postinfarction for detecting ischemic abnormalities.* Am Heart J 104:1054, 1982.

22. SCHWARTZ, KM, TURNER, JD, SHEFFIELD, LT, ET AL: *Limited exercise testing soon after myocardial infarction. Correlation with early coronary and left ventricular angiography.* Ann Intern Med 94:727, 1981.

23. FULLER, CM, RAIZNER, AE, VERANI, MS, ET AL: *Early post-myocardial infarction treadmill stress testing. An accurate predictor of multivessel coronary disease and subsequent cardiac events.* Ann Intern Med 94:734, 1981.

24. STARLING, MR, CRAWFORD, MH, RICHARDS, KL, ET AL: *Predictive value of early postmyocardial infarction modified treadmill exercise testing in multivessel coronary artery disease detection.* Am Heart J 102:169, 1981.

25. PATTERSON, RE, HOROWITZ, SF, ENG, C, ET AL: *Can noninvasive exercise test criteria identify patients with left main or 3-vessel coronary disease after a first myocardial infarction?* Am J Cardiol 51:361, 1983.

26. WEINER, DA, McCABE, CH, KLEIN, MD, ET AL: *ST segment changes post-infarction: Predictive value for multivessel coronary disease and left ventricular aneurysm.* Circulation 58:887, 1978.

27. PAINE, TD, DYE, LE, ROITMAN, DI, ET AL: *Relation of graded exercise test findings after myocardial infarction to extent of coronary artery disease and left ventricular dysfunction.* Am J Cardiol 42:716, 1978.

28. WATERS, DD, THEROUX, P, HALPHEN, C, ET AL: *Clinical predictors of angina following myocardial infarction.* Am J Med 66:991, 1979.

29. IRVING, JB AND BRUCE, RA: *Exertional hypotension and postexertional ventricular fibrillation in stress testing.* Am J Cardiol 39:849, 1977.

30. BRUCE, RA, DeROUEN, TA, PETERSON, TR, ET AL: *Non-invasive predictors of sudden cardiac death in men with coronary heart disease: Predictive value of maximal stress testing.* Am J Cardiol, 39:833, 1977.

31. DeFEYTER, PJ, VAN EENIGE, MJ, DIGHTON, DH, ET AL: *Prognostic value of exercise testing, coronary angiography, and left ventriculography 6-8 weeks after myocardial infarction.* Circulation 66:527, 1982.

32. HASKELL, WL AND DeBUSK, RF: *Cardiovascular responses to repeated exercise testing soon after myocardial infarction.* Circulation 60:1247, 1979.

33. STARLING, MR, CRAWFORD, MH, KENNEDY, GT, ET AL: *Treadmill exercise tests pre-discharge and six weeks post-myocardial infarction to detect abnormalities of known prognostic value.* Ann Intern Med 94:721, 1981.

34. MARKIEWICZ, W, HOUSTON, N, AND DeBUSK, RF: *Exercise testing soon after myocardial infarction.* Circulation 56:26, 1977.

35. TURNER, JD, SCHWARTZ, KM, LOGIC, JR, ET AL: *Detection of residual jeopardized myocardium 3 weeks after myocardial infarction with thallium-201 myocardial scintigraphy.* Circulation 61:729, 1980.

36. GIBSON, RS, TAYLOR, GJ, WATSON, DD, ET AL: *Predicting the extent and location of coronary artery disease during the early postinfarction period by quantitative thallium-201 scintigraphy.* Am J Cardiol 47:1010, 1981.

37. GIBSON, RS, WATSON, DD, CRADDOCK GB ET AL: *Prediction of cardiac events after uncomplicated myocardial infarction: A prospective study comparing predischarge exercise thallium-201 scintigraphy and coronary angiography.* Circulation 68:321, 1983.

38. WASSERMAN, AG, KATZ, RJ, CLEARY, P, ET AL: *Noninvasive detection of multivessel disease after myocardial infarction by exercise radionuclide ventriculography.* Am J Cardiol 50:1242, 1982.

39. BORER, JS, ROSING, DR, MILLER, RH, ET AL: *Natural history of left ventricular function during 1 year after acute myocardial infarction: Comparison with clinical, electrocardiographic and biochemical determinants.* Am J Cardiol 46:1, 1980.

40. CORBETT, JR, DEHMER, GJ, LEWIS, SE, ET AL: *The prognostic value of submaximal exercise testing with radionuclide ventriculography before hospital discharge in patients with recent myocardial infarction.* Circulation 64:535, 1981.

41. EPSTEIN, SE, PALMERI, ST, AND PATTERSON, RE: *Evaluation of patients after acute myocardial infarction. Indications for cardiac catheterization and surgical intervention.* N Engl J Med 307:1487, 1982.

Exercise Nuclear Imaging for the Evaluation of Coronary Artery Disease

Jay L. Meizlish, M.D., Harvey J. Berger, M.D., and Barry L. Zaret, M.D.

The first edition of this book in 1978 devoted little space to the role of noninvasive exercise nuclear techniques in the assessment of cardiac patients. In the intervening period, improved technology and subsequent clinical investigation have allowed exercise nuclear techniques to become widely used in the routine evaluation of patients with coronary artery disease. There are several reasons why they have supplemented conventional exercise electrocardiography in many instances. Exercise electrocardiographic treadmill testing alone is a reasonable means of defining the presence or absence of coronary artery disease, with approximately a 60 percent sensitivity and a 90 percent specificity. However, the 40 percent false-negative rate frequently leads to major clinical dilemmas, and the ten percent false-positive rate makes it hazardous to use as a screening procedure. In addition, exercise electrocardiograms often are impossible to evaluate in cases where the electrocardiogram is abnormal at rest, for example, bundle branch block or other conduction abnormalities, left ventricular hypertrophy, prior myocardial infarction, ST and T wave abnormalities, electrolyte imbalance, pre-excitation, hyperventilation, and therapy with digoxin, quinidine, or psychotropic drugs. Furthermore, the electrocardiogram alone often gives limited information about the location or severity of coronary artery stenosis, and it gives no information about the effects of exercise on left ventricular function.

Exercise nuclear procedures fall into two broad categories: those assessing myocardial perfusion and those assessing ventricular function. Sufficient time has elapsed since their initial description (perfusion techniques in 1973[1] and functional analysis in 1977[2]) to allow definition of many major clinical issues including (a) assessment of the patient after myocardial infarction, (b) screening for high-risk subsets of patients such as those with left main and triple vessel coronary disease, (c) assessment of the effects of physical training and cardiac rehabilitation, (d) prediction of coronary artery disease location, (e) preoperative prediction of reversible asynergy following coronary artery bypass grafting, (f) evaluation of patients with an inconclusive or negative treadmill exercise test, and (g) augmentation of the information provided by a positive exercise treadmill test.

This chapter first discusses exercise myocardial perfusion imaging and then exercise left ventricular function techniques. In both sections, the pertinent work that has been performed to date as well as likely future directions will be reviewed.

MYOCARDIAL PERFUSION

Thallium-201 (^{201}Tl), the current radionuclide of choice for clinical myocardial perfusion imaging, is a metallic element (Group IIIA of the periodic table) that is extracted by the

105

myocardium from blood in a fashion analogous to potassium. This transport is mediated via the sodium-potassium ATPase pump, as thallium activates sodium-potassium ATPase and its uptake may be altered by digoxin.[3,4] Thallium initially is distributed according to myocardial blood flow and then is extracted by cells. The heart receives approximately 4 percent of the cardiac output; and myocardial extraction efficiency is approximately 88 percent on the first pass, resulting in myocardial uptake of 3 to 4 percent of the administered dose. Normally perfused myocardium reaches a maximum ^{201}Tl uptake within minutes after its injection at peak exercise. A kinetic phase ensues during which there is slow washout of ^{201}Tl from the myocardium, especially in areas of maximal concentration. If there is a coronary artery obstruction, the myocardium supplied by this vessel may be underperfused at peak exercise and ^{201}Tl accumulation may be reduced and delayed. Likewise, the washout process may be slower, and if the ^{201}Tl concentration is sufficiently small, there may be relative regional accumulation of ^{201}Tl in the ischemic zone. This simplified explanation provides the rationale for the injection of ^{201}Tl at peak exercise, imaging as soon as possible (within approximately 10 minutes) following injection, and again 2 to 4 hours after exercise to assess for redistribution. It is also the basis for several new quantitative temporal approaches that assess regional ^{201}Tl kinetics.

Imaging Procedure

Exercise usually is performed on a treadmill according to standard exercise protocols and with routine ECG monitoring. Three ml of saline containing 2 mCi of ^{201}Tl is injected into a free-flowing intravenous line at peak exercise, and the patient is instructed to continue to exercise for 60 seconds following injection. A close geographical relation between the exercise and imaging laboratories is necessary to ensure initiation of imaging within 10 minutes following ^{201}Tl injection. Imaging is performed in the anterior, 45 degree left anterior oblique (LAO), and either left lateral (right side decubitus) or steep (70 degree) LAO views. Two hundred thousand counts are obtained in the anterior view, and the subsequent views are imaged for the same duration (usually 10 minutes). Repeat imaging in the same views is performed at 4 hours. The patient should have no more than a light breakfast prior to exercise and should not partake in major physical activity or eating except a light snack until completion of the delayed images because these activities can alter redistribution kinetics. Imaging should be performed with a single crystal Anger camera equipped with 37 photomultiplier tubes and a ¼-inch thick crystal. A 20 percent window should be centered over the ^{201}Tl peak. Computer processing is not required for visual interpretation. However, such processing involving background subtraction and image filtering, color coding, and gating can be helpful. The major role of computer analysis is in quantification and tomography, which will be discussed subsequently.

Interpretation of Qualitative Images

Visual interpretation of planar thallium-201 images is qualitative, and this is one of the major drawbacks of the technique. Extensive experience is required to discriminate defects related to inadequate myocardial perfusion from those related to position, artifact, normal variation, and soft tissue attenuation.[5,6] Exercise ^{201}Tl myocardial perfusion defects (cold spots) can be categorized as persistent, reversible, or partially reversible.

The persistent defect is comparable at 4-hour redistribution and at peak exercise and usually represents prior infarction with a myocardial scar. It correlates with irreversible resting regional wall motion abnormalities in that region.[7-9] Occasionally, a persistent defect at 4 hours is not apparent on a separate resting study. This represents severe ischemia and usually slow redistribution. If the differentiation of prior myocardial infarction from this situation is clinically important, the study should be repeated at rest with a separate ^{201}Tl injection.

Transient defects are seen on exercise images only and return to normal at the time of delayed imaging. This sequence represents exercise-induced ischemia in areas of viable myocardium. Partially reversible defects usually represent areas of infarction with superimposition of exercise-induced ischemia.

The location of the defect provides relevant anatomic information. Septal (on the LAO) and anterior (on the lateral and anterior views) defects predict left anterior descending coronary artery stenosis or obstruction; inferior defects (on the anterior or left lateral view) predict right coronary artery disease; posterolateral defects (on the LAO view) predict circumflex artery disease (Fig. 1). Optimally, defects consistent with coronary artery disease should be seen on more than one view, and this is usually the case for left anterior descending and right coronary artery lesions where the appropriate vascular beds are seen adequately on both lateral and anterior views. The left circumflex artery supply is more difficult to visualize in that its vascular bed often is seen only on the LAO view.

The possibility of false-positive image defects should be appreciated. Clues to possible false-positive ^{201}Tl scintigrams[6,10] include (a) defects seen in only one view; (b) defects without change on redistribution in the absence of known infarction; (c) defects that do not conform appropriately to a given anatomic location; (d) defects entirely related to patient position; and (e) variations caused by the normal decrease in apical uptake. The two most common examples of positioning problems are: (1) soft tissue attenuation owing to large female breasts and (2) superimposition of the diaphragm on left lateral or anterior images in the supine position. Remedies include elevation of the breast with tape if necessary and left lateral imaging in the right lateral decubitus position to avoid diaphragmatic overlap of the inferior wall.

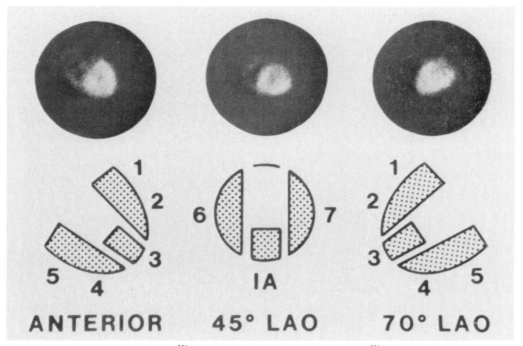

Figure 1. Regional analysis of planar ^{201}Tl myocardial perfusion images. Planar ^{201}Tl images are seen above with corresponding diagrams of left ventricular segments below. The anterior view places the anterior (1 and 2), apical (3), and inferior (4 and 5) walls into profile. The 45 degree LAO displays septum (6), inferoapical (IA), and posterolateral (7) walls. The 70 degree LAO reveals the anterior (1 and 2), apical (3), and inferior (4 and 5) segments. (From Berman, DS, Garcia, EV, and Maddahi, J,[18] with permission.)

In addition to the evaluation of the presence and pattern of perfusion defects, consideration must be given to (a) left ventricular cavity size, (b) intensity of myocardial ^{201}Tl uptake as compared with background activity in the lungs and mediastinum, and (c) left ventricular wall thickness. The issue of lung uptake is of diagnostic importance. A lung-to-myocardium ratio of greater than 0.5 is abnormal and suggests left ventricular failure at the time of exercise. When this finding is accompanied by a focal perfusion defect, it is diagnostic of coronary artery disease with ischemia-related left ventricular dysfunction with exercise.[11,12] When increased lung uptake is seen in the absence of perfusion defects, other causes of left ventricular dysfunction such as scarring from prior myocardial infarction, cardiomyopathy, and valvular heart disease also should be considered. However, ischemia may be present in the absence of visually identifiable focal defects in patients with diffuse disease and a balanced reduction in myocardial perfusion. This situation can be documented by diffuse slow washout via quantitative analysis of ^{201}Tl kinetics. Right ventricular ^{201}Tl uptake is common on exercise images. The absence of right ventricular uptake may suggest an inadequate level of exercise. Reversible right ventricular defects have been associated with proximal right coronary artery stenosis.

Clinical Use of Thallium-201 Imaging

As a means of diagnosing coronary artery disease, the presence of a defect on exercise ^{201}Tl imaging has a sensitivity of approximately 80 percent and a specificity of 90 percent.[14,16] The improved sensitivity in comparison with the exercise electrocardiogram is accounted for by the fact that imaging may be positive when the electrocardiogram is abnormal at rest or when inadequate levels of exercise do not lead to ischemic ST segment depression. The improved specificity is a result of the fact that the major cause of positive ^{201}Tl images is coronary artery

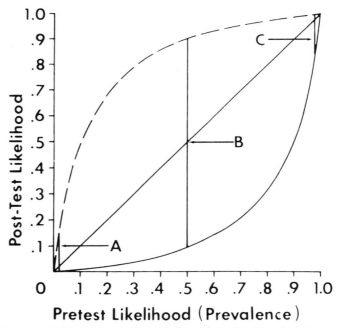

Figure 2. Impact of a test with 90 percent sensitivity and specificity. The line of identity represents the pre-test likelihood of disease and the curves portray the post-test likelihood following a positive (---) or negative (—) test. Note that the area of greatest impact of the test result is in the mid-range of probability (B), whereas least utility is found at the extremes (A and C). (From Berman, DS, Garcia, EV, and Maddahi, J,[18] with permission.)

stenosis, whereas there are a variety of causes of ST segment abnormalities with exercise other than myocardial ischemia. Although these results are uniformly better than those obtained with exercise treadmill testing using electrocardiography alone, the major impact of these studies requires the application of Bayesean analysis[17-20] and resultant individualization of the use of imaging as an adjunct to the exercise ECG (Fig. 2). For example, the middle-aged patient with a history of typical angina and a positive exercise treadmill test benefits little from imaging for diagnosis alone. In this instance, the pre-test likelihood of coronary artery disease is high, and even a negative exercise ECG would not reduce this likelihood considerably. The results of exercise ^{201}Tl testing have the greatest effect in the 30 to 70 percent range of pre-test probability. Here a positive test increases the probability to approximately 90 percent, and a negative test decreases the probability of coronary artery disease to approximately 10 percent. An understanding of how clinical history and exercise treadmill test results affect the pretest likelihood of disease is required for appropriate selection of patients for all radionuclide studies.

Inconclusive Exercise Electrocardiogram

One of the most frequent uses for ^{201}Tl exercise testing is the evaluation of the patient whose exercise treadmill ECG test is inconclusive. Extensive experience has shown that ^{201}Tl scintigraphy maintains both sensitivity (approximately 80 percent) and specificity (approximately 90 percent) in this setting.[21-24,27] A frequent cause of an inconclusive exercise treadmill ECG test is failure to reach 85 percent of the predicted maximum heart rate for age. It seems that the attainment of peak exercise is less critical with ^{201}Tl than with ECG testing alone. In fact, in a small series comparing maximal with one-half maximal exercise,[25] all patients with coronary artery disease were identified at the lower level of exercise.[25] Nevertheless, maximal exercise should be the desired end-point with imaging as well, in order to maximize the yield from these studies.

Positive Exercise Electrocardiogram in the Asymptomatic Patient

Because false-positive exercise electrocardiograms occur, there are many clinical settings where corroboration with an alternative exercise study is important in patient management. This is becoming increasingly important as exercise electrocardiogram screening of populations without symptoms has become more popular. Several studies have addressed this issue, and both sensitivity and specificity are maintained at an approximately 90 percent level in this population with positive ETT, but normal coronary arteries.[26,27] Our general impression is that this is a difficult population to assess, based on a lower diagnostic accuracy. These patients may require multiple modalities, that is, [201]Tl *and* LV function studies.

Assessment of Coronary Anatomy and Severity of Disease

The identification of patients with left main and triple vessel coronary artery disease has become important in selecting patients for angiography and coronary artery bypass surgery. In addition to this stratification between multivessel/left main disease and lesser types of stenoses, the location of coronary artery disease in each artery also is of paramount importance. For example, patients with proximal left anterior descending coronary artery stenosis have a higher morbidity than single-vessel involvement of either the right or left circumflex coronary artery.

Many studies have addressed the ability of exercise ^{201}Tl imaging to predict the site of individual coronary stenoses.[16,29-33] The site of ST segment depression during ETT is a poor means of localizing coronary artery disease, whereas reversible ^{201}Tl defects are more predictive.[28] Berman and coworkers pooled data from four such studies which included 338 patients.[18] Prediction of left anterior descending coronary artery stenosis had a sensitivity of

74 percent (174/234) and specificity of 90 percent (based on 80 normals). For the right coronary artery, sensitivity was 69 percent (124/179) and specificity 86 percent (101/117). Prediction of left circumflex artery disease had the lowest sensitivity (38 percent, 60/157), with a specificity of 91 percent. Because of frequent individual variation in areas perfused by the right and left circumflex coronary arteries, it is often difficult to specify which vessel is involved when inferolateral ^{201}Tl defects occur.

A particular pattern may be expected with left main coronary artery stenosis, that is, defects in anterior, septal, *and* lateral vascular beds. This pattern has been shown to be a highly sensitive (92 percent) pattern, but one with many false positives (specificity 15 percent).[33] The reason for the latter finding is that double or triple vessel disease is far more common and often results in similar patterns of defects in multiple vascular beds. In this setting, however, the absence of the left main pattern may be used fairly reliably to exclude the presence of significant left main coronary artery obstruction. Similarly, significant obstruction of the *proximal left anterior descending* coronary artery is associated with septal (as well as anterior) perfusion abnormalities (sensitivity 92 percent, specificity 85 percent).[34] The absence of a septal perfusion defect speaks against proximal left anterior descending coronary artery involvement.

Qualitative planar ^{201}Tl imaging defines relative differences in perfusion between vascular beds. It therefore identifies the *most severe* defect and may miss less pronounced defects. This is one of the main reasons for the less-than-perfect sensitivity to *individual* coronary artery stenoses and the much better overall sensitivity to the issue of presence vs. absence of coronary artery disease. Quantification holds great promise in this regard because it allows independent analysis of each myocardial perfusion zone irrespective of comparison to other regions (vide infra). Tomography may achieve this by avoiding wide overlap of normal and abnormal areas.

Thallium-201 myocardial perfusion imaging is generally more sensitive with increasing disease severity, that is, it has higher sensitivity in triple vessel disease than in single vessel disease.[15,34] It is also more sensitive in the setting of greater than 90 percent luminal diameter narrowing than for lesser grades of coronary artery obstruction.[17] One reason for so-called false positives is the angiographic assessment of stenosis being noncritical (usually less than 70 percent) when, in fact, it may be of major physiologic relevance. With exercise-induced ^{201}Tl perfusion defects, one must wonder whether there is not true limitation to blood flow with exercise by such a presumed noncritical lesion. In addition, there are equally large subjective errors in visual analysis of coronary arteriograms.[103]

Use of Exercise Thallium Perfusion Imaging to Predict Multivessel Disease Following Myocardial Infarction

Pre-discharge and early post-myocardial infarction exercise testing has assumed an important role in risk stratification and patient management. Several studies have assessed the role of exercise ^{201}Tl myocardial perfusion imaging in this setting. Dunn and coworkers[35] demonstrated ^{201}Tl defects in more than one vascular distribution in 37 of 40 patients with multivessel disease postinfarction. This 92 percent sensitivity was significantly better than the 72 percent sensitivity of exercise ECG testing. Dunn[35] and Massie[16] both found equal predictive accuracies whether the infarct was inferior or anterior. Rigo and associates,[34] however, showed poor sensitivity to multivessel disease in the setting of prior anterior infarction, with preserved sensitivity in the setting of prior inferior myocardial infarction.[34] It is hoped that the accuracy will be improved with quantitative and/or tomographic approaches.

Significance of Collaterals

Collateral vessels are often noted angiographically in the presence of total or subtotal (greater than 90 percent) coronary artery blockages. The physiologic effect and hemodynamic significance of collaterals remains uncertain. Thallium-201 myocardial perfusion imaging affords an opportunity to observe the impact of collateral vessels on patterns of coronary blood flow with exercise. Rigo and colleagues[36] found that 37 of 124 patients with coronary artery disease had normal exercise ^{201}Tl images. All these patients had collateral vessels. Eighty percent of these collaterals were nonjeopardized, that is, the source of the collateral itself was free of obstruction. Likewise, Tubau and coworkers[37] studied 37 patients with greater than 90 percent coronary artery stenosis in one vessel. All the 21 without collateral vessels had positive exercise ^{201}Tl images. Only 7 of 16 with large collateral vessels had exercise-induced thallium defects. These results suggest that visualized nonjeopardized collaterals afford some protection during exercise to areas perfused by critically stenosed coronary arteries. They may also be an important cause of a false-negative exercise ^{201}Tl study.

Thallium-201 imaging also may be a way to follow patients after coronary artery reperfusion, for example, after percutaneous transluminal coronary angioplasty or coronary artery bypass grafting.[106,107]

New Directions

Quantification

A major drawback to ^{201}Tl image interpretation is its subjectivity. There is a great need for standardization of readings and quantification of results. The basic approach to quantification is an assessment of ^{201}Tl uptake both spatially (the axis about the myocardial center) and temporally (exercise vs. redistribution images).[38,39]

Images are obtained in three views (anterior, 45 degree LAO, 70 degree LAO, or LLAT) immediately following exercise and at redistribution (4 hours later). Careful attention is paid to precise replication of imaging positions. The image is subjected to 9-point smoothing, and bilinear interpolative background subtraction is performed to correct for tissue cross-talk. A profile of myocardial activity then is obtained. This profile may be circumferential or linear, and it may assess average or maximal activity at each point. A curve of myocardial counts at each point in the myocardial profile is thus obtained for exercise and redistribution. Washout is calculated as [(exercise activity–redistribution activity)/(exercise activity)] and is expressed as a percentage. This parameter may also be displayed for each point along the myocardial profile.

Comparison of each of these three curves to a normal range allows definition of areas of abnormal myocardial perfusion. Transient defects on planar imaging thus will be seen as abnormalities in exercise profiles and washout curves with normal redistribution profiles. Persistent defects will reveal abnormalities in all three curves. Perhaps most important of all, the washout curve may be abnormal in areas along the profile where planar imaging or quantitation of the exercise image alone does not reveal defects. Thus, this approach adds not only standardization and quantification, it also affords a precise analysis of myocardial tracer washout which should allow identification of multiple ischemic areas heretofore impossible to assess by qualitative methods. An example of the use of quantification for the diagnosis of multivessel disease is shown in Figures 3 and 4. This patient had arteriographically documented triple vessel disease correctly identified on ^{201}Tl imaging only by diffuse slow washout. In initial studies, this approach has added to the ability to define multivessel disease and to identify patients at risk after infarction.[13,40,105]

Tomography

Routine planar ^{201}Tl images result in superimposition of myocardial regions. Small defects and/or multiple defects thus may be obscured because of overlap with normal areas. The obvious advantage afforded by tomography would be avoidance of such areas of regional overlap and opportunity for definition of lesions limited to the subendocardium.

EXERCISE

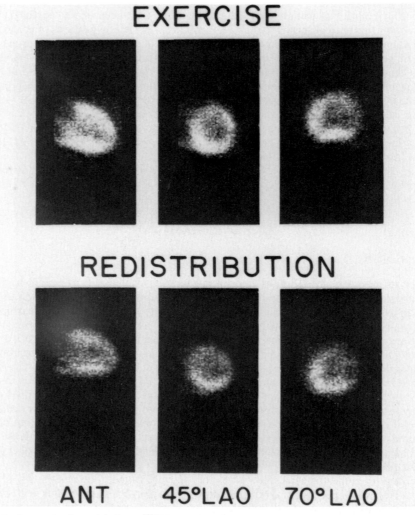

REDISTRIBUTION

ANT   45°LAO   70°LAO

Figure 3. Background subtracted planar ^{201}Tl images following exercise and at 4 hours (redistribution). There is a subtle exercise perfusion defect in the posterolateral region of the left ventricle on the 45 degree LAO image, with a suggestion of redistribution on the delayed image. The 70 degree LAO reveals possible thinning of the inferior wall but no definite defect. Impression: probably left circumflex coronary artery stenosis.

The first approach to tomography was with a seven pinhole collimator imaging along the optimal LAO long axis of the heart (usually 45 degree LAO and 10 degree caudal tilt). The seven separate images obtained may be reconstructed into 1-cm short-axis tomographic slices. Limitations include considerable overlap of segments, poor spatial resolution, and critical importance of patient positioning. The general performance of seven pinhole tomography has equaled but not exceeded planar imaging, and this approach is now largely historic.[41-44]

A more truly tomographic approach employs a camera that rotates on a gantry and acquires images at frequent intervals about the circumference. Sections are thus obtained that may be oriented in frontal, sagittal, and, most useful, transaxial (re: cardiac axis) views. It appears to have a high sensitivity (96 percent) for coronary artery disease while maintaining specificity (89 percent).[41] One concern is that the 22-minute acquisition time may allow redis-

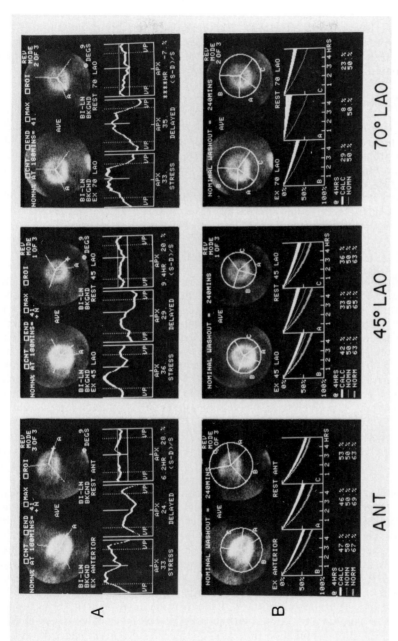

Figure 4. Quantitative analysis of exercise and redistribution ^{201}Tl images from patient in Figure 3. In A, the circumferential count profile for stress, delayed, and washout (S-D/S) is graphically displayed in each of the views (anterior, 45 degree LAO and 70 degree LAO) and reference is made to the apex (A) and valve plane (VP). In B, percent washout alone is displayed for three regions (B, A, C) distinct from VP in each view and compared with normal curves (abnormal washout 40 percent).

The posterolateral perfusion defect is confirmed on the 45 degree LAO stress count profile (indicated by vertical cursor). This is less apparent at delayed imaging consistent with redistribution. Washout is 20 percent in the center of this region, and 36 percent in the entire region and was abnormal (33 percent) in the apex as well (45 degree LAO, B). The 70 degree LAO reveals abnormal washout (B) in all three regions [B 29 percent (anterior), A 8 percent (apex), 23 percent (inferior)] despite normal stress images (Figure 3) and count profiles (A). Impression: triple vessel disease.

tribution to begin during initial post-exercise imaging and thus affect the accuracy of reconstructed data. Other concerns include the effect of attenuation, level of intrinsic resolution, ability to quantify data, and optimal use of a rotating camera versus a circumferential bank of detectors. In light of these concerns, the early results are all the more encouraging. The addition of quantitative analysis to tomographic data is a very important area. As with planar imaging, the addition of quantitation has the advantage of eliminating observer variability. The next few years should bring many advances in this area.

Nonexercise Stress Thallium-201 Imaging

There are many clinical settings where, although exercise is impossible (gait disturbance, weakness, patient cooperation, pulmonary limitations, arthritis, and so on), the assessment of coronary reserve is desirable. The best alternative approach involves coronary artery vasodilation using intravenous dipyridamole,[28,31,32] which assesses coronary flow reserve (as opposed to ischemia with exercise) and appears to equal exercise ^{201}Tl imaging in sensitivity and specificity.[29,30,44] Limitations currently include lack of wide clinical availability of the drug and occurrence of frequent side effects. Other approaches have included rapid atrial pacing and cold pressor testing, but these appear to compare less well with the exercise approach.[45,46]

EXERCISE RADIONUCLIDE ANGIOCARDIOGRAPHY (RNA)

The study of the effect of exercise on the heart has been greatly enhanced by radionuclide angiocardiographic techniques. Rapid sequential assessment of left ventricular ejection fraction, regional wall motion, ventricular volumes, and diastolic filling rates have shed light on the normal response to exercise as well as the pathophysiologic changes caused by ischemia.

The normal heart responds to exercise by increasing end-diastolic volume and maintaining or decreasing end-systolic volume, thus increasing both stroke volume and ejection fraction. Regional wall motion is maintained or improved and diastolic filling rates increase. Ejection fraction response is generally considered to increase by $\geq$ 5 percent, although if the ejection fraction at rest is $\geq$ 75 percent, no change also is considered a normal response. Ischemia generally results in increases in both end-systolic volume and end-diastolic volume. A reduction in exercise ejection fraction and the development of new regional wall motion abnormalities are the hallmarks of exercise-induced ischemia.

Procedure

Two distinct approaches to exercise radionuclide angiocardiography (RNA) are commonly employed (first-pass and gated equilibrium techniques) and both use technetium-99m as the tracer. In first-pass studies, the tracer is injected as a bolus and data are acquired with high temporal resolution as the tracer moves through the central circulation chambers. A time-activity curve is constructed, and ejection fraction is calculated (counts at end-diastole minus counts at end-systole divided by counts at end-diastole minus background) for approximately three to five cardiac cycles. Images also are presented as end-diastolic and end-systolic silhouettes, cinelike movies, and functional images to evaluate regional wall motion. Exercise is performed upright on a bicycle ergometer with the patient in the anterior or RAO position. Geometric calculations of volume and cardiac output may be obtained. Advantages of the first-pass technique include short acquisition time, ability to perform upright exercise, availability of RAO views, and minimal background. Disadvantages include limited number of studies per patient (that is, limited by the number of injections, usually at rest and peak exercise only), and pre-set patient positioning. First-pass studies ideally require multicrystal cameras or newer digital cameras to avoid excessive count rate loss because of system dead time.

114

Equilibrium blood pool imaging is performed using supine or semi-upright bicycle exercise and a single crystal camera following either in vivo or in vitro labeling of red blood cells with technetium-99m. Data are obtained by dividing each cardiac cycle into 12 to 28 frames via gating from the ECG R-wave. Data from the last 2 minutes of each 3-minute exercise stage are collected, and an endless loop cine format movie is created as well as a time-activity curve from which ejection fraction is calculated. The images are obtained in the best septal LAO view to separate right and left ventricles. The advantages of this technique include the ability to collect data at multiple points in time from a single tracer injection. Disadvantages have included necessity for supine exercise and LAO patient positioning, which make detailed regional wall motion analysis difficult. These problems may be addressed with separate studies using more than one view or computer processing techniques such as difference images designed to evaluate the function of left ventricular regions not seen in profile on the LAO view (that is, inferior and anterior walls).[2]

Whether exercise is performed upright or supine may be of major importance.[47-50] Controversy exists as to the significance and optimal choice of exercise position. Upright, as compared with supine, exercise results in loading conditions more similar to those seen during normal activity, and higher rate-pressure products are obtained. Supine exercise causes a higher preload and increases cardiac volumes, and it is possible that different exercise results may be obtained because of the altered loading state rather than intrinsic disease.[51]

The first-pass RNA, because it is performed in anterior or RAO positions and has no overlap of RV structures, affords one-view assessment of regional wall motion. This wall motion usually is scored semi-quantitatively on a scale ranging from dyskinetic to normal. It also may be quantitated using regional ejection fraction images or radial cord shortening.

Interpretation

The resting radionuclide angiocardiogram is evaluated for ejecton fraction, regional wall motion, and end-diastolic and end-systolic volumes. Regional wall motion abnormalities at rest tend to be relatively specific for coronary artery disease. Abnormal exercise responses include inability to augment ejection fraction by at least 5 percent, development of new regional wall motion abnormalities, and an increase in end-systolic volume.

Additional parameters that have been used to define abnormal response include Fourier phase analysis,[52-54] first third ejection fraction,[55] ratio of exercise systolic pressure to end-systolic volume,[56,57] changes in pulmonary blood volume,[58,59] and pulmonary volume ratio and transit time[60]

First-pass approaches are usually limited to rest and peak exercise determinations. Equilibrium gated studies also may be evaluated at submaximal points during exercise and also immediately post-exercise when an overshoot[60] in ejection fraction and improvement in regional wall motion often occur. The availability of short-lived, generator-produced tracers, for example, gold-195m,[61] allows more frequent first-pass assessments of left ventricular function without increasing the radiation dose.

Clinical Use

Diagnosis of Coronary Artery Disease

Many studies have evaluated the ability of exercise radionuclide angiocardiography to diagnose the presence of coronary artery disease.[62-70] The general range is a sensitivity of 85 percent to 90 percent, with similar specificity. Inasmuch as ventricular dysfunction is common to many cardiac diseases, diagnostic results will vary depending on the patient population studied, as well as the exercise protocol used and criteria for positivity employed. The most widely used and sensitive criterion is failure to augment ejection fraction with exercise by $\geq$

5 percent (sensitivity 87 percent).[14] Another sensitive finding is exercise-induced regional wall motion abnormalities. The most specific criterion is resting regional wall motion abnormalities (specificity 95 percent).[65] Many patients with nonischemic-induced cardiac dysfunction will fail to augment ejection fraction with exercise. These conditions include valvular heart disease,[71-74] hypertrophic cardiomyopathy,[75] chronic obstructive pulmonary disease,[76] dilated cardiomyopathy, radiation-induced myocardial fibrosis,[104] doxorubicin cardiotoxicity,[108] and iron overload.[77] Abnormal exercise responses may be common in elderly people without symptoms of coronary artery disease[78] and often are observed in females.[62] If conditions with a known association with left ventricular functional abnormalities are excluded from a study population, specificity will be maximized. Sensitivity is maximized by attainment of maximal exercise with ECG-documented ischemia[65] and increasing severity of coronary artery disease.[79] The implications of a false-positive radionuclide ventriculogram may be important. Berger and associates[80] showed that 39 percent (12/31) of patients with chest pain, abnormal exercise treadmill tests, and *normal* coronary arteries had abnormal exercise left ventricular reserve (only 3 of whom had thallium defects). One can infer that some abnormal process other than major coronary artery stenosis is causing a reduction in global left ventricular functional reserve in this patient population. There is evidence suggesting that microvascular disease may play a role.[81] The left ventricular response to exercise in the patient with low resting ejection fraction may differ from the usual circumstances. Evidence exists that further reduction in ejection fraction from a low baseline is uncommon, and the use of the exercise radionuclide ventriculogram in the assessment of this patient population may be limited.[82]

Severity and Extent of Coronary Artery Disease

In general, the severity of global dysfunction with exercise reflects the extent and severity of coronary artery disease; however, wide overlap exists. With quantitative scoring of coronary artery disease location and degree and effect of collateral flow, there seems to be a close relationship between severity and exercise ejection fraction.[83] The role of radionuclide angiocardiography in predicting severe disease appears to be predominantly in the patient with the negative or indeterminate exercise treadmill test. Campos and coworkers[84] found that 41 percent of patients with positive exercise treadmill testing had severe coronary artery disease (triple vessel or left main disease). Radionuclide angiocardiography did not greatly improve this assessment. In the patient with a negative exercise electrocardiogram, however, a positive RNA represents a 17 percent risk of coronary disease, whereas a negative RNA defines a 0 percent risk. Likewise, with indeterminate exercise electrocardiograms, a negative RNA reduced the risk of major coronary artery disease from 21 to 10 percent and a positive result increased it to 29 percent. Also, in this group of 54 patients, only 1 of 29 patients who died during followup had a negative study, whereas 8 of 29 had negative or indeterminate exercise treadmill testing, suggesting a role for exercise radionuclide angiocardiography in establishing prognosis.

Assessment of the Patient After Myocardial Infarction

Although ECG exercise treadmill testing has become the standard postinfarction prognostic assessment, several studies suggest that radionuclide angiocardiography is more useful in identifying patients with a poor prognosis.[84-86] Corbett and colleagues[86] studied 61 patients and found the exercise ECG to have a sensitivity of 54 percent and specificity of 58 percent in predicting patients with a bad outcome in six months. In contrast, using failure to improve ejection fraction with exercise by greater than 5 percent, the sensitivity was 95 percent and specificity 96 percent for detecting a poor outcome at six months. Likewise, Upton and coworkers[85] found that 20 of 42 patients after infarction decreased their ejection fraction with exercise, whereas only 9 had abnormal exercise ECGs. One of the problems with RNA assessment after infarction is the difficulty in differentiating abnormal EF responses related to exercise-induced ischemia from those reflecting the effect of scar on global left ventricular function in the absence of ischemia. The precise role of radionuclide angiocardiography in the patient after infarction remains uncertain, and its current use is probably best determined on an individual basis.

Prediction of Left Ventricular Functional Response to Coronary Artery Bypass Grafting

The presence of abnormal regional wall motion at rest does not necessarily imply irreversibility. It would be very valuable to know which regional wall motion abnormality represents a viable area with ongoing ischemia and thus may respond to revascularization. There is some evidence to suggest that this feature may be predicted by assessment of regional wall motion immediately after exercise (in addition to peak exercise as is routine). Areas that demonstrate improved function at this time are likely to demonstrate improved regional wall motion at rest after coronary artery bypass grafting.[87] In general, these are areas that on exercise ^{201}Tl imaging assessment have defects with exercise and are normal at redistribution, suggesting the presence of viable, nonscarred, but ischemic myocardium.[7]

Effect of Cardiac Rehabilitation and Training

The effect of dynamic exercise training on the normal heart involves dilation and increase in left ventricular end-diastolic volume and stroke volume with resultant higher exercise cardiac output at similar or lower heart rates.[88] The effect of cardiac rehabilitation programs in patients with coronary artery disease appears to be mediated predominantly via peripheral effects inasmuch as ejection fraction responses and regional wall motion remain basically unchanged following physical activity rehabilitation.[89-91] This is an important and difficult area to evaluate. More investigation is required to define further the effects of exercise training in the coronary patient.

Evaluation of Diastolic Left Ventricular Function With Exercise

Patients with resting systolic dysfunction often have diastolic dysfunction as well;[92] however, the role of exercise-induced diastolic functional changes has only recently been studied. A normal response is improvement of parameters of diastolic function such as peak filling rate, filling fraction, and time to peak filling rate. Ischemia causes a worsening of diastolic function, but this seems less sensitive than measurements of systolic functional reserve.[93] Exercise-induced diastolic dysfunction also occasionally occurs in normal persons and may represent the physiologic effects of rapid heart rates. Peak filling rate increases in patients with coronary artery disease as well as in normal persons during exercise; however, the absolute change is less in the former group. It does not appear thus far that study of diastolic function during exercise will add significantly to the current ability to diagnose coronary artery disease noninvasively. In addition, further work is necessary to determine if the volumetric parameters of diastolic performance obtained by radionuclide studies are of sufficient reliability to replace a more detailed invasive assessment involving pressure-volume interactions.

Assessment of Therapy

Radionuclide angiocardiography has been used to assess the effects of therapy in patients with coronary artery disease. Nitroglycerin reduces preload and improves exercise LV function.[94,95] Propranolol blocks the exercise-induced left ventricular functional effects of ischemia[96-98] and should ideally be withheld if a patient with a negative exercise treadmill test and without chest pain on exercise is to be evaluated adequately with radionuclide angiocardiography.[99]

In contrast to the limited role for monitoring exercise diastolic function in the diagnosis of coronary artery disease, RNA may play a vital role in assessing therapy. Verapamil appears to improve parameters of diastolic function such as peak filling rate, both at rest and with exercise,[100] and this drug may be an important addition to the therapy of coronary artery disease. Exercise radionuclide ventriculography also may be employed to evaluate the effects of revascularization techniques such as percutaneous transluminal coronary angioplasty and coronary artery bypass grafting.

Future Directions

The tomographic approach to radionuclide ventriculography may add greater accuracy in defining regional wall motion abnormalities. The development of new short-lived radionuclides, for example, gold-195m from a mercury-195m generator, may allow more frequent assessments of left ventricular function during exercise with first-pass evaluation at a lower radiation dosage for both patient and staff. Its ultra-short half life allows the rapid serial assessment of both left ventricular function and perfusion by enabling simultaneous ^{201}Tl myocardial perfusion imaging in a single exercise study.[101,102]

COMPARISON OF THALLIUM-201 MYOCARDIAL PERFUSION IMAGING WITH RADIONUCLIDE VENTRICULOGRAPHY

Both ^{201}Tl myocardial perfusion imaging and radionuclide angiocardiography offer the clinician valuable noninvasive ways of evaluating the cardiac response to exercise. It is important to develop an orderly and logical approach to the use of these two techniques.

Perhaps the most important consideration is the experience and training in the individual laboratory. Because the two techniques provide similar diagnostic predictive accuracy, the overriding factor is local reliability and reproducibility of each technique. On the other hand, specific issues may lead to preference of one approach over another.

Radionuclide angiocardiography is probably the more sensitive modality, and if this is paramount, RNA may be the method of choice. Thallium-201 myocardial perfusion imaging appears best for assessment of (a) a particular coronary vascular bed, (b) a patient with a very low resting ejection fraction, (c) a patient with arrhythmias in whom the technical quality of radionuclide angiocardiography might be compromised, (d) the presence of other diseases that might also lead to abnormal exercise ventricular functional responses (for example, valvular, myopathic, or systemic processes), and (e) the patient with a hypercatecholamine state in whom a high resting ejection fraction might confound interpretation of the exercise response. The assessment of the patient after myocardial infarction has been adequately accomplished with both techniques. The unresolved question of how to separate the abnormal left ventricular response to exercise secondary to scar formation from that related to exercise-induced ischemia might lead toward myocardial perfusion imaging with ^{201}Tl as the method of choice. The qualitative nature of the planar ^{201}Tl imaging might lead to a preference for radionuclide angiocardiography with its more quantitative results. However, the addition of quantitative analysis to ^{201}Tl imaging may alter this consideration.

Finally, there are circumstances in which both studies are appropriate. These are usually situations in which the goal of noninvasive testing is to classify the patient into highly likely (greater than 90 percent) or unlikely (less than 10 percent) coronary artery disease categories, and thus avoid or direct further invasive workup.[18] This may require both positive ^{201}Tl imaging and positive radionuclide angiocardiography in the patient with a negative exercise treadmill test or in one whose pretest likelihood of disease is low. Likewise, when the exercise ECG is positive and the first employed nuclear technique is conflicting, the use of the complementary modality is of great value.

CONCLUSION

Noninvasive nuclear techniques for assessing cardiac status during exercise are readily available and clinically valuable. They provide information about myocardial perfusion and left ventricular function and should continue to prove increasingly reliable with technical advances. Their role should continue to expand beyond the diagnosis of coronary artery disease into functional assessment and categorization of patients with recognized cardiovascular disease.

REFERENCES

1. ZARET, BL, STRAUSS, HW, MARTIN, ND, ET AL: *Noninvasive regional myocardial perfusion with radioactive potassium: Study of patients at rest, exercise and during angina pectoris.* N Engl J Med 288:809, 1973.

2. BORER, JS, BACHARACH, SL, GREEN, MV, ET AL: *Real time radionuclide cineangiography in the noninvasive evaluation of global and regional left ventricular function at rest and during exercise in patients with coronary artery disease.* N Engl J Med 296:839, 1977.

3. POHOST, GM, ALPERT, NM, INGWALL, JS, ET AL: *Thallium redistribution: Mechanisms and clinical utility.* Sem Nuc Med 10:72, 1980.

4. GEHRING, PJ AND HAMMOND, PB: *The interrelationship between thallium and potassium in animals.* J Pharmacol Exp Ther 155:187, 1967.

5. BOTVINICK, EH, DUNN, RF, HATTNER, RS, ET AL: *The consideration of factors affecting diagnostic accuracy of thallium-201 myocardial perfusion scintigraphy in detecting coronary artery disease.* Sem Nuc Med 10:157, 1980.

6. DUNN, RF, WOLFF, L, WAGNER, S, ET AL: *Inconsistent pattern of thallium defects: A clue to the false positive perfusion scintigram.* Am J Cardiol 48:224, 1981.

7 ROZANSKI, A, BERMAN, DS, GRAY, R, ET AL: *Use of thallium-201 redistribution scintigraphy in the preoperative differentiation of reversible and nonreversible myocardial asynergy.* Circulation 64:936, 1981.

8. JENGO, JA, FREEMAN, R, BRIZENDINE, M, ET AL: *Detection of coronary artery disease: Comparison of exercise stressed radionuclide angiocardiography and thallium stress perfusion scanning.* Am J Cardiol 45:535, 1980.

9. KIRSHENBAUM, HD, OKADA, RD, BOUCHER, CA, ET AL: *Relationship of thallium-201 myocardial perfusion to regional and global left ventricular function with exercise.* Am Heart J 101:734, 1981.

10. JOHNSTONE, DE, WACKERS, FJ, BERGER, HJ, ET AL: *Effect of patient positioning on left lateral ^{201}Tl myocardial images.* J Nuc Med 20:183, 1979.

11. GIBSON, RS, WATSON, DO, CARABELLO, BA, ET AL: *Clinical implications of increased lung uptake of thallium-201 during exercise scintigraphy 2 weeks after myocardial infarction.* Am J Cardiol 49:1586, 1982.

12. BOUCHER, CA, ZIR, LM, BELLER, GA, ET AL: *Increased pulmonary uptake of thallium-201 during exercise myocardial imaging: Clinical hemodynamic and angiographic implications with patients with coronary artery disease.* Am J Cardiol 46:189, 1980.

13. BATEMAN, TM, MADDAHI, J, GRAY, RJ, ET AL: *Diffuse slow washout of myocardial ^{201}Tl. Predictive value in the detection of unsuspected extensive coronary disease.* Circulation 66: II–62, 1982.

14. OKADA, RD, BOUCHER, CA, STRAUSS, HW, ET AL: *Exercise radionuclide imaging approaches to coronary artery disease.* Am J Cardiol 46:1188, 1980.

15. RITCHIE, JL, ZARET, BL, STRAUSS, HW, ET AL: *Myocardial imaging with thallium-201: Multicenter study in patients with angina pectoris or acute myocardial infarction.* Am J Cardiol 42:345, 1978.

16. MASSIE, BM, BOTVINICK, EH, AND BRUNDAGE, BH: *Correlation of thallium-201 scintigrams with coronary anatomy: Factors affecting region by region sensitivity.* Am J Cardiol 44:616, 1979.

17. STANILOFF, HM, DIAMOND, GA, FREEMAN, MR, ET AL: *Simplified application of Bayesean analysis to multiple cardiologic tests.* Clin Card 5:630, 1982.

18. BERMAN, DS, GARCIA, EV, AND MADDAHI, J: *Thallium-201 myocardial scintigraphy in the detection and evaluation of coronary artery disease.* IN BERMAN, DS AND MASON, DT (EDS): *Clinical Nuclear Cardiology.* Grune & Stratton, New York, 1981, pp 49–106.

19. DIAMOND, GA AND FORRESTER, JS: *Analysis of probability as an aid in diagnosis of coronary artery disease.* N Engl J Med 300:1350, 1979.

20. HAMILTON, GW, TROBAUGH, GB, RITCHIE, JL, ET AL: *Myocardial imaging with thallium-201: An analysis of clinical usefulness based on Bayes' theorem.* Sem Nucl Med 8:358, 1978.

21. ISKANDRIAN, AS AND SEGAL, BL: *Value of exercise thallium-201 imaging in patients with diagnostic and non-diagnostic exercise electrocardiograms.* Am J Cardiol 48:233, 1981.

22. ISKANDRIAN, AS, WASSERMAN, LA, ANDERSON, GS, ET AL: *Merits of stress thallium-201 myocardial perfusion imaging in patients with inconclusive exercise electrocardiograms: Correlation with coronary arteriograms.* Am J Cardiol 46:553, 1980.

23. MCCARTHY, DM, BLOOD, DK, SCIACCA, RR, ET AL: *Single dose myocardial perfusion imaging with thallium-201: Application in patients with non-diagnostic electrocardiographic stress tests.* Am J Cardiol 43:889, 1979.

24. VERANI, MS, MARCUS, ML, RAZZAK, MA, ET AL: *Sensitivity and specificity of ^{201}Tl perfusion scintigrams under exercise in the diagnosis of coronary artery disease.* J Nucl Med 19:773, 1978.

25. MCLOUGHLIN, PR, MARTIN, RP, DOUGHERTY, P, ET AL: *Reproducibility of thallium-201 myocardial imaging.* Circulation 55:497, 1979.

26. CARALIS, DG, BAILEY, I, KENNEDY, HL, ET AL: *Thallium-201 myocardial imaging in evaluation of asymptomatic individuals with ischemic ST segment depression on exercise electrocardiogram.* Br Heart J 42:562, 1979.

27. BOTVINICK, EH, TARADASH, MR, SHAMES, DM, ET AL: *Thallium-201 myocardial perfusion scintigraphy for the clinical clarification of normal, abnormal and equivocal electrocardiographic stress tests.* Am J Cardiol 41:43, 1978.

28. DUNN, RF, FREEDMAN, B, BAILEY, IK, ET AL: *Localization of coronary artery disease with electrocardiography: Correlation with thallium-201 myocardial perfusion scanning.* Am J Cardiol 48:837, 1981.

29. OKADA, RD, LIMY, L, ROTHENDLER, J, ET AL: *Split dose thallium-201 dipyrimadole imaging: A new technique for obtaining thallium images before and immediately after intervention.* J Am Coll Cardiol 1:1302, 1983.

30. JOSEPHSON, MA, BROWN, BG, HECHT, HS, ET AL: *Non-invasive detection and localization of coronary stenoses in patients: Comparison of resting dipyridamole and exercise thallium-201 myocardial perfusion imaging.* Am Heart J 103:1008, 1982.

31. REHN, T, GRIFFITH, LS, ACHUFF, SC, ET AL: *Exercise thallium-201 myocardial imaging in left main coronary artery disease: Sensitive but not specific.* Am J Cardiol 48:217, 1981.

32. PICHARD, AD, WEINER, I, MARTINEZ, E, ET AL: *Septal myocardial perfusion imaging with thallium-201 in the diagnosis of proximal left anterior descending coronary artery disease.* Am Heart J 102:30, 1981.

33. RIGO, P, BAILEY, IK, GRIFFITH, LSC, ET AL: *Value and limitations of segmental analysis of stress thallium myocardial imaging for localization of coronary artery disease.* Circulation 61:973, 1980.

34. RIGO, P, BAILEY, IK, GRIFFITH, LS, ET AL: *Stress thallium-201 myocardial scintigraphy for the detection of individual coronary arterial lesions in patients with and without previous myocardial infarction.* Am J Cardiol 48:209, 1981.

35. DUNN, R, FREEDMAN, B, BAILEY, IK, ET AL: *Non-invasive prediction of multivessel disease after myocardial infarction.* Circulation 62:726, 1980.

36. RIGO, P, BECKER, LC, GRIFFITH, LSC, ET AL: *Influence of coronary collateral vessels and results of thallium-201 myocardial stress imaging.* Am J Cardiol 44:452, 1979.

37. TUBAU, JF, CHAITMAN, BR, BOURASSA, MG, ET AL: *Importance of coronary collateral circulation in interpreting exercise test results.* Am J Cardiol 47:27, 1981.

38. GARCIA, E, MADDAHI, J, BERMAN, B, ET AL: *Space-time quantitation of thallium-201 myocardial scintigraphy.* J Nucl Med 22:309, 1981.

39. BERGER, BC, WATSON, DD, AND TAYLOR, GJ: *Quantitative thallium-201 exercise scintigraphy for detection of coronary artery disease.* J Nucl Med 22:585, 1981.

40. MADDAHI, J, GARCIA, EV, BERMAN, DS, ET AL: *Improved noninvasive assessment of coronary artery disease by quantitative analysis of regional stress myocardial distribution and washout of ^{201}Tl.* Circulation 64: 924, 1981.

41. TAMAKI, N, MUKAI, T, ISHII, Y, ET AL: *Clinical evaluation of thallium-201 emission myocardial tomography using a rotating gamma camera: Comparison with 7 pinhole tomography.* J Nucl Med 22:849, 1981.

42. BERMAN, DS, STANILOFF, H, FREEMAN, M, ET AL: *Thallium-201 stress myocardial scintigraphy: Comparison of multiple pinhole tomography with planar imaging in the assessment of patients undergoing coronary arteriography.* Am J Cardiol 45:481, 1980.

43. GREEN, A, ALDERSON, P, BERMAN, D, ET AL: *A multicenter comparison of standard and 7 pinhole tomographic myocardial perfusion imaging: ROC analysis of quantitative visual interpretation.* J Nucl Med 21:P70,1980.

44. FRANCISCO, DA, COLLINS, SM, GO, RT, ET AL: *Tomographic thallium-201 mycardial perfusion scintigrams after maximal coronary artery vasodilitation with IV dipyridamole: Comparison of qualitative approaches.* Circulation 66:370, 1983.

45. MANYARI, DE, WOLEWHAKA, AJ, PURVES, P, ET AL: *Comparative value of the cold pressor test and supine bicycle exercise to detect subjects with coronary artery disease using radionuclide ventriculography.* Circulation 65:571, 1982.

46. SLUTSKY, R: *Response of the left ventricle to stress: Effects of exercise, atrial pacing, afterload and drugs.* Am J Cardiol 47:357, 1981.

47. THADANI, U, WEST, R, MATTHEWS, T, ET AL: *Hemodynamics at rest and sitting bicycle exercise in patients with coronary artery disease.* Am J Cardiol 39:776, 1977.

48. THADANI, U AND PARKER, J: *Hemodynamics at rest during supine and sitting bicycle exercise in normal subjects.* Am J Cardiol 41:52, 1978.

49. POLINER, LR, DEHMER, GJ, LEWIS, SE, ET AL: *Left ventricular performance in normal subjects: A comparison of the responses to exercise in the upright and supine positions.* Circulation 62:528, 1980.

50. FREEMAN, MR, BERMAN, DS, STANILOFF, H, ET AL: *Comparison of upright and supine bicycle exercise in the detection and evaluation of extensive coronary artery disease by equilibrium radionuclide ventriculography.* Am Heart J 102:182, 1981.

51. MARX, P, BORKOWSKY, H, SANDS, MJ, ET AL: *Exercise left ventricular performance in aortic regurgitation: Dissimilar response in supine and upright position.* Circulation 66(Suppl II):354, 1982.

52. RATIB, O, HENZE, E, SCHON, H, ET AL: *Phase analysis of radionuclide ventriculograms for the detection of coronary artery disease.* Am Heart J 104:1, 1982.

53. BOTVINICK, EH, FRAIS, MA, SCHOSA, DW, ET AL: *An accurate means of detecting and characterizing abnormal patterns of ventricular activation by phase image analysis.* Am J Cardiol 50:289, 1982

54. DEHMER, DJ, LEWIS, SE, HILLIS, LB, ET AL: *Nongeometric determination of left ventricular volumes from equilibrium blood pool scans.* Am J Cardiol 45:293, 1980.

55. BATTLER, A, SLUTSKY, R, KARLINER, J, ET AL: *Left ventricular ejection fraction and first third ejection fraction early after acute MI: Value for predicting mortality and morbidity.* Am J Cardiol 45:197, 1980.

56. SLUTSKY, R, KARLINER, J, GERBER, K, ET AL: *Systolic blood pressure/systolic volume ratio: Assessment at rest and during exercise in normal subjects and patients with coronary heart disease.* Am J Cardiol 46:813, 1980.

57. DEHMER, DJ, LEWIS, SE, HILLIS, LD, ET AL: *Exercise induced alterations in left ventricular volumes and the pressure volume relationship: A sensitive indicator of left ventricular dysfunction in patients with coronary artery disease.* Circulation 63:108, 1981.

58. OKADA, RD, POHOST, GM, KIRSCHENBAUM, HD, ET AL: *Radionuclide determined change in pulmonary blood volume with exercise: Improved sensitivity of multigated blood scanning in detecting coronary artery disease.* N Engl J Med 301:569, 1979.

59. NICHOLS, AB, STRAUSS, HW, MOORE, RH, ET AL: *Acute changes in cardiopulmonary blood volume during upright exercise stress testing in patients with coronary heart disease.* Circulation 60:520, 1979.

60. PFISTERER, ME, SLUTSKY, RA, SCHULER, G, ET AL: *Profiles of radionuclide ventricular ejection changes induced by supine bicycle exercising in normals and patients with coronary heart disease.* Cathet Cardiovasc Diag 5:305, 1979.

61. WACKERS, FJ, GILES, RW, HOFFER, PB, ET AL: *Gold 195m: A new generator-produced short-lived radionuclide for sequential assessment of ventricular performance by first pass radionuclide angiocardiography.* Am J Cardiol 50:89, 1982.

62. JONES, RH, MCKUEN, P, NEWMAN, GE, ET AL: *Accuracy of diagnosis of coronary artery disease by radionuclide measurement of left ventricular function during rest and exercise.* Circulation 64:586, 1981.

63. RERYCH, SK, SCHOLZ, PM, NEWMAN, GE, ET AL: *Cardiac function at rest and during exercise in normals and patients with coronary heart disease.* Ann Surg 187:449, 1978.

64. BORER, JS, KENT, KM, BACHARACH, ML, ET AL: *Sensitivity, specificity and predictive accuracy of radionuclide synoangiography during exercise in patients with coronary artery disease.* Circulation 60:572, 1979.

65. BERGER, HJ, REDUTO, LA, JOHNSTONE, DE, ET AL: *Global and regional left ventricular response to bicycle exercise in coronary artery disease.* Am J Med 66:13, 1979.

66. JENGO, JA, OREN, V, CONANT, R, ET AL: *Effects of maximal exercise stress on left ventricular function in patients with coronary artery disease using first pass radionuclide angiography.* Circulation 59:60, 1979.

67. CALDWELL, J, SORENSON, S, RITCHIE, J, ET AL: *Exercise radionuclide ventriculography and thallium imaging: Comparison of sensitivity and specificity.* Am J Cardiol 43:432, 1979.

68. BORER, JS, BACHARACH, SL, AND GREEN, MV: *Sensitivity of stress radionuclide cineangiography and thallium perfusion scan in detecting coronary artery disease.* Am J Cardiol 43:431, 1979.

69. VERANI, MS, DELVENTURY, L, AND MELLER, RR: *Radionuclide ventriculograms during dynamic and isometric exercise in coronary artery disease: Comparison with thallium-201 scintigrams.* Clin Res 27:211, 1979.

70. KIRSCHENBAUM, HE, OKADA, RD, AND KUSHNER, FG: *The relation of global left ventricular function with exercise to thallium-201 exercise scintigrams.* Clin Res 27:180, 1979.

71. BORER, JS, BACHARACH, SL, GREEN, MV, ET AL: *Left ventricular function in aortic stenosis: Response to exercise and effects of operation.* Am J Cardiol 41:382, 1978.

72. BORER, JS, BACHARACH, SL, GREEN, MV, ET AL: *Exercise induced left ventricular dysfunction in symptomatic and asymptomatic patients with aortic regurgitation: Assessment with radionuclide cineangiography.* Am J Cardiol 42:351, 1978.

73. BORER, JS, GOTTDIENER, JS, ROSING, DR, ET AL: *Left ventricular function in mitral regurgitation: Determination during exercise.* Circulation 59,60(Suppl II):38, 1979.

74. GOTTDIENER, JS, BORER, JS, BACHARACH, SL, ET AL: *Left ventricular function in mitral valve prolapse: Assessment with radionuclide cineangiography.* Am J Cardiol 47:7, 1981.

75. BORER, JS, BACHARACH, SL, GREEN, MV, ET AL: *Obstructive vs non-obstructive symmetric septal hypertrophy: Differences in left ventricular function with exercise.* Am J Cardiol 41:379, 1978.

76. MATTHAY, RA, BERGER, HJ, DAVIES, RA, ET AL: *Right and left ventricular exercise performance in chronic obstructive pulmonary disease: Radionuclide assessment.* Ann Intern Med 93:234, 1980.

77. LEON, MB, BORER, JS, BACHARACH, SL, ET AL: *Detection of early cardiac dysfunction in patients with severe beta thalassemia and chronic iron overload.* N Engl J Med 301:1143, 1979.

78. PORT, S, COBB, FR, COLEMAN, RE, ET AL: *Effect of age and response of left ventricular ejection fraction to exercise.* N Engl J Med 303:1133, 1980.

79. RERYCH, SK, SCHOLZ, PM, NEWMAN, GE, ET AL: *Cardiac function at rest and during exercise in normals and in patients with coronary heart disease: Evaluation by radionuclide angiography.* Ann Surg 187:449, 1978.

80. BERGER, HJ, SANDS, MJ, DAVIES, RA, ET AL: *Exercise left ventricular performance in patients with chest pain, ischemic appearing exercise electrocardiograms, and angiographically normal coronary arteries.* Ann Intern Med 94:186, 1981.

81. OPHERK, D, ZEBE, H, WEIHE, E, ET AL: *Reduced coronary reserve and ultrastructural changes of the myocardium in patients with angina pectoris but normal coronary arteries.* Circulation 59:II-75, 1979.

82. PORT, S, MCKUEN, P, COBB, FR, ET AL: *Influence of resting left ventricular function and left ventricular response to exercise in patients with coronary artery disease.* Circulation 63:856, 1981.

83. DEPACE, NL, ISKANDRIAN, AS, HAKKI, AH, ET AL: *Value of left ventricular function during exercise in predicting the extent of coronary artery disease.* J Am Coll Cardiol 1:1002, 1983.

84. CAMPOS, CT, CHU, W, D'AGNOSTINO, HJ, ET AL: *Comparison of rest and exercise radionuclide angiocardiography and exercise treadmill testing with the diagnosis of anatomically extensive coronary artery disease.* Circulation 67:1204, 1983.

85. UPTON, MT, PALMER, ST, JONES, RH, ET AL: *Assessment of LV function by resting and exercising radionuclide angiography following acute myocardial infarction.* Am Heart J 104:1232, 1982.

86. CORBETT, JR, DEHMER, GJ, LEWIS, SE, ET AL: *The prognostic value of submaximal exercise testing with radionuclide ventriculography before hospital discharge in patients with recent myocardial infarction.* Circulation 64:535, 1981.

87. ROZANSKI, A, BERMAN, D, GRAY, R, ET AL: *Preoperative prediction of reversible myocardial asynergy by post-exercise radionuclide ventriculography.* N Engl J Med 307:212, 1982.

88. RERYCH, SK, SCHOLZ, PM, SABISTON, DC, ET AL: *Effects of exercise training of left ventricular function in normal subjects: A longitudinal study by radionuclide angiocardiography.* Am J Cardiol 45:244, 1980.

89. VERANI, MS, HARTUNG, GC, HOEPFEL-HARRIS, J, ET AL: *Effects of exercise training on left ventricular performance and in myocardial perfusion in patients with coronary artery disease.* Am J Cardiol 47:797, 1981.

90. JENSEN, D, ATWOOD, JE, FROELICHER, V, ET AL: *Improvement in ventricular function during exercise studies with radionuclide ventriculography after cardiac rehabilitation.* Am J Cardiol 46:770, 1980.

91. COBB, FR, WILLIAMS, RS, MCEWEN, P, ET AL: *Effects of exercise training on ventricular function in patients with recent myocardial infarction.* Circulation 66:100, 1982.

92. BONOW, RD, BACHARACH, SL, GREEN, MV, ET AL: *Impaired left ventricular diastolic filling in patients with coronary artery disease: Assessment with radionuclide angiography.* Circulation 64:315, 1981.

93. REDUTO, LA, WICKEMEYER, WJ, JOUNG, JB, ET AL: *Left ventricular diastolic performance at rest and during exercise in patients with coronary artery disease: Assessment with first pass radionuclide angiography.* Circulation 63:1228, 1981.

94. SLUTSKY, R, BATTLER, A, GERBER, K, ET AL: *Effect of nitrates on left ventricular size and function during exercise: Comparison of sublingual nitroglycerin and nitroglycerin paste.* Am J Cardiol 45:831, 1980.

95. BORER, JS, BACHARACH, SL, GREEN, MV, ET AL: *Effect of nitroglycerin on exercise induced abnormalities of left ventricular regional function and ejection fraction in coronary artery disease: Assessment by radionuclide cineangiography in symptomatic and asymptomatic patients.* Circulation 57:314, 1978.

96. MARSHALL, RC, WEISENBERG, G, SHELBERT, HR, ET AL: *Effect of oral propranolol on rest, exercise and post-exercise left ventricular performance in normal subjects and patients with coronary artery disease.* Circulation 3:572, 1981.

97. BATTLER, A, ROSS, J, JR, SLUTSKY, R, ET AL: *Improvement of exercise induced left ventricular dysfunction with oral propranolol in patients with coronary heart disease.* Am J Cardiol 44:318, 1979.

98. DEHMER, GJ, FALKOFF, M, LEWIS, SE, ET AL: *Effect of oral propranolol on rest and exercise left ventricular ejection fraction, volumes, and segmental wall motion in patients with angina pectoris. Assessment with equilibrium gaited blood pool imaging.* Br Heart J 45:656, 1981.

99. ISKANDRIAN, AS, HAKKI, AH, DEPACE, NJ, ET AL: *Evaluation of left ventricular function by radionuclide angiography during exercise in normal subjects and in patients with chronic coronary heart disease.* J Am Coll Cardiol 1:1518, 1983.

100. BONOW, RO, LEON, MB, ROSSING, DR, ET AL: *Effects of verapamil and propranolol on left ventricular systolic function and diastolic filling in patients with coronary artery disease: Radionuclide angiography studies at rest and during exercise.* Circulation 65:1337, 1981.

101. WACKERS, FJ, STEIN, R, LANGE, R, ET AL: *Sequential first-pass assessment of left ventricular performance during upright exercise in man with short half-life gold-195m: Combined studies with* ^{201}*Tl perfusion imaging.* J Am Coll Cardiol 1:578, 1983.

102. MENA, I, NARAHARA, KA, MAUBLANT, J, ET AL: *Ultra-short lived gold-195m: Use in simultaneous evaluation of LV function and myocardial perfusion with* ^{201}*Tl.* J Nuc Med 24:76, 1983.

103. ZIR, LM, MILLER, SW, DINSMORE, RE, ET AL: *Interobserver variability in coronary arteriography.* Circulation 53:627, 1976.

104. GOTTDIENER, JS, KATIA, MJ, BORER, JS, ET AL: *Late cardiac effects of therapeutic mediastinal irradiation.* N Engl J Med 308:569, 1983.

105. GIBSON, RS, WATSON, DD, CRAMPTON, RS, ET AL: *Comparison of pre-discharge exercise testing,* ^{201}*Tl scintigraphy and coronary angiography for identifying post-infarction patients at risk for future cardiac events.* J Nuc Med 24: P36, 1983.

106. SCHOLL, JM, CHAITMAN, BR, DAVID, PR, ET AL: *Exercise electrocardiography and myocardial scintigraphy in the serial evaluation of the results of PTCA.* Circulation 66:380, 1982.

107. PFISTERER, M, EMENNEGERLT, SCHMITT, HE, ET AL; *Accuracy of serial myocardial perfusion scintigraphy with* ^{201}*Tl for prediction of graft patency early and late after coronary artery bypass grafting.* Circulation 66:1017, 1982.

108. GOTTDIENER, JS, MATHISEN, DJ, BORER, JS, ET AL: *Doxorubicin cardiotoxicity: Assessment of late left ventricular dysfunction by radionuclide cineangiography.* Ann Intern Med 94:430, 1982.

Exercise-Induced Arrhythmias and Hypotension: Significance and Clinical Management

Myrvin H. Ellestad, M.D.

As more careful followup studies are completed, we have had to change a number of beliefs about events occurring during exercise. This chapter deals with rhythm disturbances and the blood pressure response, especially hypotension.

The atrial arrhythmias and conduction disturbances are reviewed in an abbreviated way because of their lesser importance and because less is known. The blood pressure response had been given little attention until a few years ago, but now has been shown to merit careful observation both prior to and during exercise testing.

ATRIAL ARRHYTHMIAS

It is now appreciated that the atrial transport mechanism may contribute from 10 to 30 percent of the stroke volume. Thus, the sinus node not only determines cardiac output by its chronotropic response, but the appropriately timed atrial boost to left ventricular filling is critical to function at high workloads.

Paroxysmal Atrial Tachycardia (PAT)

Although this arrhythmia, in susceptible subjects, may often be initiated by emotion and other stimuli, it only rarely occurs during exercise stress testing. Graboys and Wright reported 29 patients with sustained PAT in 3000 exercise tests.[1] These instances were from a cohort of 207 patients referred for evaluation of atrial arrhythmias. Although PAT is common in Wolff-Parkinson-White (WPW) syndrome, I have tested many patients with accelerated conduction, and I have never encountered exercise-induced paroxysmal atrial tachycardia in the WPW syndrome. In patients who do develop PAT, ST segment depression may appear, but the latter finding has less significance than when seen with sinus tachycardia.

Sick Sinus Syndrome (SSS)

An abnormally slow sinus node response will reduce exercise tolerance and the normally expected increase in cardiac output. Although we labeled subjects with this syndrome chronotropic incompetence,[2] a term that has been repeated in the literature, it now appears that some of these patients fit the category of sick sinus syndrome. It has been demonstrated that this reduced heart rate response to exercise in patients with myocardial ischemia may be reversible after successful coronary bypass surgery.[3] The mechanism of the bradyarrhythmia is somewhat obscure, but in some cases it may be related to the vagally mediated Jarish-

Bezold reflex. This reflex, which is initiated by distention of the ischemic ventricular wall, may protect the heart by preventing the short diastolic filling period associated with rapid heart rates. On the other hand, Orkin and coworkers[4] reported that some patients with SSS fail to increase their heart rate after atropine. This bradyarrhythmic response has been found to be a fairly good predictor of poor ventricular function, even in the absence of ST segment depression.[2]

Atrial Fibrillation and Flutter

The occasional occurrence of these arrhythmias during exercise testing reduces exercise capacity and ventricular filling, but no data are available to establish their significance in terms of coronary pathology or long-term prognosis. They occur more commonly in patients with rheumatic heart disease than coronary disease. Again, with these arrhythmias the accompanying ST segment depression has questionable predictive value for coronary narrowing.

CONDUCTION DISTURBANCES

First and Second Degree AV Block

These conduction disturbances are common in patients with coronary heart disease and, therefore, they are often encountered in the exercise laboratory. When rapid atrial pacing is instituted, the PR interval almost always increases. This is not so with increasing heart rates induced by exercise. Apparently the catecholamine increase or the vagal withdrawal accompanying exercise prevents PR prolongation, so that a first degree AV block may disappear with exercise and the PR interval almost never becomes prolonged. Immediately after exercise the PR interval may lengthen and transient second degree AV block may occur, probably due to return of the vagal influence. This probably has little clinical importance, however.

If second degree AV block occurs during exercise testing, it is associated with reduction in cardiac output and constitutes an indication for terminating exercise should it last for more than a few beats. No data are available about its ultimate clinical significance.

Third Degree AV Block

In contradistinction to second degree AV block, the appearance of third degree AV block not only requires immediate termination of exercise but occasionally signals severe myocardial ischemia during exercise testing.[3] Fortunately, it is rarely encountered, but when it occurs, it should be of great concern.

Wolff-Parkinson-White (WPW) Syndrome

Delta waves, reflecting conduction via bypass tracts, often occur with exercise testing and almost always are associated with ST segment depression. If the accelerated conduction is not recognized, this response may be incorrectly diagnosed as myocardial ischemia. This WPW syndrome is a recognized cause of false-positive ST segment depression.[5]

Right And Left Bundle Branch Block

The sudden appearance of bundle branch block during exercise has long been termed rate related bundle branch block. This terminology implies that any increase in heart rate could initiate the bundle branch block pattern and that it is of no clinical significance. However, approximately 70 percent of our adult male patients with this finding have significant coronary narrowing, and therefore we believe that other tests, even coronary angiography, may be indicated, especially if the patient has other risk factors.

VENTRICULAR ARRHYTHMIAS

At one time, ventricular arrhythmias at rest were believed to have ominous implications. More recently, Buckingham and associates[6] demonstrated that frequent PVCs on Holter recordings in normal subjects are usually benign. On the other hand, if they occur in subjects with significant ventricular dysfunction, they are often harbingers of serious subsequent events. The same applies to PVCs recorded during exercise testing.[7]

PVCs Initiated By Exercise

In actively employed, normal policeman[8] and airman,[9] exercise-induced PVCs have been found to have no influence on subsequent morbidity and mortality.

We have reported followup data on 1327 patients who had PVCs before, during, or after an exercise test. They were referred to our hospital primarily for chest pain syndromes.[7] In this population, PVCs were associated with a moderate increase in morbidity and mortality as compared with the normal persons even when the individuals tested did not exhibit ischemic ST segment depression. However, if they developed ST segment depression (Fig. 1), the mortality and number of coronary events almost doubled. Also, ominous PVCs increased the

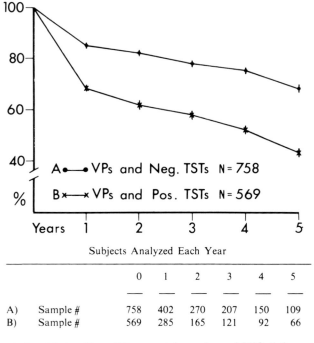

		0	1	2	3	4	5
A)	Sample #	758	402	270	207	150	109
B)	Sample #	569	285	165	121	92	66

Figure 1. Coronary events in subjects with no ST segment depression and PVCs (*A*) as compared with PVCs in conjunction with ST segment depression *(B)*. Coronary events include death, myocardial infarction, and acceleration of angina. (From Ellestad, MH: *Stress Testing: Principles and Practice,* ed 2. FA Davis, Philadelphia, 1980, with permission.)

risk even more, to about twice that of the others. Ominous PVCs were defined as multifocal, multiform, repetitive, or ventricular tachycardia. Followup data on PVCs [10] after myocardial infarction have also shown that, when associated with mild coronary disease and good left ventricular function, PVCs are of lesser clinical significance than when recorded in patients with a low ejection fraction, in whom they indicate a more serious prognosis.

PVCs Eliminated by Exercise

It seemed logical that arrhythmias at rest that disappeared on exercise were probably benign and could be discounted. However, our study revealed that patients with these arrhythmias had the same morbidity and mortality as those in whom PVCs persisted after exercise started and also had the same prognosis as those in whom the arrhythmia was initiated by exercise. We know that an increase in heart rate reduces the time for re-entry because more of the cardiac cycle is refractory; thus, re-entry type ventricular arrhythmias may be inhibited regardless of their overall severity.

PVCs During Recovery From Exercise

Inasmuch as the rate slows rapidly during recovery, PVCs occur commonly and usually have no clinical significance in our experience.

Ventricular Tachycardia

When this arrhythmia, defined as three or more consecutive PVCs, occurs during exercise it constitutes an indication for termination. Moreover, it has been associated with a high incidence of coronary events. In adult men, ventricular tachycardia is usually associated with significant coronary narrowing, and in our followup study we found it to be associated with an increased incidence of coronary events.

In summary, exercise-induced PVCs can be evaluated by the company they keep. In patients with significant coronary disease or reduced ventricular function, PVCs definitely constitute an increased risk. There is considerable evidence that ambulatory rhythm monitoring is a more satisfactory method of evaluating PVCs than an exercise test—if rhythm disturbances are of prime concern in a patient with known coronary disease. [11]

HYPOTENSION

Many complex factors are involved in the control of the blood pressure response to exercise. An understanding of these factors and how they interact with each other is necessary in order to draw conclusions concerning the responses observed in patients. The increase in blood pressure with exercise is a function of peripheral resistance and cardiac output. We have learned to expect certain blood pressure responses depending on the age and vigor of the patient (Fig. 2).

Hypotension during exercise testing has long been known to be associated with a poor prognosis. Bruce defined exertional hypotension as the inability to raise systolic pressure by at least 10 percent above resting levels. [12] He believed that this response was associated with an increased risk of sudden death and concluded that exertional hypotension was probably a manifestation of impaired cardiac function, whenever a major loss in blood volume or marked impairment of neuroregulation could be excluded. Other authors [13,14] have reported on the same response. The general thesis is that a failure to normally elevate blood pressure during the course of exercise testing or an abnormal fall in blood pressure with exercise is associated with significant impairment of left ventricular function. However, it is necessary to consider

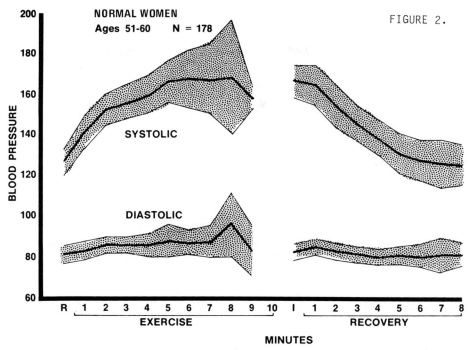

Figure 2. Blood pressure response to a standard protocol.[3] First stage (min 1–3) 1.7 mph, second stage (min 4–5) 3 mph, third stage (min 6–7) 4 mph, fourth stage (min 8–9) 5 mph. All at 10 percent grade. Note drop in blood pressure after minute 8. (From Ellestad, MH: *Stress Testing: Principles and Practice,* ed 2. FA Davis, Philadelphia, 1980, with permission.)

other possible causes of exertional hypotension and eliminate them before ischemic left ventricular dysfunction can be presumed to be responsible for the impaired response, thereby inferring a significant risk for future ischemic events (Table 1).

Reduced left ventricular contractility owing to conditions affecting the myocardium, as well as valvular heart disease, reduced blood volume, and vasomotor abnormalities, has an important effect on blood pressure response. Some antihypertensive drugs, beta blockers, sympatholytics, and peripheral vasodilators may also reduce the blood pressure response to exertion.

Table 1. Etiology of exertional hypotension

Left ventricular dysfunction
  Ischemia
  Cardiomyopathy
    Obstructive
    Congestive
Valvular heart disease
Arrhythmias
Drugs
  Antihypertensives
  Psychotropics
Exceeding anaerobic threshold

These conditions should be evaluated prior to testing so that any change encountered during the exercise test can be viewed in the proper context.

Arrhythmias

When rapid atrial arrhythmias or frequent PVCs occur, the blood pressure response is less than physiologically ideal. Thus, careful observation of the electrocardiogram, as well as repeated measurement of the blood pressure, helps the physician respond to these changes expeditiously.

Exceeding Anaerobic Threshold

The anaerobic threshold is the maximal level of work that can be sustained while the demand of peripheral tissues is met by an adequate cardiac output. If the patient exercises beyond this threshold, the peripheral tissues, primarily the skeletal muscles, are no longer able to meet their work requirements by aerobic metabolism.[15] At this point, the tissues begin to use an anaerobic pathway, with production of significant amounts of lactate and other metabolites. This response results in significant vasodilation as well as a drop in myocardial contractility, as the pH falls. This mechanism occurs in normal subjects as well as in patients with severe coronary disease, but the level of work initiating the change is lower in the latter group. The prime consideration in evaluating a drop in blood pressure is the timing. If it occurs early, when one would expect from the patient's age and apparent vigor that he or she should continue to exercise, it may represent cardiac disease. On the other hand, if it occurs near the expected maximum workload, it may well be a normal response to an energetic exercise effort.

Ischemic Left Ventricular Dysfunction

A number of studies have documented the correlation of exertional hypotension at exercise testing with severe coronary disease. As early as 1959, Bruce and coworkers[12] noted the occurrence of exertional hypotension and suggested this may be a sign of significant impairment of cardiac function. The work of Thompson and Kellerman[16] in 1975 again called attention to this blood pressure response; they reported that 14 of 15 patients with exertional hypotension had severe disease of both the left anterior descending and circumflex coronary arteries. Twelve of these 15 patients had 3-vessel coronary disease. They concluded that a fall in systolic pressure early in the exercise protocol reflects acute myocardial ischemia and usually indicates that a large mass of left ventricular muscle is ischemic. Other studies have subsequently confirmed the relationship of hypotension to coronary disease.[17,18] More recently, Weiner and colleagues[19] studied over 400 consecutive patients with exercise testing and cardiac catheterization. Forty-seven of these patients manifested a fall in blood pressure with exercise; half were randomized to medical therapy and the other half to surgical therapy. All had cardiac catheterization, and half had either 3-vessel or left main coronary artery disease. After treatment had been instituted, repeat exercise testing revealed that those who were successfully surgically revascularized had a normal blood pressure response, whereas those treated medically had no significant change and again responded to exercise with a drop in blood pressure.

In conclusion, the blood pressure response to exercise is very important and should be observed carefully. A fall in blood pressure during exercise early in the exercise protocol has particularly ominous implications. When it occurs later, the implications are less important; when exercise hypotension occurs near the expected peak exercise load, it probably indicates a normal physiologic phenomenon in which the patient has exercised beyond his aerobic capacity.

REFERENCES

1. GRABOYS, TB AND WRIGHT, RF: *Provocation of supraventricular tachycardia during exercise testing.* Cardiovasc Reviews Reports 1:57, 1980.

2. ELLESTAD, MH AND WAN, MKC. *Predictive implications of stress testing. Follow-up of 2700 subjects after maximum treadmill stress testing.* Circulation 51:363, 1975.

3. ELLESTAD, MH: *Stress testing: Principles and Practice,* ed 2. FA Davis, Philadelphia, 1980.

4. ORKIN, LR, BERGMAN, PS, AND NATHANSON, M: *Effect of atropine, scopolamine and meperidine on man.* Anesthesiology 17:30, 1956.

5. SANDBERG, L: *Studies in electrocardiogram changes during exercise tests.* Acta Med Scand 169(365),1969.

6. BUCKINGHAM, TA, LABOVITZ, AJ, AND KENNEDY, HL: *The clinical significance of ventricular arrhythmias in apparently healthy subjects.* Practical Cardiology 9(8):37, 1983.

7. UDALL, JA AND ELLESTAD, MH: *Predictive implications of ventricular premature contractions associated with treadmill stress testing.* Circulation 56:985, 1977.

8. MCHENRY, PL, FISCH, C, JORDAN, JW, ET AL: *Cardiac arrhythmias observed during maximal treadmill exercise testing in clinically normal men.* Am J Cardiol 29:331, 1972.

9. FROELICHER, VF, THOMAS, MD, PILLOW C, ET AL: *Epidemiologic study of asymptomatic men screened by maximal treadmill testing for latent coronary artery disease.* Am J Cardiol 34:770, 1974.

10. SCHULTZ, RA, STRAUSS, HW, AND PITT, B: *Sudden death in the year following myocardial infarction: Relation to ventricular premature contractions in the late hospital phase and left ventricular ejection fraction.* Am J Med 62:192, 1977.

11. POBLETE, PF, KENNEDY, HL, AND CARALIS, DG: *Detection of ventricular ectopy in patients with coronary heart disease and normal subjects by exercise testing and ambulatory electrocardiography.* Chest 74:402, 1978.

12. BRUCE, RA, COBB, LA, KATSURA, S, ET AL: *Exertional hypotension in cardiac patients.* Circulation 19:543, 1959.

13. MORRIS, S, PHILLIPS, J, JORDAN, D, ET AL: *Incidence and significance of decreases in systolic blood pressure during graded treadmill exercise testing.* Am J Cardiol 41:221, 1978.

14. SAN MARCO, M, PONTIUS, S, AND SELVESTER, R: *Abnormal blood pressure response and marked ischemic ST segment depression as predictors of severe coronary artery disease.* Circulation 61:572, 1980.

15. WASSERMAN, K, WHIPP, BJ, KOYAL, SN, ET AL: *Anaerobic threshold and respiratory gas exchange during exercise.* J Appl Physiol 35:230, 1973.

16. THOMPSON, P AND KELLERMAN, M: *Hypotension accompanying the onset of exertional angina.* Circulation 52:28, 1975.

17. IRVING, J, BRUCE, RA, AND DEROUEN, T: *Variations in and significance of systolic pressure during maximal exercise (treadmill) testing.* Am J Cardiol 40:841, 1977.

18. HAMMERMEISTER, MD, DEROUEN, TA, DODGE, HT, ET AL: *Prognostic and predictive value of exertional hypotension in suspected coronary heart disease.* Am J Cardiol 51:1261, 1983.

19. WEINER, D, MACABE, C, CUTLER, D, ET AL: *Decrease in systolic blood pressure during exercise testing: Reproducibility, response to coronary bypass surgery, and prognostic significance.* Am J Cardiol 49:1627, 1982.

Cardiovascular Drugs: Effects on Exercise Testing and Exercise Training of the Coronary Patient*

Nanette K. Wenger, M.D.

EXERCISE TESTING

Exercise testing, in clinical practice and in the research setting, may be performed for a variety of reasons, including the assessment of functional capacity; the identification of myocardial ischemia (suggesting that atherosclerotic coronary heart disease may be present); prescription of rehabilitative exercise; recommendations for return to work; obtaining of prognostic information in patients known to have coronary disease; evaluation of the efficacy of drug, exercise, or surgical therapy; and so forth. All these evaluations depend variably on the heart rate and blood pressure responses to graded exercise and on the associated symptomatic and electrocardiographic abnormalities, which are typically prominently related to the rate-pressure product. Thus, any cardiovascular medication that alters the balance of myocardial oxygen supply and demand by influencing any of its components is likely to modify the results obtained at exercise testing. The effects of cardiovascular drugs on any of the determinants of myocardial oxygen demand—heart rate, myocardial wall tension (ventricular volume, ventricular filling pressure, systolic blood pressure), ventricular ejection time, and myocardial contractile state—require careful assessment; to date, pharmacotherapy has not been demonstrated to significantly alter myocardial oxygen supply.

Changes in the exercise electrocardiogram associated with pharmacotherapy may reflect either the hemodynamic changes due to drug administration or the direct effects of the drug on the myocardium, or both.[1]

EXERCISE TRAINING

Individualized prescriptive exercise is the hallmark of rehabilitative physical activity for patients with atherosclerotic coronary heart disease—patients with angina pectoris and those recovered from myocardial infarction or following coronary bypass surgery. The physiologic goal of rehabilitative exercise training for patients with symptomatic coronary disease is an improvement in cardiorespiratory fitness. The trained patient will exhibit a modest decrease in the resting heart rate and systolic blood pressure; of greater importance, there will be a lesser increase in heart rate and systolic blood pressure at any level of submaximal work (Table 1). Improvement in arteriovenous oxygen extraction (increased A-V O_2 difference) by trained skeletal muscle is the major determinant of this change, resulting in a lesser demand

---

*Adapted in part from Wenger, NK: The Coronary Patient: Interactions of Cardiovascular Drugs and Exercise. Drug Therapy, 13:59, 1982, with permission.

Table 1. Effect on major determinants of myocardial oxygen demand

	Nitrate Drugs	Propranolol	Exercise Training
Myocardial Wall Tension (Stress)			
Systolic Blood Pressure	↓	↓	SL ↓
L. V. Filling Pressure or Volume (Preload)	↓↓	O → SL ↑	O → SL ↑
Ejection Time (Time of Wall Stress)	↓	SL ↑	SL ↑
Heart Rate (Frequency of Wall Stress)	SL ↑	↓↓	↓
Myocardial Contractility (dp/dt)	SL ↑	↓	?

(Reproduced from Wenger, N. K.: Rehabilitation of the Patient with Symptomatic Coronary Atherosclerotic Heart Disease, Part II. In *Cardiology Series,* edited by H. D. McIntosh, Continuing Education, Baylor College of Medicine, Houston, 1980, p. 15, with permission).

for increased blood flow to exercising muscle; this decreases the myocardial oxygen demand relative to the total body oxygen demand. Maximal oxygen uptake also increases. Heart rate and systolic blood pressure—the rate pressure product—are major determinants of myocardial oxygen demand. Thus the decrease in myocardial oxygen demand enables the trained coronary patient to do more work before the onset of angina pectoris and before the appearance of ECG evidence of myocardial ischemia (ST-T changes). Exercise-trained patients, in performing usual daily activities, function farther from their ischemic threshold; patients describe this decrease in perceived exertion as increased stamina or endurance. Exercise training thus decreases symptoms and improves the patient's functional capacity.

The dosage of exercise prescribed is a function of its intensity, duration, and frequency. The intensity of prescriptive exercise is typically guided by the heart rate range. During dynamic exercise, the increases in heart rate and in cardiac output parallel the increase in oxygen consumption, that is, the progressive increase in exercise intensity. This underlies the use of pulse monitoring to gauge exercise intensity. Exercise testing is the basis for determining the intensity component of the exercise prescription, with the recommendation usually based on the highest heart rate safely achieved at exercise testing, that is, the heart rate attained before the appearance of any adverse signs or symptoms. Because it is inadvisable for rehabilitative physical activity for coronary patients to entail a myocardial oxygen demand (as estimated by the heart rate) greater than that demonstrated to evoke an appropriate cardiovascular response in the controlled setting of the exercise testing laboratory, a target heart rate range of 70 to 85 percent of this value is typically chosen. As patients check their heart rate response only intermittently during exercise, this prescriptive concept makes it likely that a training effect will be achieved while safety is assured. Using this approach, patients are unlikely to exceed the 100 percent heart rate level, the threshold at which adverse signs or symptoms appeared at exercise testing. The 70 to 85 percent heart rate range corresponds to 60 to 78 percent of the peak oxygen uptake, an effective yet safe range within which to stimulate aerobic metabolism and achieve the training effect. It is unwise to use age-predicted maximal heart rates to prescribe the exercise intensity for patients with atherosclerotic coronary heart disease—those with angina pectoris, myocardial infarction, or following coronary bypass surgery—because the underlying cardiac disease, the resultant impairment of the conduction system, as well as the pharmacotherapy, may alter the heart rate response to exercise.

Cardiovascular drugs that alter any of the major determinants of myocardial oxygen demand (see above) can comparably alter the ability to exercise. In contradistinction, then, to the virtually drug-free state desirable for exercise testing done to establish the diagnosis of myocardial ischemia (in an attempt to reduce the drug-related false-positive exercise ECG responses), exercise testing for exercise prescription should be performed with the patient on an optimal medical regimen, receiving all the drugs and at the approximate dosages that will be continued during exercise training. Indeed, a significant alteration in the drug regimen should be an indication for repeated exercise testing for revision of the exercise prescription;[2] this is because the new drug regimen may necessitate a change in the target heart rate range and because a major therapeutic alteration is usually made in response to a change in clinical status. Just as any drug altering the determinants of myocardial oxygen demand may influence the results of the exercise test used to prescribe exercise training levels, so may cardiovascular drug therapy alter the response to the exercise training.

APPLICATION TO CLINICAL PRACTICE

Physicians are increasingly using exercise testing and exercise training in their management of patients with atherosclerotic coronary heart disease. A recent survey[3] designed to assess changes in clinical practice during the past decade in the management of patients with uncomplicated myocardial infarction revealed that most general practitioners, internists, and cardiologists routinely recommended a progressive exercise regimen for patients recovered from an uncomplicated myocardial infarction. Physician-supervised group exercise programs and unsupervised individual home exercise were advised with about equal frequency; the choice was dictated primarily by availability and cost considerations. In addition, there was a significant increase in the routine use of exercise testing by all physician groups; the reasons cited for this change included increased familiarity with the procedure, greater availability of exercise testing in the local community, and less concern about potential adverse effects in the exercise testing of coronary patients.

In the 1980s, most coronary patients presenting for exercise testing for exercise prescription and/or participating in a prescriptive exercise regimen are likely to be taking a variety of cardiovascular drugs. During the period of recruitment of patients recovered from myocardial infarction for the National Exercise and Heart Disease Project[4] over five years ago, 43 percent of the men enrolled were receiving nitrate drugs, 19 percent a variety of diuretic preparations, 16 percent were taking digitalis, 13 percent beta-adrenergic blocking drugs, 13 percent antiarrhythmic drugs, particularly procainamide or quinidine, and 8 percent nondiuretic, non-beta-blocking antihypertensive drugs. Today, an increased percentage of patients is likely to be taking beta-blocking drugs; the current use of the newly available antiarrhythmic and vasodilator drugs is far more prevalent; and a new class of antianginal compounds, calcium entry blocking drugs, has been licensed for clinical use in the U.S.

ANTIANGINAL DRUGS

Nitrate Preparations

A variety of short- and long-acting nitrate preparations—sublingual nitroglycerin; swallowed, chewable, or sublingual long-acting nitrate tablets; nitroglycerin ointments or pastes; or the newer transdermal patch long-acting nitrate preparations—uniformly improve exercise tolerance in patients with angina, increasing the duration of exercise before the onset of chest pain and/or ECG evidence of myocardial ischemia. Typically, one sublingual nitroglycerin tablet may improve the treadmill exercise capacity by as much as one MET. Nitroglycerin administration reduces the elevation in left ventricular end-diastolic pressure characteristically associated with the angina induced by dynamic exercise. Indeed, in some patients with mild to moderate angina pectoris, the administration of long-acting nitrate drugs may reduce or eliminate the symptomatic and electrocardiographic abnormalities of myocardial ischemia at exercise testing.[5] Clinically, patients can perform more activity before the onset of angina pectoris. Isometric exercise may induce (reversible) left ventricular dysfunction, with elevation of the left ventricular filling pressure in patients with atherosclerotic heart disease. Nitroglycerin appears to improve left ventricular function during isometric exercise in these coronary patients with compromised left ventricular function by reducing both left ventricular preload and afterload.[6]

Nitrate drugs decrease myocardial oxygen demand by a combination of several mechanisms. They act primarily as vasodilator agents, producing an important decrease in myocardial oxygen demand owing to reduction of the left ventricular filling pressure and volume (preload). Nitrate drugs are also arteriolar vasodilators, decreasing peripheral vascular resistance (systemic arterial pressure) and thereby left ventricular work. Additionally, because collateral vessels appear to predominate in the subendocardial plexus, the decrease in left ventricular end-diastolic pressure favors coronary collateral flow. Coronary vasodilatation has also been described, but its clinical importance remains uncertain. Nitrate drugs also decrease ejection time. The resultant decrease in myocardial ischemia is often evident as an improvement in ventricular wall motion and an increase in ejection fraction.

It is the arteriolar vasodilation property, the decrease in peripheral vascular resistance, that may limit the use of nitrate drugs or cause adverse drug responses. A baroreceptor-mediated reflex tachycardia often results from systemic vasodilatation. The combination of tachycardia and a decreased diastolic blood pressure may actually decrease coronary blood flow despite the coronary vasodilatation. Patients taking sublingual nitroglycerin to relieve chest pain associated with exercise should be carefully instructed to use the medication while seated, particularly if a series of tablets are taken; acute vasodilation and hypotension may result in lightheadedness or syncope when upright; this may be even more pronounced with exercise-induced angina, when the effects of nitroglycerin are superimposed on the prominent arteriolar vasodilatation that occurs with high-level exercise.

The predominant beneficial effect of nitrate drugs appears related to the decrease in myocardial oxygen demand[7] rather than to an increased delivery of oxygen to ischemic myocardium;[8,9] both before and after nitrate administration, angina pectoris occurs at the same triple product (heart rate × blood pressure × systolic ejection time). After nitrate administration, however, this triple product is reached only after application of an increased workload, that is, nitrate drugs raise the work threshold for angina. [10]

Although they both decrease myocardial oxygen demand, nitrate therapy and exercise training do so by eliciting different hemodynamic changes (Table 1). An additional important difference is that nitrate therapy does not improve peripheral oxygen extraction by muscle, as occurs after training. Nevertheless, as exercise training progresses and the patient's fitness improves, the nitrate dosage required may be decreased.

Research studies define a difference in the acute and long-term effects of nitrate therapy on exercise capacity. The administration of a single dose of a nitrate drug to patients with left ventricular failure related to ischemic heart disease resulted in a decrease in the rest and exercise pulmonary capillary wedge pressure, pulmonary and systemic arterial pressures, and pulmonary and systemic vascular resistances, and an increase in cardiac output; despite these changes, there was no improvement in the maximal exercise capacity or the exercise hemodynamics at peak exercise.[11] Long-term nitrate therapy, however, improved both the clinical status and the exercise capacity; although tolerance seemed to develop to the systemic arterial vascular effects, the improvement in the venous and pulmonary vascular parameters remained. These patients had a documented increase in their physical activity.[11] In another study, the increase in arteriovenous oxygen difference in patients receiving chronic nitrate therapy alone suggested that a peripheral training effect may have occurred, in that the now less-symptomatic patients were spontaneously more physically active during their course of therapy,[12] with resultant exercise-induced physical conditioning.

Other Vasodilator Drugs

In patients with congestive heart failure, the acute administration of other vasodilator drugs such as hydralazine and prazosin typically results in symptomatic relief and in improvement in hemodynamic measurements at rest; pulmonary arterial and venous pressures decrease and the cardiac output improves. As with nitrate drugs, there is no comparable improvement in the patient's exercise performance acutely.[13]

However, in a number of studies, exercise capacity has been shown to increase both with long-term vasodilator therapy alone and with long-term vasodilator therapy in association with exercise training.[14,15] Exercise training significantly improved the results of treadmill exercise testing, suggesting that deconditioning of the peripheral musculature owing to prolonged inactivity prior to therapy may have contributed to the initial exercise intolerance after the acute administration of vasodilator therapy.

Beta Adrenergic Blocking Drugs

The demonstration that appropriately selected patients, recovered from myocardial infarction, have an improved prognosis when treated with beta adrenergic blocking drugs[16-18] has greatly increased the number of coronary patients treated with these drugs undergoing exercise testing and/or exercise training.

Both cardioselective and nonselective beta adrenergic blocking drugs decrease myocardial oxygen requirements at rest and with exercise, with a resultant decrease in angina pectoris and an improvement in exercise tolerance; there is a decrease in the electrocardiographic evidence of ischemia. This enables the patient receiving beta-blocking drugs to perform an increased intensity and/or duration of work with a similar myocardial oxygen consumption, that is, before the attainment of the ischemic threshold and before the onset of the signs and symptoms of myocardial ischemia.[19]

The major effect of this class of compounds is to limit the response to catecholamine stimulation; as a result there is a decrease in the resting heart rate and blood pressure and a lessening of the usual exercise-induced increases in heart rate and blood pressure.[19] Therapy with beta-blocking drugs thus enables the patient to exercise at an increased intensity and/ or for a longer duration before achieving the same heart rate or rate-pressure product. There is also a decrease in myocardial contractility, reflecting the decreased responsiveness to catecholamine stimulation in the beta-blocked patient (Table 1).

The decrease in heart rate in the patient receiving beta-blocking drugs reflects both the degree of beta blockade and the underlying vagal tone. Isometric exercise (for example, handgrip) has been suggested as valuable in estimating the contribution of vagal tone to the bradycardia; vagal withdrawal causes cardioacceleration with isometric exercise.[20]

The decrease in heart rate is the major contributor to the decrease in myocardial oxygen demand for the patient with symptomatic coronary atherosclerotic heart desease; the prolonged diastolic time increases coronary blood flow and myocardial perfusion, as well as increasing coronary collateral flow in the subendocardial plexus. The clinical corollary is that patients with rapid pre-treatment heart rates typically have a more dramatic response to beta blockade than individuals with slower initial heart rates, in whom the percent of change is likely to be small. The contribution of the decreased systemic arterial pressure and myocardial contractility appears of lesser importance.

However, the depression of myocardial contractility, if excessive, may paradoxically worsen the angina and limit the patient's activity. Impaired myocardial contractility may result in an increase in left ventricular filling pressure and pulmonary capillary pressure at rest and with exercise. As cardiac dilatation develops as a compensatory mechanism, the resultant increases in myocardial wall tension and thereby in myocardial oxygen requirements may result in myocardial ischemia that will limit the ability to exercise. This is more likely to occur in patients with pre-existing borderline ventricular function, or in those receiving concomitant therapy with drugs having negative inotropic properties.

The theoretical adverse effect of coronary arterial vasoconstriction (owing to an unopposed alpha adrenergic effect) in decreasing coronary blood flow and oxygen delivery, if it occurs, appears overshadowed when compared with the beneficial effects of the decrease in myocardial oxygen demand and the increased coronary blood flow related to the reduction in heart rate. Theoretically, beta blockade may worsen variant (Prinzmetal) angina by causing coronary vasospasm by this mechanism.

A number of extracardiac effects of the nonselective beta-blocking drugs may also potentially limit the ability to exercise. Prominent among these effects are peripheral arterial constriction with resultant leg claudication and bronchoconstriction. The effect of the beta-blockade-induced increase in plasma epinephrine on the alpha adrenergic receptors has been proposed as the mechanism producing the increase in peripheral vascular resistance; however, the use of cardioselective beta blockade does not appear to elicit a superior response to exercise by lessening leg claudication.[21] Two alternate explanations for the leg claudication seem more likely: a beta-blockade-mediated decrease in cardiac output may limit perfusion of an atherosclerotic peripheral arterial bed; and/or the increased activity enabled by the reduction in angina pectoris may render more prominent the symptoms related to the peripheral arterial obstructive disease. Cardioselective and nonselective beta-blocking drugs also effected a comparable reduction in the exercise tachycardia and the systolic blood pressure response to short-term dynamic exercise in normal subjects; there was no significant drug effect on the anaerobic threshold or on maximal oxygen consumption. Thus a cardioselective beta-blocking drug (metoprolol) did not appear superior to a nonselective drug (propranolol) in its effect on exercise capacity or on the response to short-term maximal exercise.[21] The use of selective beta-blocking drugs, however, can limit the bronchoconstriction in susceptible subjects with reactive airway disease.

An important feature documented in recent years is that patients taking long-term beta-blocking drugs can participate in exercise training[22] and that, despite their lessened heart rate and blood pressure response to exercise, they can increase their exercise capacity.[2,23,24] Heart rate and systolic blood pressure responses to exercise are reduced with exercise training.[25] Early reports described a failure of the maximal oxygen uptake (maximal physical work capacity) to increase during short-term dynamic exercise training in patients receiving selective and nonselective beta-blocking drugs. However, an elegant experimental design by Ewy and associates[26] demonstrated the training effect. Twelve normal subjects, treated with beta-blocking drugs, participated in an exercise training regimen for 13 weeks with a resultant significant decrease in heart rate response and improvement in treadmill time as compared with a control group; however, their maximal oxygen uptake did not improve. When beta-blocking drugs were withdrawn, the increased heart rate response enabled demonstration of an increased oxygen uptake (physical work capacity) as compared with pre-exercise training levels—evidence of a training effect. An increase in stroke volume or peripheral oxygen extraction or both may be needed to maintain physical work capacity in normal individuals receiving beta blockade; these adaptations may be limited in coronary patients. Nevertheless, in a small group of patients recovered from myocardial infarction and treated with beta adrenergic blocking drugs, four months of endurance training significantly decreased the heart rate and increased the exercise duration and workload achieved; the maximal oxygen uptake, oxygen pulse, and respiratory exchange ratio all improved.[27] Thus, hemodynamic determinants of the training effect are seen in beta-blocked persons; the heart rate and systolic blood pressure responses to exercise decrease and the peak oxygen uptake increases.[28] Stated another way, the usual physiologic adaptations of training occur in patients receiving beta adrenergic blocking drugs; their heart rate response remains a useful guide for physical activity recommendations and for assessing the effects of training.[25]

The effect on endurance exercise is less well defined in that blockade of the beta-receptor-mediated mobilization of free fatty acids and muscle glycogen may potentially limit the ability to perform long-term exercise.[29]

Inhibition of the exercise-induced stimulation of glucose metabolism by beta-blocking drugs has been postulated to alter the respiratory exchange ratio and thereby to potentially impair exercise training, [30] but these data are controversial.[25,27] The decreases in maximal exercise duration and maximal oxygen uptake described in some studies may be related to the specific beta-blocking drug studied or may be dose dependent.[22,31] Selective and nonselective beta blockade did not limit maximal physical performance during short-term dynamic exercise in mildly hypertensive men.[32]

Recommendations for the heart rate range, that is, the intensity of exercise to be attained during training for patients receiving beta-blocking drugs, are based on the highest heart rate safely achieved at exercise testing. In prescribing exercise for patients receiving beta-blocking drugs, the exercise test from which the training heart rate range is determined should be performed while the patient receives the dose of the beta-blocking drug to be taken during training.[2]

The combined use of nitrate or other vasodilator agents and beta-blocking drugs for patients with angina negates some of the undesirable effects of each class of drugs (Table 1). For example, beta blockade may limit the nitrate-induced reflex tachycardia and increased myocardial contractility, whereas nitrate or other vasodilator preparations may limit the increases in ventricular volume, filling pressure, and end-diastolic pressure caused by beta blockade.

Calcium Entry Blocking Drugs

These relatively new compounds available for clinical use in the United States act as potent coronary and peripheral vasodilators, with variable negative inotropic effects and electrophysiologic properties (Table 2). The drugs currently available (1983) are verapamil, nifedipine, and diltiazem. Although these drugs are believed to act by selectively blocking the calcium-dependent excitation-concentration coupling process in the myocardium and in vascular smooth muscle, as well as by inhibiting calcium entry into the cardiac conduction system cells, it remains uncertain whether all the pharmacologic effects of these drugs with heterogeneous clinical structures are related entirely to inhibition of calcium entry via the so-called slow channel.[33,34] Because of the effect of these drugs on the myocardium and on conduction tissue, their variable negative inotropic properties and impairment of atrioventricular conduction are not unexpected. The predominant antianginal effect of calcium entry blocking drugs is related to the vasodilator-mediated decrease in myocardial oxygen demand, although they may increase oxygen supply to the myocardium (increased coronary flow) as well. Reduction of afterload, with the resultant decrease in cardiac work, is probably the most important antianginal effect of calcium antagonist drugs. Beneficial effects of exercise training can be documented in patients receiving calcium entry blocking drugs during their training.[35]

Verapamil, a potent peripheral and coronary vasodilator, improves exercise tolerance and decreases nitroglycerin usage. It results in the most pronounced depression of atrioventricular conduction and myocardial contractility, mandating that concomitant administration with beta-blocking drugs be undertaken with great caution. Although verapamil increases serum levels of digitalis and decreases the renal clearance of digitalis, major digitalis toxicity is unusual with concomitant therapy.

Table 2. Effects of calcium channel blocking drugs

	Verapamil	Nifedipine	Diltiazem
Peripheral (systemic) vasodilation	+	+ +	+
Coronary vasodilation	+ +	+ + +	+ + +
↓ AV conduction	+ +	±	+
↓ Myocardial contractility	+ +	±	+
Side effects	+ +	+ + +	+
↑ Heart rate	±	+	−

Nifedipine is a potent long-acting vasodilator with little antiarrhythmic and atrioventricular conduction depressant effects; there is no major depression of myocardial contractility because of the unloading effect. It thus may be used in combination with beta blockade therapy without deleterious consequence and even to advantage.[36] Propranolol may limit nifedipine-induced tachycardia. Coronary vasodilatation and an increase in coronary blood flow have been described with nifedipine administration. Although nifedipine typically increases exercise capacity, on occasion excessive tachycardia or excessive hypotension or both may paradoxically worsen the angina and limit activity in patients receiving the drug. Because it is a potent long-acting vasodilator, nifedipine may cause prominent ankle edema; this may be pronounced enough to require discontinuation of therapy. The inappropriate addition of diuretic drugs for this problem may cause hypovolemia with resultant lightheadedness or syncope, particularly when the patient exercises. Nevertheless, exercise conditioning has been documented in subjects receiving nifedipine.[35]

Diltiazem increases exercise duration; this results, at least in part, from a drug-related decrease in the rate-pressure product,[37] although some studies suggest that the increase in coronary blood flow may also be contributory. There is little reflex tachycardia, despite the significant vasodilatation; the explanation for the lack of tachycardia is not readily apparent. Diltiazem seems to have little significant negative inotropic effects on the myocardium, either at rest or with exercise; indeed, exercise performance appears to improve in patients with angina and left ventricular dysfunction treated with diltiazem. The effect on atrioventricular conduction is negligible.

Calcium blocking drugs are of particular value in patients with bronchospastic pulmonary disease and those with labile insulin-dependent diabetes in whom beta-blocking therapy is contraindicated; they may be important alternative therapy in patients who complain of fatigue from beta-blocking drugs.

ANTIARRHYTHMIC AGENTS

Although beta-blocking drugs used as antiarrhythmic agents may significantly alter the response to exercise, this effect is less marked with many other antiarrhythmic compounds.

Quinidine

In a group of 17 normal subjects,[38] quinidine increased the heart rate at rest and at low levels of exercise, owing both to the vagolytic effect of quinidine and the alpha-receptor blocking effect of the drug, with a reflex increase in sympathetic activity. However, quinidine effected no significant change in the systolic blood pressure response to any workload. The investigators cautioned that, because of the cardioacceleratory effects of quinidine, a heart rate-limited exercise test would entail a lesser workload compared with a test in which the subject was not receiving quinidine.

Procainamide and Disopyramide

Despite the anticholinergic properties of procainamide and disopyramide and the prominent negative inotropic effect of disopyramide, neither drug exerted significant effects on the heart rate or blood pressure response to treadmill exercise in 9 healthy volunteers.[39] It is not known whether exercise responses may differ in coronary patients receiving these antiarrhythmic drugs.

Other Antiarrhythmic Drugs

Exercise tolerance[40] did not change significantly after the administration of encainide, ethmozine, lorcainide, tocainide, or mexilitine; peak heart rate, peak blood pressure, exercise duration, and peak rate-pressure product remained comparable. The non-beta adrenergic blocking antiarrhythmic drug that appeared to alter myocardial oxygen demand, as reflected by exercise test parameters, was aprindine; aprindine significantly limited exercise performance as evidenced by a decrease in the peak heart rate and blood pressure and thus the peak rate pressure product.

ANTIHYPERTENSIVE DRUGS

A major exercise-related benefit of antihypertensive therapy is that drugs that control the blood pressure at rest in hypertensive patients also limit the excessive hypertensive response to exercise as well. An undue exercise-induced increase in peripheral vascular resistance may limit the capacity to exercise.

The clinician must also appreciate the potential exercise-related complications of antihypertensive therapy. Excessive diuresis with thiazides or other diuretic drugs may accentuate the exercise-induced tachycardia and the post-exercise hypotension and may even cause syncope. Because the cardiac output is maintained in the patient taking thiazide drugs, tachycardia does not occur unless the patient is hypovolemic. In the exercise testing laboratory, thiazide-induced hypokalemia may produce or accentuate electrocardiographic ST segment abnormalities, mimicking the change of myocardial ischemia.

The decrease in vasomotor tone secondary to adrenergic blocking antihypertensive drugs such as guanethidine allows dependent pooling of blood. Orthostatic hypotension may result from the abrupt decrease in cardiac output on standing.

CATECHOLAMINES

Although catecholamines are not generally routinely administered to patients with symptomatic atherosclerotic coronary heart disease, an increase in epinephrine and norepinephrine concentrations occurs from cigarette smoking. Because heart rate, blood pressure, and myocardial contractility are enhanced by catecholamine stimulation, cigarette smoking acutely decreases the ability to exercise and produces ST segment abnormalities on the exercise ECG at lower workloads than in the nonsmoking state; these changes were not eliminated by pretreatment with propranolol.[41] The decrease in oxygen transport related to elevated blood carboxyhemoglobin levels may also be contributory.[42]

DIGITALIS

Digitalis, administered to patients with heart failure, improves their ability to exercise and may increase myocardial perfusion as well.[43] The positive inotropic action of digitalis increases myocardial contractility and decreases both left ventricular filling pressure and pulmonary capillary pressure in the failing heart. The decrease in left ventricular diastolic volume lessens the myocardial oxygen demand; exercise tolerance is thereby improved.[44]

Although concern has been voiced about the increase in myocardial contractility, because digitalis increases myocardial oxygen demand in patients with symptomatic coronary disease and thereby worsens their angina, this modest increase in myocardial oxygen requirement is encountered only in the normal, nonfailing heart. In patients with heart failure, the decrease in myocardial oxygen demand related to the decrease in left ventricular diastolic volume predominates, improving exercise capacity.

Nevertheless, both in normal people[45] and in patients with a variety of cardiovascular diseases, digitalis (even in therapeutic doses and in the absence of hypokalemia) may alter the ST segment of the electrocardiogram or augment a baseline ST segment abnormality; this change is accentuated with exercise.[46] The mechanism of the ST segment alteration remains uncertain.

141

SUMMARY

The exercise test response and exercise capacity of patients with atherosclerotic coronary heart disease may be significantly altered by a number of commonly used cardiovascular drugs, alone or in combination, via complex interactions of hemodynamic and electrophysiologic changes. The clinician must assess the effects of pharmacotherapy when evaluating the results of exercise testing as well as when prescribing a rehabilitative exercise training regimen.

ACKNOWLEDGMENT

I appreciate the help of Jeanette Zahler and Julia Wright in the preparation and typing of the manuscript.

REFERENCES

1. SIMOONS, ML AND BALAKUMARAN, K: *The effects of drugs on the exercise electrocardiogram.* Cardiology 68 (Suppl 2):124, 1981.

2. HOSSACK, KF, BRUCE RA, AND CLARK LJ: *Influence of propranolol on exercise prescription of training heart rates.* Cardiology 65:47, 1980.

3. WENGER, NK, HELLERSTEIN, HK, BLACKBURN, H, ET AL: *Physician practice in the management of patients with uncomplicated myocardial infarction—Changes in the past decade.* Circulation 65:421, 1982.

4. NAUGHTON, J: *The National Exercise and Heart Disease Project: Development, recruitment, and implementation.* In WENGER, NK (ED): *Exercise and the Heart.* FA Davis, Philadelphia, 1978, p 205.

5. MARKIS, JE, GORLIN, R, MILLS, RM, ET AL: *Sustained effect of orally administered isosorbide dinitrate on exercise performance of patients with angina pectoris.* Am J Cardiol 43:265, 1979.

6. FLESSAS, AP AND RYAN, TJ: *Effects of nitroglycerin on isometric exercise.* Am Heart J 105:239, 1983.

7. GILES, TD, ITELD, BJ, QUIROZ, AC, ET AL: *The prolonged effect of pentaerythritol tetranitrate on exercise capacity in stable effort angina pectoris.* Chest 80:142, 1981.

8. GOLDSTEIN, RE AND EPSTEIN, SE: *Medical management of patients with angina pectoris.* Prog Cardiovasc Dis 14:360, 1972.

9. MOSKOWITZ, RM, KINNEY, EL, AND ZELIS, RF: *Hemodynamic and metabolic responses to upright exercise in patients with congestive heart failure,* Chest 76:640, 1979.

10. KATTUS, AA: *Treadmill exercise protocols to demonstrate effectiveness of nitrate drugs in relief of angina pectoris: Duration of action and degree of functional enhancement.* Cardiology 68 (Suppl 2):161, 1981.

11. LEIER, CV, HUSS, P, MAGORIEN, RD, ET AL: *Improved exercise capacity and differing arterial and venous tolerance during chronic isosorbide dinitrate therapy for congestive heart failure.* Circulation 67:817, 1983.

12. FRANCIOSA, JS, GOLDSMITH, SR, AND COHN, JN: *Contrasting immediate and long-term effects of isosorbide dinitrate on exercise capacity in congestive heart failure.* Am J Med 69:559, 1980.

13. RUBIN, SA, CHATTERJEE, K, AND PARMLEY, WW: *Metabolic assessment of exercise in chronic heart failure patients treated treated with short-term vasodilators.* Circulation 61:543, 1980.

14. AWAN, NA, MILLER, RR, DeMARIA, AN, ET AL: *Efficacy of ambulatory systemic vasodilator therapy with oral prazosin in chronic refractory heart failure.* Circulation 56:346, 1977.

15. GOLDSMITH, SR, FANCIOSA, JA, AND COHN, JN: *Contrasting acute and chronic effects of nitrates on exercise capacity in heart failure.* Am J Cardiol 43:404, 1979.

16. β-*Blocker Heart Attack Study Group: The β-Blocker Heart Attack Trial.* National Heart, Lung, and Blood Institute. JAMA 246:2073, 1981.

17. HJALMARSON, A, ELMFELDT, D. HERLITZ, J, ET AL: *Effect on mortality of metroprolol in acute myocardial infarction. A double-blind randomised trial.* Lancet, 2:823, 1981.

18. THE NORWEGIAN MULTICENTER STUDY GROUP: *Timolol-induced reduction in mortality and reinfarction in patients surviving acute myocardial infarction.* N Engl J Med 304:801, 1981.

19. THADANI, U AND PARKER, JO: *Propranolol in angina pectoris: Duration of improved exercise tolerance and circulatory effects after acute oral administration.* Am J Cardiol 44:118, 1979.

20. FLESSAS, AP AND RYAN, TJ: *Atropine-induced cardioacceleration in patients on chronic propranolol therapy: Comparison with the positive chronotropic effect of isometric exercise.* Am Heart J 105:230, 1983.

21. SKLAR, J, JOHNSTON. GD, OVERLIE, P, ET AL: *The effects of a cardioselective (metoprolol) and a nonselective (propranolol) beta-adrenergic blocker on the response to dynamic exercise in normal men.* Circulation 65:894, 1982.

22. EPSTEIN, SE, ROBINSON, BF, KAHLER, RL, ET AL: *Effects of beta-adrenergic blockade on the cardiac response to maximal and submaximal exercise in man.* J Clin Invest 44:1745, 1965.

23. SCHNEIDER, MS, KANAREK, DJ, AND NELSON, KM: *Positive training effects on anaerobic threshold during β-adrenergic blockade in cardiac rehabilitation.* Circulation 66 (Suppl II):186 , 1982.

24. BRUCE, RA, HOSSACK, KF, KUSUMI, F, ET AL: *Acute hemodynamic effects of propranolol during symptom-limited maximal exercise.* Am J Cardiol 44:132, 1979.

25. VANHEES. L, FAGARD, R, AND AMERY, A: *Influence of beta adrenergic blockade on effects of physical training in patients with ischaemic heart disease.* Br Heart J 48:33, 1982.

26. EWY, GA, WILMORE, JH, MORTON, AR, ET AL: *The effect of beta-adrenergic blockade on obtaining a trained exercise state.* J Cardiac Rehab 3:25, 1983.

27. GORDON, NF, KRUGER, PE, HONS, BA, ET AL: *Improved exercise ventilatory responses after training in coronary heart disease during long-term beta-adrenergic blockade.* Am J Cardiol 51:755, 1983.

28. PRATT, CM, WELTON, DE, SQUIRES, WG, JR, ET AL: *Demonstration of training effect during chronic beta-adrenergic blockade in patients with coronary artery disease.* Circulation 64: 1125, 1981.

29. FRISK-HOLMBERG, M, JORFELDT, L, AND JUHLIN-DANFELDT A: *Influence of alprenolol on hemodynamic and metabolic responses to prolonged exercise in subjects with hypertension.* Clin Pharmacol Ther 21:675, 1977.

30. HOSSACK, KF, BRUCE, RA, and KUSUMI, F: *Altered exercise ventilatory responses by apparent propranolol-diminished glucose metabolism: Implications concerning impaired physical training benefit in coronary patients.* Am Heart J 102:378, 1981.

31. FRANCIOSA, JA, JOHNSON, SM, AND TOBIAN, LJ: *Exercise performance in mildly hypertensive patients.* Chest 78:291, 1980.

32. LEENEN, FHH, COENEN, CHM, ZONDERLAND, M, ET AL : *Effects of cardioselective and nonselective β-blockade on dynamic exercise performance in mildly hypertensive men.* Clin Pharmacol Ther 28:12, 1980.

33. HENRY, PD: *Comparative pharmacology of calcium antagonists: Nifedipine, verapamil, and diltiazem.* Am J Cardiol 46:1047, 1980.

34. ZELIS, RF AND SCHROEDER, JS (EDS): *Calcium, calcium antagonists, and cardiovascular disease.* Chest 78 (Suppl):121, 1980.

35. DUFFEY, DJ, HORWITZ, LD, AND BRAMMELL, HL: *Nifedipine and the conditioning response.* Circulation 66 (Suppl II) :184, 1982.

36. DEPONTI, C, DEBIASE, AM, PIRELLI, S, ET AL: *Effects of nifedipine, acebutolol, and their association on exercise tolerance in patients with effort angina.* Cardiology 68 (Suppl 2):195, 1981.

37. POOL, PE, SEAGREN, SC, BONANNO, JA, ET AL: *The treatment of exercise-inducible chronic stable angina with diltiazem. Effect on treadmill exercise.* Chest 78:234, 1980.

38. FENSTER, PE, DAHL, C, MARCUS, FI, ET AL: *Effect of quinidine on the heart rate and blood pressure response to treadmill exercise.* Am Heart J 104:1244, 1982.

39. FENSTER, PE, COMESS, KA, AND HANSON, CD: *Effect of antidysrhythmic drugs on the heart rate and blood pressure response to treadmill exercise.* Cardiology 69:366, 1982.

40. LAMPERT, S AND LOWN, B: *Drug effects on the hemodynamic response to exercise.* Circulation 66 (Suppl II):186, 1982.

41. DEANFIELD, J, JONATHAN, A, SELWYN, A, ET AL: *Treatment of angina pectoris with propranolol: The harmful effects of cigarette smoking.* Cardiology 68 (Suppl 2):186, 1981.

42. CRYER, PE HAYMOND, MW, SANTIAGO, JV, ET AL: *Smoking, catecholamines and coronary heart disease.* Cardiovasc Med 2:471, 1977.

43. VOGEL, R, KIRCH D, LEFREE, M, ET AL: *Effects of digitalis on resting and isometric exercise myocardial perfusion in patients with coronary artery disease and left ventricular dysfunction.* Circulation 56:355, 1977.

44. LEWINTER, MM, CRAWFORD, MH, O'ROURKE, RA, ET AL: *The effects of oral propranolol, digoxin and combination therapy on the resting and exercise electrocardiogram.* Am Heart J 93:202, 1977.

45. TONKON, MJ, LEE, G, DEMARIA, AN, ET AL *The effect of digitalis on the exercise electrocardiogram in normal adult subjects.* Chest 72:714, 1977.

46. DEGRE, S, LONGO B, THIRION, M, ET AL: *Analysis of exercise-induced R-wave-amplitude changes in detection of coronary artery disease in patients with typical or atypical chest pain under digitalis treatment.* Cardiology 68 (Suppl 2):178, 1981.

Exercise Regimens
After Myocardial Infarction:
Rationale And Results

Roy J. Shephard, M.D. (Lond.), Ph.D.

This chapter examines some of the mechanisms whereby an exercise-centered cardiac rehabilitation program might enhance prognosis after myocardial infarction, assesses their relative importance, and examines the overall response to exercise therapy as commonly administered. A more detailed bibliography can be found in a recent monograph.[1]

RATIONALE OF EXERCISE THERAPY

There is no way in whch an exercise rehabilitation program can effect the replacement of damaged myocardium in a patient who has sustained a myocardial infarction. However, a graded exercise prescription can maximize utilization of the individual's residual potential through (1) group influences associated with the exercise class, (2) an increase of daily energy expenditure, (3) the development of endurance training, and (4) renewed habituation to intensive effort.

Group Influences

Many of the benefits of an exercise-centered rehabilitation program can be traced to the group support found in an exercise class. Myocardial infarction commonly precipitates a severe reactive depression,[2] and in countering this problem, it is helpful for the patient to share the support and camaraderie of other class members who have conquered similar feelings. A regular exercise class allows the physician to establish a warm, human contact not only with the patient but also with the spouse. In this way, various practical challenges (such as life on a reduced income, shelved personal or business responsibilities, and any necessary adjustments of sexual behavior) can be faced jointly by husband and wife, in consultation with the medical team.[3] Attendance at a regular class allows much informal psychiatric therapy to be given by the staff of a rehabilitation center, and, where necessary, the patient can be referred for such specific modalities of treatment as hypnosis[4] and stress relaxation therapy.[5]

Advice on other health issues can be provided during class attendance. Continued cigarette smoking doubles the risk of a recurrence of infarction,[6] and exercise rehabilitation offers a chance of continued counselling. Some 35 percent of cardiac patients referred to the Toronto Rehabilitation Centre (TRC) are persistent smokers[6] (although many of this group have reduced their cigarette consumption in the 2 to 3 months following myocardial infarction). A longitudinal study[6] showed little change in the proportion of smokers over an average of three years of graded exercise rehabilitation; although superficially disappointing, this contrasts favorably with the recidivism usually encountered in a smoking withdrawal program. A small proportion of the TRC subjects have progressed to marathon distance running; and in keeping with other reports,[7] a very low percentage of this group are current smokers. All patients attending the Rehabilitation Centre can also be given information regularly on diet and drug therapy. There is an opportunity to discuss any unusual symptoms that have developed, and early warning is often obtained if there is an extension of the coronary vascular disease; this approach allows early referral for detailed clinical and laboratory examination, with the possibility of modifying drug dosage or instituting coronary bypass surgery if necessary.

Daily Energy Expenditure

A second obvious advantage of an exercise-centered rehabilitation program is that daily energy expenditure can be increased substantially. If a matching increase of food intake can be avoided, the augmented energy usage will inevitably help to counter the usual middle-aged accumulation of body fat. Inasmuch as the energy cost of many tasks is almost directly proportional to body mass,[8] the loss of fat reduces the work that must be undertaken by the damaged myocardium. A negative energy balance provides a natural mechanism for the correction of hypertension if present,[1] reduces serum cholesterol level,[9] and diminishes insulin requirements in patients with maturity-onset diabetes.[10,11]

In practice (Table 1), the average member of a post-coronary exercise class loses relatively little body fat over a year of observation.[12] Again, this is disappointing to the conscientious physician. However, the patients concerned have often undergone stringent dieting while in the hospital, and maintenance of their improved physique may in itself be a significant achievement, particularly if there has been recent smoking withdrawal.

If the exercise class generates a sufficiently large energy expenditure, there may be an increase of HDL cholesterol (Table 2). The protective value of HDL cholesterol is problematic once myocardial infarction has occurred, but it seems likely that the plentiful presence of this scavenger molecule will at least avoid extension of the disease process. Unfortunately, the threshold activity needed to induce any appreciable increase of HDL cholesterol seems to be a weekly jogging distance of at least 20 km, and many patients require a substantial period of exercise rehabilitation before they can reach this threshold.[13]

Endurance Training

Many of the benefits of an exercise class are associated with the development of endurance training. This requires substantial (20 to 30 min) periods of exercise at > 60 percent of the individual's maximum oxygen intake, performed three to five times per week. Again, weeks

Table 1. Initial body composition of post-coronary patients and changes over one year of either vigorous or homeopathic exercise*

Variable	Vigorous Exercise		Homeopathic Exercise	
	Initial Value	Δ 1 yr	Initial Value	Δ 1 yr
Body mass (kg)	74.6	+0.1	75.6	+1.5
Average of 3 skinfold measurements (mm)	16.5	−1.0	16.2	+1.6
Estimated body fat (%)	27.3	−0.4	26.2	+1.2

*Based on data of Shephard, RJ, et al[12]

Table 2. Changes of lipid profile among post-coronary distance runners initially covering 68 km·wk⁻¹

Variable	Increased Distance Run		Decreased Distance Run	
	Initial Value	Δ 1 year	Initial Value	Δ 1 year
Body mass (kg)	69.4	+1.2	70.0	+1.1
Plasma cholesterol (mg·dl⁻¹)	205.2	−5.2	207.0	−10.9
HDL cholesterol (mg·dl⁻¹)	46.3	+5.6	59.9	−4.9
LDL cholesterol (mg·dl⁻¹)	139.1	−9.8	124.6	−5.2
HDL/LDL (%)	37.9	+4.2	51.4	−3.1
Plasma triglycerides (mg·dl⁻¹)	101.8	−2.5	112.5	−8.4

*Based on data of Kavanagh, T and Shephard, RJ[13] for (a) 11 patients who increased running distance by 15 km·wk⁻¹ and (b) 10 patients who decreased running distance by 23 km·wk⁻¹ over a one-year period.

or even months of more gentle preliminary conditioning are advisable for a severely disabled patient[1] (Fig. 1).

The immediate response of the cardiac patient to endurance training is a decrease of the heart rate induced by a given work rate. As the peripheral muscles become strengthened, there may also be a lesser rise of systemic blood pressure for a given power-output. Both of these changes reduce the myocardial workload, as gauged by the rate-pressure product. There is also a training-induced increase of maximal arteriovenous oxygen difference.[14–16] Some authors once attributed the latter to an increase of skeletal muscle enzyme concentrations, but most investigators now agree that muscle enzyme concentrations are not the rate-limiting factor during aerobic exercise. An alternative and more reasonable explanation is that the

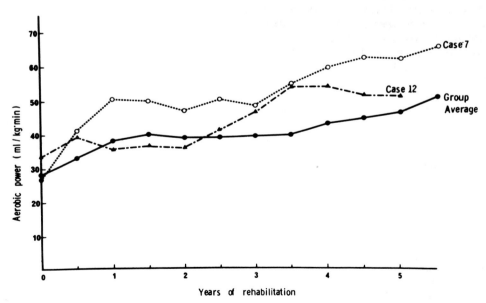

Figure 1. Illustrated time course of increase in maximum oxygen intake. (From Shephard, RJ: Cardiac rehabilitation in prospect. In Pollock, ML and Schmidt, DH (eds): *Heart Disease and Rehabilitation.* Houghton Mifflin, Boston, 1979, with permission.)

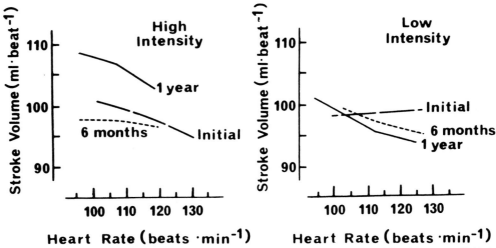

Figure 2. Influence of prolonged endurance training on the stroke volume of patients following myocardial infarction. (Based on data of Paterson, DH et al,[14] presented in Shephard, RJ: *Ischaemic Heart Disease and Exercise.* Croom Helm, 1981, with permission.)

strengthened muscles are more readily perfused while they develop a substantial force;[17] certainly, peripheral oxygen extraction cannot occur unless the heart is able to pump blood through the working muscles.

A number of investigators have concluded that training does not increase the stroke volume of the coronary patient.[18,19] There may be some truth to this paradox in cases in which a large sector of the normal myocardium has been replaced by functionless scar tissue, but it is also worthy of comment that many longitudinal studies of changes in stroke volume have been limited to quite short periods of exercise rehabilitation. If observations are continued for as long as one year, the average exercise class member shows a significant gain of stroke volume (Fig. 2).[14,15] Some of the post-coronary marathon runners studied by Kavanagh and coworkers[20] increased their maximum oxygen intake from 25 to 30 ml·kg^{-1} min^{-1} to more than 60 ml·kg^{-1}min^{-1}; it is inconceivable that a change in oxygen transport of this magnitude could have come about in the absence of a substantial increase in maximal stroke volume. An increase of stroke volume further reduces the heart rate, and thus, the myocardial work rate needed to sustain any given external power output.

Other possible beneficial effects of endurance training include an increase of red cell mass (not an obvious response in most post-coronary programs) and hormonal responses aimed at a greater mobilization and utilization of body fat during exercise (an increased output of growth hormone and thyroid hormone; neither change is particularly likely with the intensity and duration of activity attained by the average post-coronary program).

Intense Exercise

In general, post-coronary programs have avoided intense exercise, and indeed many physicians have prescribed an essentially homeopathic regimen. Nevertheless, it is increasingly recognized that with appropriate supervision most patients referred to rehabilitation programs can progress quite safely to brief bouts of maximum aerobic exercise,[21] and a fair number can train to the level needed for completion of a marathon run.[20]

The main justification for suggesting a patient should engage in vigorous exercise is that sooner or later some emergency will demand an equivalent expenditure of energy by the individual. If such exercise is unaccustomed and is accompanied by the emotional stress of the emergency itself, there is a real risk that myocardial infarction may recur. However, participation in regular bouts of intensive exercise habituates the subject to vigorous effort[22] while moving what was previously a maximal or supramaximal task within the submaximal range. It is also likely that the regular experience of intense physical activity diminishes the catecholamine response to such effort.[23,24] The acute effect of hard work upon the coagulability of the blood is an enhancement of clotting, but the more long-term reaction to the same stimulus is an increase of fibrinolysis.[25]

There has been much discussion as to the extent that intensive training can stimulate the development of coronary collateral vessels, thus enhancing oxygen delivery to the myocardium. In general, the conclusion seems to be that the vigor of training possible in a post-coronary patient is insufficient to stimulate the growth of collateral vessels.[26-30] Nevertheless, training does reduce the liability to anginal pain at any given intensity of effort.[31] Among the suggested mechanisms of benefit, we may note (1) a placebo-mediated increment of pain threshold,[24,32,33] (2) a reduction of the cardiac work-rate at any given external power output (owing to decreases of heart rate,[35,36] blood pressure,[37] and end-diastolic dimensions[38]), (3) an increase of coronary blood flow associated with a longer diastolic period, (4) a redistribution of coronary blood flow from superficial to deeper parts of the myocardial wall as intramural tension falls,[39] and (5) increases of myocardial oxygen extraction (associated with an increase of hemoglobin level, a shift of the oxygen dissociation curve, and possibly some augmentation of myocardial enzyme activity[40,41]).

Training also increases myocardial contractility. In an isolated muscle preparation such a change would augment myocardial oxygen consumption, thus worsening the situation of the individual with rigid, sclerosed vessels. In vivo, the potential increase of oxygen usage due to a speeding of myocardial contraction is offset by other factors, including a reduction of ventricular size and a decreased output of catecholamines at any given external power output. Thus, when patients with angina pectoris have been investigated before and after participation in an exercise-centered rehabilitation program, the changes in ventricular function have been minimal.[42,43]

SPECIFIC PROBLEMS OF THE PATIENT WITH SEVERE ANGINA

In patients with severe angina, due account must be taken of the possibility that the acute myocardial hypoxemia induced by vigorous physical activity will provoke left ventricular failure. A high proportion of fatalities in post-coronary rehabilitation programs occurs among patients with angina and/or deep ST segment depression.[44] Moreover, such patients seem particularly vulnerable to death during periods of physical activity (Table 3).

There is less evidence (Table 4) that the overall prognosis of the patient with angina pectoris is worsened by an increase in daily physical activity.[6] Nevertheless, it is important to recognize that, when first seen, many patients with angina have a stiff ventricular wall with poor myocardial contractility.[26,45]

Thus, if activity is pursued too vigorously in the presence of anginal pain, a vicious cycle of diminishing stroke volume, increasing end-diastolic volume, increased tension work, and left ventricular failure may develop.[46,47]

Beta adrenergic blocking drugs are frequently administered to post-coronary patients, particularly if there is a tendency to anginal pain or cardiac dysrhythmia. These agents reduce both the positive inotropic response (increase of contractility) and the chronotropic response (increase of heart rate) during exercise. Beta blockers may also exert a negative inotropic effect in their own right.[48] The end result is usually a reduction of myocardial oxygen consumption for a given external power output, with a curtailing of both PVCs and anginal pain. However, if dysfunction of the ventricular wall is so extensive that the patient is already close

Table 3. Risk factors in patients sustaining recurrence of myocardial infarction during physical activity compared with risk factors in those sustaining reinfarction at other times*

| | Frequency of Occurrence | | |
| | Recurrence During Exercise | Recurrence at Other Times | |
Risk Factor	%	%	P
Exercise non-compliance	61.6	37.6	0.2 > P > 0.1
Current smoking	60.0	64.5	n.s.
Angina	60.0	58.1	n.s.
Systemic hypertension	0	11.1	n.s.
Serum cholesterol > 270 mg·dl^{-1}	0	9.1	n.s.
Persistent resting ECG abnormalities	83.3	53.3	0.2 > P > 0.1
Exercise ST segment depression > 0.2 mV	50.0	22.6	0.1 > P > 0.05
Premature ventricular contractions	0	4.9	n.s.

*Based on data from Southern Ontario Multicentre Exercise-Heart Trial[44]

to cardiac failure, a combination of exercise and beta-blocking drugs may precipitate the vicious cycle of increasing end-diastolic volume, augmented cardiac work, and left ventricular failure discussed above.[49] In such individuals, exercise tolerance may be helped by administration of digitalis, the direct energy cost of an increase in myocardial contractility being more than offset by a decrease in heart size and wall stress.[50]

Several recent reports have examined the modifications of exercise and training responses in patients who are treated with beta-blocking agents.[51,52] Low exercise heart rates cause some difficulty in regulating the exercise prescription, but there is general agreement that the increase of maximum oxygen intake and other benefits associated with endurance training proceed unimpaired. This finding is not surprising because patients who are being treated

Table 4. A comparison of simple risk ratios for active and sedentary patients following myocardial infarction*

| | Simple Risk Ratio† | |
Risk Factor	Active Patients	Sedentary Patients*
Current smoking	1.30	2.00
Angina	1.93	1.93
Systemic hypertension	0.98	2.55
Serum cholesterol > 270 mg·dl^{-1}	1.98	1.49
		0.80
		1.09
Persistent resting ECG abnormalities	1.02	2.47
Exercise ST segment depression > 0.2 mV	1.82	1.23
Multifocal PVCs	1.53	1.61
Enlarged heart	2.40	2.32
Ventricular aneurysm	2.05	1.80

*See Kavanagh et al[6] for references.
†Ratio of incidence in group with risk factor to incidence in group without risk factor.

with beta-blocking agents must meet the blood flow demands of exercise by a larger increase of cardiac stroke volume than would be encountered in an individual who was not receiving such treatment.

RESPONSE TO EXERCISE THERAPY

Choice of End-Point

The majority of clinical trials to date have sought answers to the question: Will progressive exercise rehabilitation diminish the chances that the post-coronary patient will suffer a fatal or a nonfatal recurrence of myocardial infarction? This has reflected in part a traditional concern with vital statistics and in part a commendable desire to ensure that the end-points used in any trial are relatively clear-cut and unequivocal events. The latter point has particular importance when evaluating exercise-centered rehabilitation programs, inasmuch as exercise cannot be administered in a double-blind fashion.

Unfortunately, the answers possible from this type of clinical trial have only limited practical value.[53] The average entrant in a post-coronary rehabilitation program has an age of about 45 years. The infarction is generally mild and even in the absence of prescribed exercise mortality (1.5 to 3.0 percent per annum [54-56]) is only a little above the expected figure for a person of this age (Table 5). Considerations of trial organization, expense, and sample attrition have held experiments to a length of 1 to 3 years, with the expectation that mortality might be halved over this period. Given a 1.5 percent mortality among control subjects, a halving of mortality would require a *total* reversal of the effects of infarction (Table 5). If this somewhat unrealistic goal could be realized for each of two years, then an additional 1.5 percent of patients would enjoy their expected longevity of 30 years. The average increase of life span would be 1.5/100 × 30, or half a year. The saving to society is usually reckoned as the added value of 20 years additional work, assumed to be some 25 percent of the individual's net earnings for the same period. Given a working year of 220 days, the gain of productivity from the reduction of mortality is thus about 110 × $\frac{20}{30}$ × $\frac{25}{100}$ or 18 person-days of work per patient. The impact of any change in nonfatal recurrence rates is even less exciting. Let us suppose that nonfatal recurrences of 3 percent per year are halved. Over two years, 3 percent of the sample thus escapes a nonfatal recurrence that would have caused an average of 3 months incapacity. The consumption of goods and services remains approximately the same whether the patient is working or not, so that society is spared an expense of 220 × $\frac{3}{12}$ × $\frac{3}{100}$,

Table 5. Mortality of older adults in the absence of myocardial infarction*

Age (Years)	Mortality (Deaths per 1000)
45–49	5.7
50–54	9.3
55–59	14.6
60–64	22.9
65–69	34.7
70–74	51.9
75–79	79.0
80–84	118.8
85+	198.5

*Based on data of Statistics Canada for 1971

or 1.7 person-days of work per patient.* The two-year impact of a 50 percent reduction in both fatal and nonfatal infarctions is therefore less than 20 person-days of work per patient, not greatly different from the normal amount of industrial absenteeism for a two-year period. Moreover, equal benefit could have been obtained by any treatment shortening by 4 weeks the average period of absence from work following the initial infarction.

Plainly, the average patient is more interested in the happiness of his or her remaining years than in a 1.5 percent increase in longevity. Equally, the physician is making a greater contribution to society by promoting an early return to work than by ensuring an 18 to 20 day reduction of long-term mortality.

Clearly, if it could be established that exercise halved mortality throughout the remaining 30-year life span, the proposed program would have a much greater importance for both the individual and society. However, practical constraints of expense and sample attrition would appear to preclude any formal testing of this hypothesis.

Fatal and Nonfatal Recurrence

The world literature now contains details of several randomized controlled trials, each of which has sought to test the value of exercise-centered rehabilitation in reducing the recurrence of fatal and nonfatal infarctions.[54-56] However, differences in statististics for treated and control patients have generally been insignificant.

Some authors have rashly concluded from such data that there was no exercise effect. In fact, the limitation lies not in the therapy itself but in its experimental evaluation. Most published trials have shown a substantial (approximately 30 percent) advantage of survival to the exercised group; among reasons why this finding is statistically insignificant,[57] I may note:

(1) A substantially lower mortality in the control population than the figure anticipated by the trial organizers (this may reflect the referral of low-risk patients to rehabilitation centers, general improvements in therapy, a contamination of the control sample by an interest in physical activity, and the general phenomenon that volunteers for any clinical trial are health-conscious individuals with a lower than expected mortality).

(2) Recruitment of an insufficient sample (the necessary sample size to ensure a 90 percent probability of detecting a 50 percent reduction in mortality over a 3-year trial is in the range 1500 to 5000, compared with actual samples of 100 to 750 patients who were followed for 1 to 3 years).

(3) Frequent defections from the exercise program (for example, the Southern Ontario Multicentre Exercise-Heart Trial initially anticipated 25 percent sample attrition over a 4-year trial, but in practice losses were as large as 10 percent of the residual sample for each 6 months of observation—a final loss of about 60 percent).

(4) Delays in the appearance of an exercise response (because the patient and the supervising physician are at first hesitant about undertaking vigorous exercise, and time is needed for healing of the infarction, an increase of cardiac stroke volume is a relatively late response to training. Gains of oxygen transport develop slowly over 1 to 4 years of exercise therapy, and many patients show no training response if the trial lasts only 1 to 2 years).

(5) Contamination of the supposed control group with an interest in exercise.

Individual exercise trials have differed substantially in protocol, including criteria for diagnosis and acceptance into the trial, the entry period after infarction, and the pattern and

---

*This calculation ignores direct costs for medical and hospital services; although the patient *could* have incurred substantial charges for intensive care, other recent cost/effectiveness analyses indicate that recovery following a mild infarction is enhanced if the intensive care unit is avoided.

Table 6. The impact of exercise-centered rehabilitation upon the recurrence of fatal myocardial infarction as assessed by the pooling of results from several randomized control trials*

Period of Observation (Years)	Cumulative Survival		Significance of Difference in Survival for Interval (P)
	Exercise Group	Control Group	
0–1	0.956	0.932	0.031
1–1½	0.939	0.919	0.079
1½–2	0.933	0.897	0.011
2–3	0.911	0.875	0.024
3–4	0.879	0.840	0.075

*Based upon an analysis of Shephard[58]

intensity of the required training. Nevertheless, if results from several of the trials are combined,[58] a statistically significant benefit of exercise therapy becomes apparent (Table 6).

Evidence concerning the more long-term effects of exercise therapy rests upon a quasi-experimental approach,[59] inferences being drawn from (1) intrasample comparisons, and (2) comparisons with matched control populations.

Data obtained at the Toronto Rehabilitation Centre now include up to 12 years of exercise-centered therapy.[59,60] During the first year of observation, the recurrence rate is relatively low (3.11 percent yearly), implying *either* referral of a relatively low-risk group or some immediate benefit from the program. More interesting, recurrences drop to 2.58 percent in year 2, 1.50 percent in years 3 to 5, and 0.81 percent (all fatal) in years 6 to 8, in contrast with normal post-coronary experience, in which both recurrences and mortality remain relatively constant from one year to the next. Moreover, the benefit is closely linked to sustained exercise participation[61] in both low- and high-risk patients (Table 7).

Anticipated mortality was synthesized for the Toronto Rehabilitation Centre patients, based upon risk ratios determined in a New York Health Insurance Plan study of patients with ischemic heart disease.[59] A total of 63.5 deaths was predicted for a 3-year interval (3.42 percent yearly), compared with an observed total of 35 deaths (1.88 percent yearly); this difference was statistically significant.

Table 7. Impact of exercise-centered rehabilitation upon odds-ratio* for recurrence of myocardial infarction†

	Odds Ratio	
	Risk Factor Present	Risk Factor Absent
Smoking	7.87	3.34
Angina	5.87	4.91
ST segment depression	4.12	7.48
Enlarged heart	16.00	5.00

*Odds ratio = (Number of recurrences in noncompliant group/number without recurrences in noncompliant group) × (number without recurrences in compliant group/number of recurrences in compliant group).

†Data from Toronto Rehabilitation Centre, grouped in terms of several major risk factors

Soft End-Point Responses

Soft end-point measures of benefit following myocardial infarction include the period of absence from work, the proportion of subjects making a successful return to full-time employment with or without modification of the nature of work, the ability to engage in normal sexual activity, symptom scores, and the usage of drugs to control anginal pain or abnormal cardiac rhythms.[62-64] Regarding each of these criteria, patients enrolled in an exercise-centered rehabilitation program show benefit relative to patients not receiving such treatment. It is less clear how much of the observed benefit is causally related to the enhanced physical activity and how much is due rather to a group therapy effect that includes (1) counselling of patient and spouse with respect to smoking, diet, attitudes to work, and other aspects of lifestyle, (2) mutual support from other patients with similar problems, and (3) early detection, evaluation, and treatment of any complications.

Mood Changes

Many patients remain unimpressed by either hard or soft end-points. They comment that the main reason they exercise is in order to feel better.

Certainly, a substantial proportion of patients are very anxious and develop a severe reactive depression in the period immediately following their infarction.[65-67] There is furthermore some evidence that recovery from depression is linked to exercise participation (Table 8).[2] Nevertheless, certain tests of mood state such as Taylor's Manifest Anxiety Scale[68] and the Profile of Mood States[69] show remarkably little change over one to two years of exercise therapy. It remains unclear how much this reflects a lack of sensitivity of the psychologic test instrument, and how much the patient has an inherent abnormality of mood-state that remains uncorrected by the exercise program.

Contraindications to Exercise

Contraindications to exercise in the post-coronary patient are surprisingly few. One simple method of identifying patients who need a modified training regimen is to calculate the risk of a recurrence for various complications,[6] relating the risk-ratio to that reported for subjects not enrolled in an exercise program (see Table 4). Two groups stand out as having an adverse prognosis—those with deep exercise-induced ST segment depression, and those with incipient left ventricular failure, as indicated by aneurysmal bulging or treatment by digitalis and/or diuretics.

As noted previously, exercise can provoke both left ventricular failure and death in the first category of patients if severe myocardial ischemia develops. The risk ratio relative to patients

Table 8. The association between compliance with exercise-centered rehabilitation and relief of MMPI depression (raw score) in patients with a history of myocardial infarction*

	Compliant Subjects	Non-compliant Subjects
Initial depression score (16–18 months postinfarction)	29.2 ± 3.6	27.1 ± 4.5
Final depression score (4 years later)	25.3 ± 5.5	27.1 ± 2.3
Change of score	−4.0 ± 6.4	0.0 ± 4.0

*Based upon data of Kavanagh et al[2]

without persistent ST segment abnormalities is somewhat greater in exercised than in control subjects; but because exercise has a substantial impact upon recurrence rates in the uncomplicated patient, the patient with angina is still well advised to undertake a program of modified interval training. If there is continuing ischemic pain, coronary angiography may also be required with a view to possible surgical treatment.

If there is evidence of left ventricular failure, stabilization of the patient is a necessary prelude to an exercise program. Drug therapy should be evaluated critically to see how much this contributes to myocardial dysfunction, and scintigraphy and/or echocardiography can be used to assess both regional and overall ventricular performance. If there is a large ventricular aneurysm, surgical treatment may be required. However, if the main basis of ventricular failure is myocardial ischemia, it seems likely that the condition can be improved by cautious yet progressive exercise.

CONCLUSION

There are sound physiologic reasons why exercise should help the patient who has sustained a myocardial infarction. In terms of fatal and nonfatal recurrence, activity must be sustained for many years to generate significant benefits to the patient or to society, and it is difficult to offer convincing experimental proof of benefit over such a long period. However, exercise also yields important short-term gains of mood and adjustment to life, and many patients find such dividends the main justification for their participation in an exercise-centered rehabilitation program.

REFERENCES

1. SHEPHARD, RJ: *Ischemic Heart Disease and Physical Activity.* Year Book, Chicago Medical Publishers, 1982.
2. KAVANAGH, T, SHEPHARD, RJ, TUCK, JA, ET AL: *Depression Following myocardial infarction: The effects of distance running.* Ann NY Acad Sci 301:1029, 1977.
3. SHEPHARD, RJ AND KAVANAGH, T: *Patient reactions to a regular conditioning programme following myocardial infarction.* J Sports Med Phys Fitness 18:373, 1978.
4 KAVANAGH, T, SHEPHARD, RJ, AND DONEY, H: *Hypnosis and exercise—A possible combined therapy following myocardial infarction.* Am J Clin Hypnosis 16:160, 1974.
5. JACOBSEN, E: *Progressive Relaxation.* University of Chicago Press, Chicago, 1938.
6. KAVANAGH, T, SHEPHARD, RJ, CHISHOLM, AW, ET AL: *Prognostic indexes for patients with ischemic heart disease enrolled in an exercise-centered rehabilitation program.* Am J Cardiol 44:1230, 1979.
7. MORGAN, R, GILDINER, M, AND WRIGHT, GR: *Smoking reduction in adults who take up exercise: A survey of a running club for adults.* CAHPER Journal 42:39, 1976.
8. GODIN, G AND SHEPHARD, RJ: *Body weight and the energy cost of activity.* Arch Environ Health 27:289, 1973.
9. GOODE, RC, FIRSTBROOK, JB, AND SHEPHARD, RJ: *Effects of exercise and a cholesterol free diet on human serum lipids.* Canad J Physiol Pharm 44:575, 1966.
10. DEVLIN, J: *The effect of training and acute physical exercise on plasma insulin-like activity.* Irish J Med Sci 6:423, 1963.
11. GRODSKY, GM AND BENOIL, F: *Effect of massive weight-reduction on insulin secretion in obese subjects.* International Diabetes Symposium, Stockholm, 1967.
12. SEPHARD, RJ, COX, M AND KAVANAGH, T: *Post-coronary rehabilitation and risk factors, with special reference to diet.* Canad J Appl Sports Sci 5:250, 1980.
13. KAVANAGH, T AND SHEPHARD, RJ: *Influence of exercise and lifestyle variables upon HDL cholesterol following myocardial infarction.* Atherosclerosis (in press), 1983.
14. PATERSON, DH, SHEPHARD, RJ, CUNNINGHAM, D, ET AL: *Effects of physical training upon cardiovascular function following myocardial infarction.* J Appl Physiol 47:482, 1979.
15. EHSANI, AA. MARTIN, WH, HEATH, GW, ET AL: *Cardiac effects of prolonged and intensive exercise training in patients with coronary artery disease.* Am J Cardiol 50:246, 1982.
16. DETRY, JR, ROUSSEAU, M, VANDENBRONCHE, G, ET AL: *Increased arteriovenous oxygen difference after physical training in coronary heart disease.* Circulation 44:109, 1971.

17. KAY, C AND SHEPHARD, RJ: *On muscle strength and the threshold of anaerobic work.* Int Z Angew Physiol 27:311, 1969.

18. SIM, DN AND NEIL, WA: *Investigation of the physiological basis for increased exercise threshold for angina pectoris after physical conditioning.* J Clin Invest 54:763, 1974.

19. LETAC, B, CRIBIER, A, AND DESPLANCHES, JF: *A study of left ventricular function in coronary patients before and after physical training.* Circulation 56:375, 1977.

20. KAVANAGH, T, SHEPHARD, RJ, AND KENNEDY, J: *Characteristics of post-coronary marathon runners.* Ann NY Acad Sci 301:656, 1977.

21. KAVANAGH, T AND SHEPHARD, RJ: *Maximum exercise tests on 'post-coronary' patients.* J Appl Physiol 40:611, 1976.

22. SHEPHARD. RJ: *Learning, habituation and training.* Int Z Angew Physiol 26:272, 1969.

23. BLOOM, SR, JOHNSON, RH, PARK, DM, ET AL: *Differences in the metabolic and hormonal response to exercise between racing cyclists and untrained individuals.* J Physiol 258:1, 1976.

24. WINDER, WW, HAGBERG, JM, HICKSON, RC, ET AL: *Time course of sympatho-adrenal adaptation to endurance exercise training in men.* J Appl Physiol 45:370, 1978.

25. ÅSTRUP, P: *The effects of physical activity on blood coagulation and fibrinolysis.* In NAUGHTON, JP, HELLERSTEIN, HK, and MOHLER, IC (EDS): *Exercise Testing and Exercise Training in Coronary Heart Disease.* Academic Press, New York, 1973, pp 169–192.

26. ELLERSTAD, MH: *Stress Testing: Principles and Practice.* FA Davis, Philadelphia, 1975.

27. WENGER, NK: *Does exercise training enhance collateral circulation?* In KELLERMAN, J AND DENOLIN, H (EDS): *Critical Evaluation of Cardiac Rehabilitation.* Karger, Basel, 1977, pp 143–145.

28. FERGUSON, RJ, PETITCLERC, CHOQUETTE, G, ET AL: *Effect of physical training on treadmill exercise capacity, collateral circulation and progression of coronary disease.* Am J Cardiol 34:764, 1974.

29. KATTUS, A AND GROLLMANN, J: *Patterns of coronary collateral circulation in angina pectoris: Relation to exercise training.* In RUSSEK, HI AND ZOHMAN, BL (EDS): *Changing Concepts in Cardiovascular Disease.* Williams & Wilkins, Baltimore, 1972.

30. BARMEYER, J: *Physical activity and coronary collateral development.* Adv Cardiol 18:104, 1976.

31. SHEPHARD, RJ: *Rationale for physical training in angina pectoris.* World Congress of Cardiac Rehabilitation, Jerusalem, 1981.

32. BERGMAN, H AND VARNAUSKAS, E: *Placebo effect in physical training of coronary heart disease.* In LARSEN, OA AND MALMBORG, RO: *Coronary Heart Disease and Physical Fitness.* Munksgaard, Copenhagen, 1971.

33. ZOHMAN, LR AND TOBIS, JS: *The effect of exercise training on patients with angina pectoris.* Phys Med 48:525, 1967.

34. KELLERMANN, JJ, BEN-ARI, E, CHAYET, M, ET AL: *Cardiocirculatory response to different types of training in patients with angina pectoris.* Cardiology 62:218, 1977.

35. SIM, DN AND NEIL, WA: *Investigation of the physiological basis for increased exercise threshold for angina pectoris after physical conditioning.* J Clin Invest 54:763, 1974.

36. KENNEDY, CK, SIEKERMAN, RE, LINDSAY, MI, ET AL : *One-year graduated exercise program for men with angina pectoris. Evaluation by physiological studies and coronary arteriography.* Mayo Clin Proc 51:231, 1976.

37 DRESSENDORFER, RH, AMSTERDAM, EA, AND MASON, DT: *Therapeutic effects of exercise training in angina patients.* In COHEN, LS, MOCK, MB, AND RINGQVIST, I (EDS): *Physical Conditioning and Cardiovascular Rehabilitation.* John Wiley & Sons, New York, 1981, pp 121–138.

38. MIRSKY, I, GHISTA, EN, AND SANDLER, H: *Cardiac Mechanics: Physiological, Clinical and Mathematical Considerations.* Wiley/Interscience, New York, 1974.

39. McGREGOR, M: *Coronary steal: A review.* In ROSKAMM, H AND REINDELL, W (EDS): *Das chronische Kranke Herz.* Schattauer, Stuttgart, 1973, p 69.

40. VARNAUSKAS, E AND HOLMBERG, S: *Myocardial blood flow during exercise in patients with coronary heart disease. Comments on training effects.* In LARSEN, OA AND MALMBORG, RO (EDS): *Coronary Heart Disease and Physical Fitness.* University Park Press, Baltimore, 1971, pp 102–104.

41. BARNARD, RJ: *Long-term effects of exercise on cardiac function.* Exercise Sports Sci Rev 3:113, 1975.

42. DETRY, JM, ROUSSEAU, RL, VANDENBROUCKE, M, ET AL: *Increased arteriovenous oxygen difference after physical training in coronary disease.* Circulation 44:109, 1971.

43. BATTLER, A, FROELICHER, V, SLUTSKY, R, ET AL: *Initial observations of changes in ventricular function after exercise in coronary disease patients.* Circulation 59 and 60 (Suppl II): 21, 1979.

44. SHEPHARD, RJ: *Recurrence of myocardial infarction in an exercising population.* Br Heart J 42:133, 1979.

45. FOGELMAN, M, ABBASI, AS, PEARCH, ML, ET AL: *Echocardiographic study of the abnormal motion of the posterior left ventricular wall during angina pectoris.* Circulation 46:905, 913, 1972.

46. PARKER, JO, DiGIORGI, S, AND WEST, RO: *A haemodynamic study of acute coronary insufficiency precipitated by exercise. With observations on the effects of nitroglycerin.* Am J Med 17:470, 1966.

47. MOIR, TW AND DEBRA, DW: *Effect of left ventricular hypertension, ischemia and vasoactive drugs on the myocardial distribution of coronary flow.* Circ Res 21:65, 1967.

48. EPSTEIN, SE, AND BRAUNWALD, E: *Beta-adrenergic receptor blocking drugs.* N Engl J Med 275:1106, 1175, 1966.

49. ROBIN, E, COWAN, C, PURI, P, ET AL: *A comparative study of nitroglycerin and propranolol.* Circulation 36:175, 1967.

50. COVELL, JW, BRAUNWALD, E, ROSS, J, ET AL: *Studies on digitalis XVI. Effects on myocardial oxygen consumption.* J Clin Invest 45:1535, 1966.

51. SKLAR, J, JOHNSTON, GD, OVERLIE, P, ET AL: *The effects of a cardio-selective (metoprolol) and a non-selective (propranolol) beta adrenergic blocker on the response to dynamic exercise in normal men.* Circulation 65:894, 1982.

52. MORRISON, SC, ET AL: *Selective and non-selective beta-adrenoceptor blockade in hypertension: Responses to changes in position, cold and exercise.* Circulation 65:1171, 1982.

53. SHEPHARD, RJ: *Editorial—Are we asking the right questions?* J Cardiac Rehab 2:21, 1982.

54. WILHELMSEN, L, SANNE, H, ELMFELDT, D, ET AL: *A controlled trial of physical training after myocardial infarction. Effects on risk factors, non-fatal reinfarction.* Prev Med 4:491, 1975.

55. HAKKILA, J: *Morbidity and mortality after myocardial infarction.* In KELLERMAN, JJ AND DENOLIN, H (EDS): *Evaluation of Cardiac Rehabilitation.* Karger, Basel, 1977, pp 159–163.

56. SHAW, LW: *Effects of a prescribed supervised exercise program on mortality and cardiovascular morbidity in patients after a myocardial infarction. The national exercise and heart disease project.* Am J Cardiol 48:39, 1981.

57. SHEPHARD, RJ: *Evaluation of earlier studies: Canada.* In COHEN, LS, MOCK, MB, AND RINGQUIST, I (EDS): *Physical Conditioning and Cardiovascular Rehabilitation.* John Wiley & Sons, New York, 1981, pp 271–288.

58. SHEPHARD, RJ: *The value of exercise in ischaemic heart disease—A cumulative analysis.* J Cardiac Rehab 3:294, 1983.

59. SHEPHARD, RJ, KAVANAGH, T, KENNEDY, J, ET AL: *Prognosis in myocardial infarction—The benefits of exercise as seen in non-randomized trials.* J Sports Med 15:6, 1981.

60. KAVANAGH, T: *Twelve year follow-up experiences with an out-patient community-based exercise program in Toronto.* Proceedings II World Congress on Cardiac Rehabilitation, Jerusalem, December 1981.

61. SHEPHARD, RJ, COREY, P, AND KAVANAGH, T: *Compliance and the prevention of myocardial infarction.* Med Sci Sports 13:1, 1981.

62. HAYES, JR, GAU, GT, AND O'BRIEN, PC: *The effect of intensive cardiac rehabilitation on long term morbidity and mortality after myocardial infarction.* Proceedings II World Congress on Cardiac Rehabilitation, Jerusalem, December 1981.

63. BUCHWALSKY, R, KAUDERER, M, AND TANCZOS P: *Four years study of mortality, morbidity and social outcome in 530 MI patients in relation to left ventricular function.* Proceedings II World Congress on Cardiac Rehabilitation, Jerusalem, 1981.

64. CODY, DV, MAUMILL, D, DUNN, E, ET AL: *The effect of an integrated cardiac rehabilitation programme on return to work following myocardial infarction.* Proceedings II World Congress on Cardiac Rehabilitation, Jerusalem, 1981.

65. KAVANAGH, T, SHEPHARD, RJ, AND TUCK, JA: *Depression after myocardial infarction.* Canad MAJ 113:23, 1975.

66. RUSKIN, HD, STEIN, LL. SHELSKY, IM, ET AL: *MMPI comparison between patients with coronary heart disease and their spouses and other demographic data.* Scand J Rehab Med 2: 99, 1970.

67. HACKETT, TP AND CASSEM, NH: *Psychological adaptation to convalescence in myocardial infarction patients.* In NAUGHTON, JP AND HELLERSTEIN, HR (EDS): *Exercise Testing and Exercise Training in Coronary Heart Disease.* Academic Press, New York 1973, pp 253–262.

68. MCPHERSON, BD, PAIVIO, A, AND YUHASZ, MS: *Psychological effects of an exercise program for post-infarct and normal adult men.* J Sports Med 7:95, 1967.

69. MORGAN, WP: *Psychological aspects of heart disease.* In POLLOCK, ML AND SCHMIDT, DH (EDS): *Heart Disease and Rehabilitation.* Houghton Mifflin, Boston, 1979, pp 105–119.

Exercise Regimens
After Myocardial Revascularization Surgery:
Rationale and Results

Michael L. Pollock, Ph.D.

In individuals who have had prior manifestations of coronary heart disease, including myocardial revascularization surgery, cardiac rehabilitation can be considered the process of restoring psychologic, physical, and social function to optimal levels.[1,2] During recent years there has been a profound shift away from the conservative approach that previously discouraged patients with angina pectoris and myocardial infarction (MI) from becoming as active as their symptoms and medical status might have permitted. Many were told to resign from the golf club and some to stop driving their cars and climbing stairs. Six weeks of bed rest after an MI was the common practice.[3] Fortunately, many cardiologists questioned this pessimistic and conservative approach.[1,4−8] Since the 1940s, the safety of activity for the patient with angina, the early use of bedside chair for stabilized patients with MI, and progressive endurance exercises for those recovering from an MI have all been demonstrated.[1,4−8]

Another chapter outlines exercise regimens recommended for patients after an MI. The purpose of this chapter is to describe exercise regimens after myocardial revascularization surgery, with the emphasis on differences in programs for patients with MI and after coronary bypass surgery. The rehabilitation process will be described for the acute stage, that is, in-hospital cardiac rehabilitation (Phase I), the intermediate stage (usually the first 8 to 12 weeks after discharge) (Phase II), and the long-term program usually conducted in a community-based exercise facility (Phase III).

Although this chapter will emphasize the exercise aspects of cardiac rehabilitation, it should be noted that the multidisciplinary staff and intervention approach to cardiac rehabilitation is characteristic of most cardiac rehabilitation programs.[2,9,10] Multiple intervention would include exercise, diet, smoking cessation, and stress management. The purpose of the multi-intervention approach with a multidisciplinary team is to attempt to make life-style changes that will control the various risk factors related to the further progression of CHD, that is, smoking, hyperlipidemia, hypertension, lack of exercise, diabetes mellitus, obesity, and stress.

EXERCISE PRESCRIPTION FOR THE CARDIAC PATIENT

It has been suggested that the principles of exercise prescription for noncardiac patients are appropriate for use with the cardiac patient.[2] The major differences are related to the application of the principles to the patient and how they affect the regulation of frequency, intensity, and duration of training, the rate of progression, and selection of mode of training. The basic components of the training session include a warm-up, a muscular conditioning period, an aerobic exercise, and a cool-down. In comparison with the healthy noncardiac person, the cardiac patient may need a longer warm-up period and require modifications of the aerobic exercise phase, depending on current medical status and the phase of training. The various phases will be discussed in more detail later.

For improvement in cardiorespiratory endurance and weight control, the American College of Sports Medicine has recommended that the average aerobic phase of the endurance training program for noncardiac patients should be approximately 300 to 500 kilocalories (Kcal) per exercise session.[11] These guidelines support the concept that the total energy cost is an important factor and that the intensity and duration of the training program can vary as long as a certain intensity threshold and Kcal expenditure are achieved.[12-14] The guidelines recommend that the frequency of training should be between 3 and 5 days per week, the intensity a minimum of 60 percent of the maximum heart rate (HR max) reserve, and the duration of training between 15 and 60 minutes. They also suggest that, depending upon frequency, intensity, and duration of training, most aerobic activities will accomplish similar results. For example, when running, walking, and stationary cycling were performed at similar frequencies (3 days per week), intensities (85 percent HR max reserve), and durations (30 minutes), aerobic capacity and body composition improved equally among groups of individuals performing these activities.[15] In a fast walking program, in which intensity of training is less than the intensity of running, similar results can often be accomplished by increasing the duration of walking to 40 to 60 minutes.[16-18] The initial level of fitness has also been shown to be important in eliciting a training effect.[19,20] Persons who are low in fitness, such as cardiac patients, have an intensity threshold for improving aerobic fitness lower than 60 percent HR max reserve. The reverse is true for persons in the higher than average level of fitness.[20] Therefore, frequency, intensity, and duration of exercise should be adjusted to meet the needs of the participant/patient.

The initial training load is lower and the progression rate slower in training the cardiac patient than in training the healthy noncardiac individual.[2] Figure 1 shows the general rate of progression in Kcal per training session of cardiac and noncardiac groups. The figure suggests average values because the rate of progression will depend on the participant's age, phase of rehabilitation, level of fitness, and health status. It has been estimated that the noncardiac participant starts at 150 to 200 Kcal per exercise session and progresses to the 300

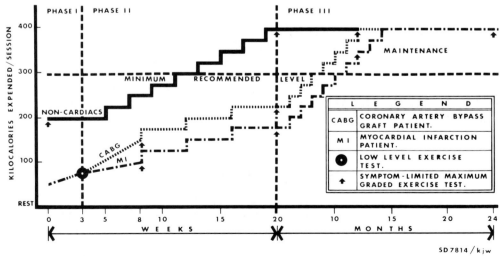

Figure 1. Progression in aerobic training in noncardiac and cardiac patients. (From Pollock, ML, Foster, C, and Ward, A,[21] with permission.)

Table 1. Guidelines for exercise prescription for cardiac patients as recommended and practiced at Mount Sinai Medical Center, Milwaukee, Wisconsin*

Prescription	Phase I (Inpatient Program)	Phase II (Discharge → 3 mo)	Phase III (3 mo →)	Healthy Adults
Frequency	2–3 times/day	1–2 times/day	3–5 times/wk	3–5 times/wk
Intensity	MI: RHR + 20	MI: RHR + 20,† RPE 13	70–85% max	60–90% max
	CABG: RHR + 20	CABG: RHR + 20,† RPE 13	HR reserve	HR reserve
Duration	MI: 5–20 min CABG: 10–30 min	MI: 20–60 min CABG: 30–60 min	30–60 min	15–60 min
Mode-activity, sports	ROM, TDM, bike, 1 flight of stairs, Wgt Trg	ROM, TDM (walk, walk-jog), bike, arm erg, endurance sports	Walk, bike, jog, swim, cal, Wgt Trg, cal	Walk, jog, run, bike, swim, endurance sports

Abbreviations: MI, myocardial infarction patient; CABG, coronary artery bypass graft surgery patient; HR, heart rate, beats/min; RHR, standing resting HR; ROM, range of motion exercise; TDM, treadmill; arm erg, arm ergometer; cal, calisthenics; Wgt Trg, weight training; RPE, rating of perceived exertion.
*Modified from Pollock, M, Foster, C, and Ward, A.[21]
†After 6–8 weeks postsurgery or event, a symptom-limited exercise test is performed. Heart rate intensity is then based on 70 percent of maximum heart rate reserve.

Kcal level by 8 to 10 weeks of training.[21] In contrast, the cardiac patient begins the in-hospital program at a level below 50 Kcal per session and requires several weeks to months longer to reach the 300 Kcal level.[21–23] The slightly slower rate of progression for the MI patient compared with the coronary artery bypass graft (CABG) surgery patient is a result of the slower progression normally used for the MI patient during the first 4 to 8 weeks of recovery. Although progression in ambulation is usually faster with patients following CABG surgery than with patients following MI in the early phase of rehabilitation, practitioners should be cautious with both groups for up to 6 to 8 weeks. Generally by 6 to 8 weeks scar tissue has adequately developed and the healing process is nearly complete for the MI and the sternum is healed following the surgery.[24,25] Depending on test results (medical status), a more normal type of progression can take place after this time, both for patients recovering from CABG surgery and MI.

The suggested rates and level of progression for cardiac and noncardiac groups shown in Figure 1 are realistic estimates. Whether patients can progress at faster rates without added risk is not known at this time. Research by DeBusk and coworkers[26] suggests that during the first 12 weeks of rehabilitation, patients after uncomplicated MI can progress at a rate faster than that shown in the illustration, but more research is necessary to clarify this issue.

A healthy noncardiac individual usually reaches the maintenance level of training after 6 to 8 months.[11,27] At that time the participant has attained a satisfactory level of fitness and may no longer be interested in increasing the training load. Once the maintenance level is reached, additional development is minimal and the emphasis of the program becomes that of maintaining fitness rather than seeking its further development. Progression for the cardiac patient is slower and may take from 6 to 18 months longer than for the noncardiac patient. Kavanagh and associates[28] have shown that younger cardiac patients continue to improve their aerobic capacity for up to 2 years.

The general guidelines for exercise prescription for cardiac patients are shown in Table 1. Phases I and II show the slower progression and intensity levels for cardiac patients in their earlier stages of training and coincides with the Kcal progression shown in Figure 1. As the patient reaches Phase III, the program begins to resemble the guidelines recommended for noncardiac patients.

It is believed by many that uncomplicated cardiac patients should be encouraged to attain the 300 Kcal expenditure in their training program, as recommended for noncardiac patients. Thus the slow, gradual approach suggested in Figure 1 and Table 1 is recommended. It has been shown that progression of intensity as compared with frequency and duration may be more dangerous for the cardiac patient. Hossack and Hartwig[29] found that in a Phase III program significantly more cardiac events occurred among patients who had above average fitness, had ST segment depression during training, and whose intensity exceeded their upper limit target heart rate.

INPATIENT CARDIAC REHABILITATION—PHASE I

The purpose of the Inpatient Exercise Program is to offset problems associated with bed rest.[30] Once the patient is considered stable, the rehabilitation process should begin. Many of the dramatic changes found with bed rest are a result of the loss of use of the postural reflexes associated with keeping the body upright.[30–32] With bed rest, patients lose cardiovascular efficiency more in the upright position than when tested in the supine position.[31,32] Thus, the earlier that patients can be allowed in the upright postural position and started in range of motion (ROM) activities, the less the potential for deterioration of various biochemical and physiologic factors.

Usually a 24-hour stabilization period is recommended prior to initiation of the cardiac rehabilitation program. A survey of cardiac rehabilitation programs revealed that most patients with MI begin low level rehabilitation approximately 3 days after the event. In comparison, the surgery patients were usually started 1 to 2 days after surgery.[21]

Other important goals of the inpatient cardiac rehabilitation are to reduce anxiety and depression, develop patient confidence, give patient education regarding risk factor modification, increase the chance of earlier hospital discharge, and enhance patient management prior to hospital discharge.[22,23,33–41]

The contraindications to exercise for the patient following coronary bypass surgery are similar to those for patients following MI. More specific information is published elsewhere.[2,42,43] The surgery patient will be extubated, but chest tubes are normally still in place when they are initially referred for cardiac rehabilitation. An exception to the generally described, absolute contraindications to exercise is the patient's body temperature. Although a body temperature of 100°F is used under most conditions, 102°F is used for surgery patients in the critical care unit. Other relative contraindications used for surgery patients are sinus tachycardia greater than 120 beats/min at rest; symptomatic anemia (hematocrit < 30 percent); wound infection; and unstable sternum. In the case of an unstable sternum, only upper extremity ROM exercises may be contraindicated.

Once the patient is accepted into the program, the activity schedule and guidelines listed in Table 2 for patients after open heart surgery are initiated. Similar guidelines for use with patients after MI are also available.[2] The guidelines are designed in three parts: (a) the activity program when the cardiac rehabilitation staff is supervising the patient; (b) the ward activity when the primary nurse or patient supervises the program; and (c) patient education. These guidelines were designed so that at step 5 of the post CABG protocol, the patient goes to an inpatient exercise center once a day for the activity part of the program. The inpatient exercise center contains treadmills, cycle ergometers, a special set of stairs with a handrail for initiating stair climbing, and a mat area for ROM exercises. Although the use of treadmills at this stage of rehabilitation may not be feasible for most institutions, it is believed that it helps give better quantification of training and increases the confidence of the patient.[2,36] Having known distances measured in the hospital area also aids in quantifying the patient's training level. Generally the patient progresses 1 step each day. The rate of progression is

Table 2. Post open heart surgery inpatient rehabilitation program guidelines

Step/Date	Cardiac Rehab/Physical Therapy	*Ward Activity	Patient Education
1 1.5 MET __/__/__	AM WARD TX: SITTING with feet supported: active-assistive to active ROM to major muscle groups, active ankle exercises, active scapular elevation/depression, retraction/protraction, 3–5 Reps; deep breathing. Monitored ambulation of 100 ft as tolerated. PM WARD TX: SITTING with feet supported: Active ROM to major muscle groups, 5 Reps; deep breathing. Monitored ambulation 100–200 ft with assistance as tolerated.	1. Begin sitting in chair (when stable) several times/day for 10–30 min. 2. May ambulate 100–200 ft with assistance, 1–2× daily.	Orient to CVICU. Reinforce purpose of physical therapy and deep breathing exercises. Orient to exercise component of rehabilitation program. Answer patient and family questions regarding progress.
2 1.5 MET __/__/__	WARD TX: SITTING: repeat exercises from Step 1 and increase repetitions to 5–10; deep breathing BID. Monitored ambulation of 200 ft with assistance as tolerated (stress correct posture) BID.	Continue activities from Step 1.	Continue above.
3 1.5–2 MET __/__/__	WARD TX: STANDING: Begin active upper extremity and trunk exercises bilaterally without resistance (shoulder: flexion, abduction, internal/external rotation, hyperextension, circumduction backwards; elbow flexion; trunk: lateral flexion: rotation), knee extension (if appropriate); ankle exercises; 5–10 Reps; BID. Monitored ambulation of 300 ft BID.	Increase ambulation to 300 ft or approximately 3 corridor lengths at slow pace with assistance, BID.	Begin pulse-taking instruction when appropriate and explain RPE scale. Answer questions of patient and family. Reorient patient and family to ICCU. Encourage family attendance at group classes.
4 1.5–2 MET __/__/__	WARD TX: STANDING: Active exercises from Step 3, 10–15 Reps; BID. Monitored ambulation of 424 ft BID.	Increase ambulation to 1 Lap† (424 ft or once around square) at slow pace with assistance BID.	
5 1.2–2.5 MET __/__/__	WARD TX: STANDING: Active exercises from Step 3, 15 Reps; once daily. Monitored ambulation for 5–10 min (424–848 ft) as tolerated. EXERCISE CENTER: Walk to Inpatient Exercise Center (IEC) for monitored ROM/strengthening exercises from Step 3, 15 Reps; leg stretching (posterior thigh muscles, gastrocenemius), 10 Reps; treadmill and/or bicycle 5–10 min (refer to treadmill/bicycle protocol) with physician approval.	1. Increase ambulation up to 3 Laps (up to 1320 ft) daily as tolerated. 2. Begin participating in daily ADL and personal care as tolerated. 3. Encourage chair sitting with legs elevated.	Orient to IEC. Continue instruction in pulse-taking and use of RPE scale. Explain value of exercise. Present T-shirt and activity log.

Table 2. (*Continued*)

Step/Date	Cardiac Rehab/Physical Therapy	*Ward Activity	Patient Education
6 1.5–2.5 MET __/__/__	*WARD TX:* STANDING: Active exercises from Step 3 with 1-lb weight each upper extremity, 15 Reps; once daily. Monitored ambulation for 10–15 min (up to 1980 ft) if appropriate. *EXERCISE CENTER:* Walk to IEC for monitored ROM/strengthening exercises from Step 5 with 1-lb weight each upper extremity, 15 Reps; leg stretching, 10 Reps; treadmill and/or bicycle 15–20 min; and stair-climbing (6–12 stairs) with assistance.	1. Increase ambulation up to 5 Laps (up to 1980 ft) daily. 2. Encourage independence in ADL. 3. Encourage chair sitting with legs elevated.	Give discharge booklet and general discharge instructions to patient and family. Encourage group class attendance. Individual instruction by physical therapist, nutritionist, pharmacist.
7 2–3 MET __/__/__	*WARD TX:* STANDING: Active exercises from Step 3 with 1-lb weight each upper extremity, 15 Reps; once daily. Monitored ambulation for 15–20 min (up to 3300 ft) if appropriate. *EXERCISE CENTER:* Walk to IEC for monitored ROM/strengthening exercises from Step 5 with 1-lb weight each upper extremity, 15 Reps; leg stretching, 10 Reps; treadmill and/or bicycle 20–30 min; and stair-climbing (up to 14 stairs) with assistance.	1. Continue activities from Step 6. 2. Increase ambulation up to 8 Laps (up to 3300 ft) daily.	Discuss referral to Phase 2 program if appropriate.
8 2–3 MET __/__/__	*WARD TX:* STANDING: Exercises from Step 3 with 2-lb weight each upper extremity, 15 Reps; once daily. Monitored ambulation if appropriate. *EXERCISE CENTER:* Walk to IEC for monitored ROM/strengthening exercises from Step 5 with 2-lb weight each upper extremity, 15 Reps; leg stretching, 10 Reps; treadmill and/or bicycle 20–30 min; and stair-climbing (up to 16 stairs).	1. Continue activities from Step 7. 2. Increase ambulation up to 9 Laps (up to 3746 ft) daily.	Reinforce prior teaching. Explain pre-discharge graded exercise test (PDGXT) and upper limit heart rate. Continue with possible referral to Phase 2.
9 2–3 MET __/__/__	*WARD TX:* STANDING: Exercises from Step 3 with 2-lb weight each upper extremity, 15 Reps; once daily. Monitored ambulation if appropriate. *EXERCISE CENTER:* Walk to IEC for monitored ROM/strengthening exercises from Step 5 with 2-lb weight each upper extremity, 15 Reps; leg stretching, 10 Reps; treadmill and/or bicycle 20–30 min; and stair-climbing (up to 18 stairs).	1. Continue activities from Step 8. 2. Increase ambulation up to 12 Laps (up to 5060 ft) daily.	Give final dicharge instructions. Complete referral to Phase 2.

Table 2. (*Continued*)

Step/Date	Cardiac Rehab/Physical Therapy	*Ward Activity	Patient Education
10 2–3 MET _/_/_	*WARD TX:* STANDING: Exercises from Step 3 with 3-lb weight each upper extremity, 15 Reps; once daily. Monitored ambulation if appropriate. *EXERCISE CENTER:* Walk to IEC for monitored ROM/strengthening exercises from Step 5 with 3-lb weight each upper extremity, 15 Reps; leg stretching, 10 Reps; treadmill and/or bicycle 20–30 min; and stair-climbing (up to 24 stairs). A pre-discharge graded exercise test (PDGXT) is recommended at this time.	1. Continue activities from Step 9. 2. Increase ambulation up to 14 Laps (up to 5940 ft) daily.	

*Ward Activity = Activities performed alone, with family, or primary nurse.
†Lap = Distance of approximately 424 feet or once around square.
Heart rates, blood pressures, and comments are recorded on Inpatient Data Record or Exercise Log.

individualized and depends upon how successfully the patient adapts to each stage of the program.

The program for patients after MI and after CABG surgery differs in the following ways. Surgery patients begin sooner and usually ambulate on the first treatment day (approximately 65 percent of surgery patients); surgery patients progress at a slightly higher intensity (approximately 0.5 mph), and duration of ambulation is more accelerated; and upper extremity ROM exercise is emphasized for the surgical patient.[22,23] Most inpatient programs include ROM exercise, ambulation, and stair climbing activities.[2,10] One exception for surgery patients is the reluctance of some surgeons to allow surgical patients to do upper extremity ROM exercise. Since 1977, Mount Sinai Medical Center, Milwaukee, Wisconsin, has used active ROM exercise with surgical patients. Their experience shows that approximately 95 percent of surgical patients can do upper extremity ROM exercise without overt problems.[22,23] Patients who experience sternal movement or have postsurgical sternal wound complications will not receive these exercises.

Why are upper extremity ROM exercises important in the early recovery from open heart surgery? Significant soft tissue and bone damage to the chest wall and anterior-superior regions of the arms occurs during surgery. If these areas do not receive ROM exercise, adhesions may develop and the musculature can become weaker and foreshortened. Patients will also favor these areas, which tends to accentuate later problems of poor posture and difficulties in attaining their previous strength and full ROM. Thus, it appears that the longer the delay in receiving upper extremity ROM exercise, the more discomfort the open heart surgery patient will experience during the recovery period, thereby extending the period for reaching full recovery.

The ROM exercises used in the inpatient program for the surgery patient typically include shoulder flexion, abduction, internal and external rotation; elbow flexion; hip flexion, abduction, internal and external rotation; and ankle plantar and dorsal flexion, inversion and eversion. Once the patient leaves the critical care areas, ROM exercises for the upper extremity are often completed with the help of a stick or cane. (See Pollock, Wilmore, and Fox[2] for more details on upper body exercises for the surgery patient.)

The intensity of exercise for the inpatient is within the 2 to 3 MET level.[22,23] The exercise heart rate usually increases no more than 5 to 10 beats/min above standing rest for either

ROM exercise or ambulation in the early phases of rehabilitation for the surgical patient. During the latter phases of the program (approximately 10 to 11 days post surgery), heart rates average 13 to 14 beats/min above standing rest. Systolic blood pressure rises no more than 5 mm Hg for ROM exercise and stair climbing. During the initial ambulation period, systolic blood pressure will rise approximately 5 to 10 mm Hg, and during the last few days prior to discharge approximately 15 mm Hg.[22,23] Use of the psychologic perception scale developed by Borg[44,45] shows that patients rate ROM exercise, ambulation, and stair climbing at approximately the same level, that is, 11 to 12 (between fairly light and somewhat hard).[22,23] This rating of perceived exertion (RPE) scale is used extensively as an adjunct to signs/symptoms and heart rate in exercise prescription. This psychologic scale relates well to physiologic variables such as blood lactate, pulmonary ventilation, heart rate, and oxygen uptake.[46] The use of the RPE scale also appears valid for use with arm work[47] and for patients on a beta-blocking drug.[48-50]

In summary, in comparison with the post-MI patient, the surgery patient usually starts earlier in both ROM exercise and ambulation. Upper extremity ROM exercises are emphasized more with the surgery patient. The surgery patient progresses faster in both the intensity and duration of exercise. Although the upper limit target heart rate (20 beats/min above standing rest) is used for both patient populations, the surgery patient is exercised at a level approximately 0.5 mph greater than that of the MI patient, which raises the heart rate 3 to 4 beats/min. The ambulation period is such that the surgery patient starts earlier and progresses slightly faster and thus ambulates approximately 5 to 10 minutes longer at hospital discharge (Table 2).

Patients who experience a perioperative infarction are progressed slower than the usual patient after CABG surgery and follow the progression rate suggested for the patient after MI.

Rationale for Exercise Intensity

There is no set answer as to the best manner in which to determine the safe upper limit target/training heart rate. A survey of experts in cardiac rehabilitation from 18 inpatient centers showed that training intensity was low in all programs and below the level of producing symptoms; but the means of determining an upper limit was quite varied.[21] The two most common guidelines were (a) the use of fixed low-level heart rate, or (b) a defined heart rate above standing resting heart rate. In the former method, the upper-limit heart rates were usually between 110 and 120 beats/min. In the latter method, 10 to 20 beats/min above resting level was most commonly used.

In lieu of significant signs or symptoms, 20 beats/min above standing resting heart rate may be most appropriate for use as the upper limit target/training exercise heart rate for both medical and surgical inpatients. Unless a predischarge exercise test is performed, this same standard is recommended for use until an exercise test is performed (usually at 6 to 8 weeks after the MI or surgery).

Why use 20 beats/min above standing resting and why not use a fixed low level heart rate? As shown earlier, most inpatient activities are performed at a heart rate of 10 to 15 beats/min above standing rest (RPE approximately 11 to 12).[22,23] In addition, because of the generally wide range of resting heart rates in cardiac patients, that is, 50 to 120 beats/min, a fixed heart rate seems inappropriate. Surgical patients generally exhibit tachycardia, and many have resting heart rates of 110 to 120 beats/min.

Pollock, Foster, and Ward[21] originally recommended 30 beats/min above standing rest as the upper limit heart rate for patients after CABG surgery, but subsequent data have resulted in a lowering of this limit to 20 beats/min above standing rest.[2,51] Rod and coworkers[51] found that a heart rate of 30 to 40 beats/min above standing rest was near maximum for most surgical patients at hospital discharge, and 13 on the RPE scale (somewhat hard) was approximately 20 beats/min above standing rest.

MEDICAL PROBLEMS

Dion and associates[22] and Silvidi and associates[23] showed that patients after CABG surgery can safely participate in a cardiac rehabilitation program as described above. Their studies documented many significant medical problems, but none was catastrophic in nature, and many were not necessarily associated with the rehabilitation program itself. The study of Dion and colleagues[22] was conducted on 521 patients who had undergone CABG surgery. The most common medical problems found during rehabilitation were angina pectoris (4 percent); incisional pain (14 percent); claudication (3 percent); lightheadedness (14 percent); hypotension (8 percent); hypertension (1 percent); ST segment changes (2 percent); and supraventricular (17 percent) and ventricular (44 percent) dysrhythmias. These results showed that the medical problems encountered after myocardial revascularization surgery are somewhat different from those after MI. Surgical patients appear to have a greater incidence of hypotension, lightheadness, and musculoskeletal chest-shoulder discomfort. Conversely, the successfully revascularized surgical patient experiences significantly less angina pectoris than the patient after MI. An interesting observation of the study of Dion and colleagues was the significant number of medical problems that were first detected while patients were being supervised in the cardiac rehabilitation program. Approximately 25 percent of all medical problems were first detected by the inpatient cardiac rehabilitation staff. Identification of these problems resulted in a significant number of medical interventions by the primary physician. Thus, the added surveillance of the cardiac rehabilitation program may be important in improving patient care and management prior to hospital discharge.

Because of the significant number of episodes of hypotension encountered in surgical patients, the following guidelines were developed for use by patients starting a cardiac rehabilitation program. All patients have orthostatic blood pressure measurements prior to beginning exercise. The following protocol is observed in regard to orthostatic or exercise-induced hypotension.

1. Symptomatic patient will not be exercised.
2. If the standing blood pressure is below 90 mm Hg (without symptoms), the attending physician will be notified and the patient will not be allowed to exercise until consulting with the medical director or attending physician.
3. If the patient exhibits a 10 to 20 mm Hg orthostatic drop in the systolic blood pressure (without symptoms), the medical director will be consulted prior to the patient being exercised.
4. If the patient exhibits more than a 20 mm Hg orthostatic drop in the systolic blood pressure (without symptoms), the attending physician will be notified. Usually the patient will not be exercised.

OUTPATIENT CARDIAC REHABILITATION—PHASE II

The outpatient program can begin when the patient is discharged from the hospital. It is generally organized as a hospital-based or free-standing program, as a home program with specific recommendations, or as a program based in a community gymnasium-type facility.[2,9,10] The outpatient phase of cardiac rehabilitation is the intermediate phase during which the patient progresses from a restricted low-level training program and a condition of unknown stability to a less restricted, moderate level program and a more stable status. As shown in Figure 1 the activity progression remains slow, with the program beginning at a level at which the patient left the inpatient program. Table 1 outlines the general aspects of exercise prescription for the outpatient program.

Table 3. Results from a pre-discharge graded exercise test and determination of upper limit target/training heart rate*

PATIENT NO. 1	Age: 44	HT: 6′2″	WT: 193 lb	
SEX: M	PREVIOUS MI: YES		SURGERY: 3 GRAFTS 7–23–80	
MEDICATION: COUMADIN				
TYPE OF TEST: PRE-DISCHARGE 8–7–80		PROTOCOL: MODIFIED NAUGHTON		
Time	MET	HR	BP	RPE
Rest	—	110	116/70	—
1		111		6
2	2	108	124/60	7
3		115		8
4	3	112	132/60	8
5		119		8
6	4	127	140/60	9
7		132		11
8	5	136	154/60	12
9		143		13
10	6	147	160/60	15
11		152		16
12	7	157	160/60	17

NORMAL RECOVERY   REASON FOR STOPPING: FATIGUE
  RECOMMENDED UPPER LIMIT HR 143
HIGHEST TRAINING HR INPATIENT CENTER 133, WORKLOAD 2.5–3 mph, 30 min

*Patient was recovering from CABG surgery and had an above average MET capacity. (From Pollock, ML, Wilmore, JH, and Fox, SM,[2] with permission.)

Particularly in the early stages of the outpatient program and prior to the patient going back to work, the frequency of training may be twice daily. This will vary somewhat depending upon the patient's medical status and ease of fatigability.

Initially, intensity of training is based upon the results of a predischarge exercise test or, if this was not done, the target level is 20 beats above standing resting heart rate. Table 3 shows the results from a predischarge graded exercise test and the subsequent prescribed upper limit target/training heart rate. Many factors are taken into consideration: the patient's medical status and symptoms, what was previously accomplished during the patient's inpatient exercise program, and, if used, the RPE on the exercise test. As with the case of most patients after CABG surgery, the patient illustrated in Table 3 did not have symptoms of ischemia but stopped because of fatigue.[51] He had a slightly higher than average MET capacity,[51] and his training level in the inpatient exercise center was above average.[22,23] His exercise test heart rate at an RPE of 13 (somewhat hard) was 143 beats/min. This heart rate is what the patient was assigned based on the test and was approximately 10 beats/min higher than his highest training heart rate in the inpatient program. In combination with other factors, the RPE rating has been shown to be helpful in designating the proper exercise training heart rate. Studies have shown that 13 on the RPE scale correlates well with 70 percent of HR max reserve.[47,50,52] Patients who are symptomatic (angina pectoris) are usually given an upper limit target heart rate 5 to 10 beats/min below their angina threshold.

The duration of training starts where the inpatient exercise program ended. Table 1 shows the patient after MI beginning at 20 minutes duration and the patient after CABG surgery at 30 minutes. Again these time limits are individualized, depending upon the patient's medical status and fitness level. Normally, during the first 6 weeks after hospital discharge, the surgery patient still progresses at a slightly faster rate than the post-MI patient.

At 6 to 8 weeks after discharge, many programs have their patients perform symptom-limited maximum graded exercise tests. At this time the exercise intensity is based on a certain percentage of maximum HR, usually 70 to 85 percent. In our experience, the calculation of 70 percent HR max reserve from the 6 to 8 week exercise test raises the training heart rate intensity approximately 5 to 10 beats/min.[53]

During the earlier stages of rehabilitation the program is progressed first by duration and then by intensity. Although many programs limit their duration to approximately 30 minutes, some believe 45 minutes is more appropriate.[21] The rationale for the longer duration is based on the belief that the cardiac patient should exercise at a more moderate intensity than the noncardiac patient. If one of the purposes of the cardiac rehabilitation program is to eventually have the patient reach the 300 Kcal level of exercise, then longer exercise duration may be necessary.

Initially the mode of activity is similar to that done in the inpatient program. If patients have a cycle ergometer at home, some cycle activity will be included. Some programs use circuit training in which patients rotate among 4 to 6 stations.[54] The various stations usually include both arm and leg activities. For example, a circuit may include treadmill ambulation, stationary cycling, bench stepping, rowing, and use of an arm ergometer or shoulder wheel. Because of the importance of developing the entire body, some strength exercises should begin as early as the first few weeks after discharge. Some programs use dumbbells or other types of light weights for upper body strength training.[10] These activities are integrated as a part of a total fitness program and may be necessary for preparing a patient to return to work or leisure time activities. How safe is this type of training? Traditionally, weight training exercises, particularly with the upper body, have not been recommended for cardiac patients, especially coronary patients. It has been shown that moderate to heavy static exercise significantly increases blood pressure.[55] The increase in blood pressure seems to be related to the size of the muscle group involved and not just whether the exercise is isometric or dynamic in nature.[56,57] For example, using a similar weight for the muscles involved in palmar flexion of the hand as compared with elbow flexion causes a significantly higher increase in blood pressure with the former. Thus, strength training should be dynamic with as little an isometric component as possible and should emphasize the use of large muscle groups. When possible, hand gripping activities should be avoided. As far as safety is concerned, the use of rhythmic arm activity at similar heart rate levels as used for leg work has not been associated with an increase in ischemia, dysrhythmia, or incidence of cardiac events.[58,59] Usually a combination of calisthenic and weight lifting exercises can be incorporated into the program.

Regarding other activities for the surgery patient, it has been estimated that it takes approximately 6 to 8 weeks for the sternum to heal completely. Therefore, only ROM exercise and light strength training (usually less than 10 pound weights) should be used during this period of recovery. After this time, more traditional strength training, twisting, pushing, and pulling can be slowly initiated. After this healing period has taken place, many programs recommend that their patients use the Airdyne ergometer (Excelsior Fitness Corp., Chicago, Illinois), which trains both arms and legs. The arm activity is a push and pull action that helps strengthen the large muscle groups of the arms, shoulders, back, and chest. More research is necessary to further determine the safe limits for weight training using moderate to heavier weights (resistance). It seems probable that many patients without cardiac complications can train with heavier weights. Possibly, weight training without the hand grip component will safely allow patients to do more.

The duration of training varies and depends upon the patient's level of fitness and available time. As mentioned earlier, the ultimate goal is to have the patient progress in such a way that a minimum of 300 Kcal per session or 1000 Kcal per week are expended. Therefore, at a slow to moderate walking speed, patients must eventually walk 45 to 60 minutes per session and/or increase the training frequency. Although patients are not necessarily expected to reach these Kcal levels during the outpatient program (many do), those patients who have lower exercise tolerance or are limited in their time to visit an outpatient exercise center may be encouraged to train twice a day, once at the center and once at home. Once the patient returns to work, it is difficult to recommend exercise more than once per day.

As patients improve, and depending on their medical status, higher levels of exercise intensity may be prescribed. This can include activities such as jogging. For both post-MI and postsurgical patients, jogging is not recommended until after the estimated 6 to 8 week healing period. Prior to initiating a jogging program, it is important to have a symptom-limited graded exercise test. Usually, patients without complications who have a MET capacity above 8 or who can walk on a treadmill at 3.5 mph, 5 percent grade can jog.[2] Jogging is usually started by the use of interval training, that is, alternating between a walking speed (3 to 4 mph) and a jogging speed (4.75 to 5.5 mph). It is difficult to jog at 70 percent of HR max reserve, and thus, as patients get into higher intensity programs, their upper limits can be raised to 80 percent and eventually 85 percent of HR max reserve. This intensity can occur at the latter stages of Phase II and certainly in the Phase III community programs. Once the intensity reaches 80 to 85 percent of HR max reserve, then frequency and duration can be reduced.

Although swimming can be introduced in the Phase II program, it is not recommended until after the 6 to 8 week healing period. This allows adequate time for the sternum and leg incisions to heal for the surgical patient and the heart tissue for the patient after MI. The advantages of a swimming program are many: it is an aerobic activity involving both arms and legs; it puts patient in a nongravity situation, helping venous return; it keeps heart rate lower (may allow symptomatic patients to do more exercise); it causes less musculoskeletal injuries; and it can be therapeutic for patients with arthritis, intermittent claudication, limb amputations, or paralysis.[60-62] Swimming or other water activities such as jogging or walking in water (using arms to paddle in combination with legs) can be the best alternative aerobic conditioner for the aforementioned patients. The disadvantages of swimming lie in the wide variation in skill level and the energy costs of swimming among patients.[63,64] For nonswimmers or those with poor swimming skills, swimming would most likely be an anaerobic activity and is not recommended.

COMMUNITY BASED CARDIAC REHABILITATION PROGRAM—PHASE III

A supervised Phase III program is generally conducted at a YMCA, Jewish Community Center, community or private rehabilitation/preventive center, or university campus facility.[10] These programs are also based on physician referral. Patients attending the Phase III programs are normally 8 to 12 weeks after surgery or MI and in many cases have returned to work. Inasmuch as the distance traveled to and from exercise facilities correlates well with program adherence,[65] patients should be encouraged to attend programs that are most convenient to their office or home.

Because Phase III patients have had more time to recover from their surgery or MI, they are generally more medically stable and physically stronger. The same contraindications to exercise and the same guidelines for modifying the training program as described earlier are also appropriate for use in the Phase III program.

Usually the exercise prescription at this phase of training will be no different for patients after surgery or after MI. One exception is that if a patient after surgery had not been involved in any prior rehabilitative exercise for the upper body, then ROM and strengthening exercises recommended for Phase II would be appropriate. Table 1 shows that the exercise program for Phase III appears much like that recommended for the noncardiac patient. The major difference is how the exercise prescription is applied. At this stage in rehabilitation the cardiac patient normally works at the lower end of the intensity scale, 70 to 75 percent HR max reserve, and thus a greater frequency and duration of exercise is recommended. If a patient participates in higher intensity activities such as jogging/running in which the heart rate reaches 80 to 85 percent of HR max reserve, then the frequency and duration of training can be modified appropriately. The rate of progression of training and the level of intensity is dependent on medical status and level of fitness.

Many of the activities recommended for the Phase III program are similar to those used in Phase II, the major difference being that higher intensity training and more vigorous strength routines can be incorporated for patients without complications. It is unwise to recommend game type activities that require twisting and turning and short sprints without the patient having proper preparation. Thus, the more rigorous game type activities are not recommended until 6 months after beginning rehabilitation and after proper preparatory activities have been completed.

MORBIDITY, MORTALITY, AND PHYSIOLOGIC FACTORS ASSOCIATED WITH REHABILITATION AFTER MYOCARDIAL REVASCULARIZATION SURGERY

In general, the benefits of myocardial revascularization surgery include improved cardiovascular function and mortality in patients with left main and/or multivessel atherosclerotic disease.[66-68] There have been no randomized trials conducted to evaluate the effect of exercise training or risk factor reduction on the graft patency, morbidity, and mortality after CABG surgery. Until more information is available for patients after CABG surgery, it appears that the conclusions of the randomized and nonrandomized exercise rehabilitation trials and multiple intervention risk factor trials conducted on patients after MI should be applied to patients after CABG surgery.[38,69-72] Conceivably, graft patency should be maintained and mortality improved with exercise training and multiple intervention.

The effects of exercise training on patients after CABG surgery have shown results similar to those found with patients after MI.[73-76] Thus, similar results would normally be expected for both groups of patients in all physiologic and psychologic variables, if training is conducted at similar levels of frequency, intensity, and duration.

Data concerning the return to work of patients after CABG surgery were recently reviewed at an NIH concensus conference.[77] The results from various studies have been discouraging concerning the effect of CABG surgery on work resumption. Factors most related to return to work include age, working status prior to surgery, medical and emotional status, being a blue or white collar worker, financial compensation, and various social attitudes. Data suggest that several psychobehavioral-cultural factors (for example, patient expectations about work and attitude toward illness, possibly physician encouragement to return to work, and formal cardiac rehabilitation programs) may significantly affect return to work.[77]

SUMMARY

Although the exercise prescription for the patient after myocardial revascularization surgery has unique differences from the regimen for the patient after infarction, there are many similarities. Most differences between the two patient groups apply during the initial weeks of rehabilitation (approximately 6 to 8 weeks). In the inpatient program the patient after CABG surgery usually begins ROM exercise and ambulation earlier. Upper extremity ROM exercises are emphasized more with the surgery patient, and the rate of progression of the intensity and duration of training is faster. Most data concerning morbidity, mortality, physiologic and psychologic factors, and return to work show similar results for patients after coronary bypass surgery and after MI.

REFERENCES

1. HELLERSTEIN, HK AND FORD, AB: *Rehabilitation of the cardiac patient.* JAMA 164:225, 1957.

2. POLLOCK, ML, WILMORE, JH, AND FOX, SM: *Exercise in Health and Disease: Evaluation, Prescription, and Rehabilitation.* WB Saunders, Philadelphia, 1984.

3. LEWIS, T: *Diseases of the Heart.* Macmillan, New York, 1933, pp 41–49.

4. LEVINE, SA AND LOWN, B: *The chair treatment of acute coronary thrombosis.* Trans Ass Am Physicians 64:316, 1951.

5. CAIN, HD, FRASHER, WG, AND STIVELMAN, R: *Graded activity program for safe return to self-care after myocardial infarction.* JAMA 177:111, 1961.

6. WENGER, NK: *The use of exercise in the rehabilitation of patients after myocardial infarction.* J South Carolina Med Ass Suppl. 1-12, 65:66, 1969.

7. NAUGHTON, J, BRUHN, JG, AND IATEGOLA, MT: *Effects of physical training on physiologic and behavioral characteristics of cardiac patients.* Arch Phys Med Rehabil 49:131, 1968.

8. ZOHMAN, LR: *Early ambulation of post-myocardial infarction patients: Montefiore Hospital.* In NAUGHTON, JP AND HELLERSTEIN, HK (EDS): *Exercise Testing and Exercise Training in Coronary Heart Disease.* Academic Press, New York, 1973, 329.

9. WILSON, PK, FARDY, PS, AND FROELICHER, VF: *Cardiac Rehabilitation, Adult Fitness, and Exercise Testing.* Lea & Febiger, Philadelphia, 1981.

10. FROELICHER, VF AND POLLOCK, ML (EDS): *Cardiac Rehabilitation Programs: State of the Art 1983.* J Cardiac Rehab 2:429, 1982.

11. AMERICAN COLLEGE OF SPORTS MEDICINE: *The recommended quantity and quality of exercise for developing and maintaining fitness in healthy adults.* Med Sci Sports 10:vii, 1978.

12. OLREE, HD, CORBIN, B, PENROD. J, ET AL: *Methods of achieving and maintaining physical fitness for prolonged space flight.* Final Progress Rep. to NASA, Grant No. NGR-04-002-004, 1969.

13. SHARKEY, BJ: *Intensity and duration of training and the development of cardiorespiratory endurance.* Med Sci Sports 2:197, 1970.

14. POLLOCK, ML, BROIDA, J, KENDRICK, Z, ET AL: *Effects of training two days per week at different intensities on middle-aged men.* Med Sci Sports 4:192, 1972.

15. POLLOCK, ML, DIMMICK, J, MILLER, HS, ET AL: *Effects of mode of training on cardiovascular function and body composition of middle-aged men.* Med Sci Sports 7:139, 1975.

16. SHARKEY, BJ AND HOLLEMAN, JP: *Cardiorespiratory adaptations to training at specified intensities.* Res Quart 38:698, 1967.

17. POLLOCK, ML, MILLER, H, JANEWAY, R, ET AL: *Effects of walking on body composition and cardiovascular function of middle-aged men.* J Appl Physiol 30:126, 1971.

18. LEON, AS, CONRAD, J, HUNNINGHAKE, DB, ET AL: *Effects of vigorous walking program on body composition, and carbohydrate and lipid metabolism of obese young men.* Am J Clin Nutr 32:1776, 1979.

19. SALTIN, B, HARTLEY, L, KILBOM, A, ET AL: *Physical training in sedentary middle-aged men, II.* Scand J Clin Lab Invest 24:323, 1969.

20. GLEDHILL, N AND EYNON, RB: *The intensity of training.* In TAYLOR, AW AND HOWELL, ML (EDS): *Training Scientific Basis and Application.* Charles C Thomas, Springfield, Illinois, 1972, p 97.

21. POLLOCK, ML, FOSTER, C, AND WARD, A: *Exercise prescription for rehabilitation of the cardiac patient.* In POLLOCK, ML AND SCHMIDT, DH (EDS): *Heart Disease and Rehabilitation.* John Wiley & Sons, New York, 1979, p 413.

22. DION, FW, GREVENOW, P, POLLOCK, ML, ET AL: *Medical problems and physiologic responses during supervised inpatient cardiac rehabilitation: The patient after coronary bypass grafting.* Heart Lung 11:248, 1982.

23. SILVIDI, GE, SQUIRES, RW, POLLOCK, ML, ET AL: *Hemodynamic responses and medical problems associated with early exercise and ambulation in coronary artery bypass graft surgery patients.* J Cardiac Rehab 2:355, 1982.

24. MALLORY, GK, WHITE, PD, AND SALCEDO-SALGAR, J: *The speed of healing of myocardial infarction: A study of the pathologic anatomy in seventy-two cases.* Am Heart J 18:647, 1939.

25. WENGER, NK: *The physiological basis for early ambulation after myocardial infarction.* In WENGER, NK (ED): *Exercise and the Heart.* FA Davis, Philadelphia, 1978, pp 107–116.

26. DEBUSK, RF, HOUSTON, N, HASKELL, W, ET AL: *Exercise training soon after myocardial infarction.* Am J Cardiol 44:1223, 1979.

27. POLLOCK, ML: *The quantification of endurance training programs.* In WILMORE, JH (ED): *Exercise and Sport Sciences Reviews,* Vol. 1. Academic Press, New York, 1973, pp 155–188.

28. KAVANAGH, T, SHEPHARD, RJ, DONEY, H, ET AL: *Intensive exercise in coronary rehabilitation.* Med Sci Sports 5:34, 1973.

29. HOSSACK, KF AND HARTWIG, R: *Cardiac arrest associated with supervised cardiac rehabilitation.* J Cardiac Rehab 2:402, 1982.

30. SALTIN, B, BLOMQVIST, G, MITCHELL, J, ET AL: *Responses to exercise after bed rest and after training.* Circulation 37 and 38 (Suppl 7):1, 1968.

31. CONVERTINO, V, HUNG, J, GOLDWATER, D, ET AL: *Cardiovascular responses to exercise in middle-aged men after 10 days of bed rest.* Circulation 65:134, 1982.

32. HUNG, J, GOLDWATER, D, CONVERTINO, VA, ET AL: *Mechanisms for decreased exercise capacity after bed rest in normal middle-aged men.* Am J Cardiol 51:344, 1983.

33. CASSEM, NH AND HACKETT, TP: *Psychological rehabilitation of myocardial infarction patients in the acute phase.* Heart Lung 2:382, 1973.

34. MORGAN ,WP AND POLLOCK, ML: *Physical activity and cardiovascular health: Psychological aspects.* In LANDRY, F AND ORBAN, WAR (EDS): *Physical Activity and Human Well-being.* Symposium Specialists, Incorporated, Miami, 1978, pp 163–181.

35. BLOCK, A, MAEDER, JP, HASSILY, FC, ET AL: *Early mobilization after myocardial infarction. A controlled study.* Am J Cardiol 34:152, 1974.

36. EWART, CK, TAYLOR, B, REESE, LB, ET AL: *Effects of early myocardial infarction exercise testing on self-perception and subsequent physical activity.* Am J Cardiol 51:1077, 1983.

37. AMERICAN HEART ASSOCIATION: *Risk factors and coronary heart disease—A statement for physicians.* Circulation 62:445, 1980.

38. KELLERMAN, JJ (ED): *Comprehensive Cardiac Rehabilitation.* Karger, Basel, 1982.

39. NAUGHTON, JP, HELLERSTEIN, HK, AND MOHLER, LC (EDS): *Exercise Testing and Exercise Training in Coronary Heart Disease.* Academic Press, New York, 1973.

40. LEON, AS AND BLACKBURN, H: *Exercise rehabilitation of the coronary heart disease patient.* Geriatr 32:66, 1977.

41. POLLOCK, ML AND SCHMIDT, DH (EDS): *Heart Disease and Rehabilitation.* John Wiley & Sons, New York, 1979.

42. AMERICAN HEART ASSOCIATION: *Exercise Testing and Training of Individuals with Heart Disease or at High Risk for its Development: A Handbook for Physicians.* American Heart Association, Dallas, 1975.

43. AMERICAN COLLEGE OF SPORTS MEDICINE: *Guidelines for Graded Exercise Testing and Exercise Prescription,* ed 2. Lea & Febiger, Philadelphia, 1980.

44. BORG, G: *Physical Performance and Perceived Exertion.* Gleerup, Lund, Sweden, 1962, pp 1–63.

45. BORG, GAV: *Psychological bases of perceived exertion.* Med Sci Sports Exer 14:377, 1982.

46. MORGAN, WP AND POLLOCK, ML: *Psychological characterization of the elite distance runner.* Ann NY Acad Sci 301:382, 1977.

47. POLLOCK, ML, FOSTER, C, AND HARE, J: *Metabolic and perceptual responses to arm and leg exercise.* Med Sci Sports Exer 15:140, 1983.

48. DAVIES, CTM AND SARGEANT, AJ: *The effects of atropine and practolol on the perception of exertion during treadmill exercise.* Ergonomics 22:1141, 1979.

49. SQUIRES, RW, ROD, JL, POLLOCK, ML, ET AL: *Effect of propranolol on perceived exertion soon after myocardial revascularization surgery.* Med Sci Sports Exer 14:276, 1982.

50. POLLOCK, ML AND FOSTER, C: *Exercise prescription for participants on propranolol.* J Am Coll Cardiol 2:624, 1983.

51. ROD, JL, SQUIRES, RW, POLLOCK, ML, ET AL: *Symptom-limited graded exercise testing soon after myocardial revascularization surgery.* J Cardiac Rehab 2:199, 1982.

52. POLLOCK, ML, FOSTER, C, ROD, JL, ET AL: *Comparison of methods for determining exercise training intensity for cardiac patients and healthy adults.* In KELLERMANN, JJ (ED): *Comprehensive Cardiac Rehabilitation.* Karger, Basel, 1982, pp 129–133.

53. GUTMANN, MC, SQUIRES, RW, POLLOCK, ML, ET AL: *Perceived exertion-heart rate relationship during exercise testing and training in cardiac patients.* J Cardiac Rehab 1:52, 1981.

54. NAUGHTON, J: *The national exercise and heart disease project: development, recruitment, and implementation.* In WENGER, NK (ED): *Exercise and the Heart.* FA Davis, Philadelphia, 1978, pp 205–222.

55. LIND, AR AND McNICOL, GW: *Muscular factors which determine the cardiovascular responses to sustained and rhythmic exercise.* Canad Med Ass J 96:706, 1967.

56. BEZUCHA, GR, LENSER, MC, HANSON, PG, ET AL: *Comparison of hemodynamic responses to static and dynamic exercise.* J Appl Physiol 53:1589, 1982.

57. BLOMQVIST, CG, LEWIS, SF, TAYLOR, WF, ET AL: *Similarity of the hemodynamic responses to static and dynamic exercise of small muscle groups.* Circ Res Suppl II 48:87, 1981.

58. MARKIEWICZ, W, HOUSTON, N, AND DEBUSK, R: *A comparison of static and dynamic exercise soon after myocardial infarction.* Israel J Med Sci 15:894, 1979.

59. DEBUSK, RF, VALDEZ, R, HOUSTON, N, ET AL: *Cardiovascular responses to dynamic and static effort soon after myocardial infarction. Application to occupational work assessment.* Circulation 58:368, 1978.

60. ASTRAND, PO AND RODAHL, K: *Textbook of Work Physiology.* McGraw-Hill, New York, 1977.

61. MAGDER, S, LINNARSSON, D, AND GULLSTRAND, L: *The effect of swimming on patients with ischemic heart disease.* Circulation 63:979, 1981.

62. THOMPSON, DL, BOONE, TW, AND MILLER, HS: *Comparison of treadmill exercise and tethered swimming to determine validity of exercise prescription.* J Cardiac Rehab 2:363, 1982.

63. HOLMER, I, STEIN, EM, SALTIN, B, ET AL: *Hemodynamic and respiratory responses compared in swimming and running.* J Appl Physiol 37:49, 1974.

64. FLETCHER, GF, CANTWELL, JD, AND WATT, EW: *Oxygen consumption and hemodynamic response of exercises used in training of patients with recent myocardial infarction.* Circulation 60:140, 1979.

65. OLDRIDGE, NB, WICKS, JR, HANLEY, C, ET AL: *Non-compliance in an exercise rehabilitation program for men who have suffered a myocardial infarction.* Canad Med Ass J 118:361, 1978.

66. STARCK, PJU: *Effects of coronary artery surgery on early and late survival.* Cardiovasc Rev Rep 4:551, 1983.

67. FAVALORO, RG: *Direct myocardial revascularization: A ten year journey, myths and realities.* Am J Cardiol 43:109, 1979.

68. NEWMAN, GE, RERCH, SK, JONES, RH, ET AL *Noninvasive assessment of the effects of aorta-coronary by-pass grafting on ventricular function during rest and exercise.* J Thorac Cardiovasc Surg 79:617, 1980.

69. KALLIO, V, HAMALAINEN, H, HAKKILA, J, ET AL: *Reduction in sudden deaths by a multifactorial intervention programme after acute myocardial infarction.* Lancet 2(8152):1091, 1979.

70. HJERMANN, I, VELVE DYRE, K, AND HOLME, I: *Effect of diet and smoking intervention on the incidence of a randomized trial in healthy men.* Lancet 2(8259):1303, 1981.

71. SHEPARD, RJ, COREY, P, AND KAVANAGH, T: *Exercise compliance and the prevention of a recurrence of myocardial infarction.* Med Sci Sports Exer 13:1, 1981.

72. NAUGHTON, J: *Physical activity for myocardial infarction patients.* Cardiovasc Rev Rep 3:237, 1982.

73. OLDRIDGE, NB, NAGLE, FJ, BALKE, B, ET AL: *Aorto coronary bypass surgery: Effects of surgery and 32 months of physical conditioning on treadmill performance.* Arch Phys Med Rehabil 59:268, 1978.

74. HARTUNG, GH AND RANGEL, R: *Exercise training in post-myocardial infarction patients: Comparison of results with high risk coronary and post-bypass patients.* Arch Phys Med Rehabil 62:147, 1981.

75. POLLOCK, ML, FOSTER, C, ANHOLM, J, ET AL: *Randomized exercise and relaxation trials with myocardial revascularization surgery patients: Cardiorespiratory and hemodynamic effects.* Med Sci Sports Exer 13:133, 1981.

76. WAITES, TF, WATT, DW, AND FLETCHER, GF: *Comparative functional and physiologic status of active and dropout coronary bypass patients of a rehabilitation program.* Am J Cardiol 51:1087, 1983.

77. ELIASTAM, M AND GASTEL, E (EDS): *Technology assessment forum on coronary bypass surgery: Economic, ethical, and social issues.* Circulation 66 (Suppl 3):III, 1982.

Upper Extremity Exercise Testing and Training

C. Gunnar Blomqvist, M.D.

Standard clinical exercise testing is based on dynamic leg exercise (treadmill, bicycle, or step test). Therapeutic exercise programs also emphasize dynamic leg exercise. Activity patterns during daily life are more varied. Many tasks require static or isometric efforts, sometimes in combination with dynamic exercise and often involving the arms rather than the legs. The acute cardiovascular and metabolic responses to dynamic leg exercise have been well characterized in normal subjects and in patients with various forms of heart disease. There is also a large amount of data on the effect of physical training based on various forms of locomotion (walking, running, bicycling, swimming, and so on). Much less is known about the effects of other forms of exercise. The purpose of this chapter is to review acute and chronic responses to alternate modes of physical activity, particularly arm exercise.

ACUTE RESPONSES

Static or Isometric Exercise

Arm exercise often includes a static component. Sustained static efforts produce a marked increase in systolic and diastolic arterial pressures with a modest increase in heart rate and cardiac output. Peripheral resistance changes little in normal subjects, but vasoconstriction is the principal mechanism of the pressor response in patients with severe cardiac dysfunction.[1] A pressor response mediated by vasoconstriction is also present in normal subjects after combined beta-adrenergic and parasympathetic blockade[2] and in patients with transplanted, that is, denervated hearts.[3]

According to classical concepts[1] the magnitude of the pressor and heart rate responses is independent of muscle mass and absolute force development but closely linked to relative effort, or developed force as a fraction or percentage of the force during a maximal voluntary contraction (MVC). Recent studies have demonstrated that the magnitude of the cardiovascular response (Fig. 1) is greatly influenced not only by relative load but also by active muscle mass and absolute force development.[4] The relationship is nonlinear, with decreasing effects of increasing active muscle mass at high levels of force development.

The normal left ventricle is able to maintain stroke volume at resting levels with little or no increase in end-diastolic pressure despite the marked increase in systolic blood pressure and afterload. Stroke work increases markedly. These findings are consistent with enhanced myocardial contractility. A large number of invasive and noninvasive studies of left ventricular function in patients with heart disease, recently reviewed by Perez-Gonzales and associates[5] and Krayenbuehl and coworkers,[6] have shown that, during isometric forearm exer-

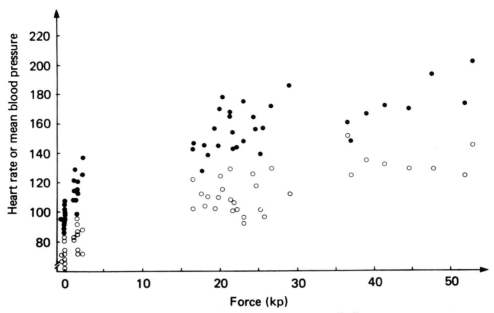

Figure 1. Individual values of heart rate and mean blood pressure between 1^{40}-1^{50} min of sustained contractions at 40 percent MVC performed with the fingers, forearm, thigh, and forearm plus thigh. ●, mm Hg; ○, beats/min. (From Mitchell, JH, et al,[4] with permission.)

cise (handgrip), patients with myocardial dysfunction respond with a larger increase in filling pressures than normal subjects but are nevertheless unable to maintain a normal stroke volume. Left ventricular ejection fraction and velocity of fiber shortening decrease.[6] The degree of ventricular dysfunction during isometric exercise can be quantitated by noninvasive techniques, for example, echocardiography,[5] or during cardiac catheterization,[6] and the results have prognostic significance.

Systolic blood pressure may increase by more than 50 mm Hg during handgrip at 30 to 50 percent MVC, but high force levels can be maintained only for short periods, for example, typically less than 5 minutes at 30 percent and less than 3 minutes at 50 percent MVC. The heart rate increase is modest, usually less than 25 beats/min at 30 percent MVC. The short duration of the hemodynamic response and the relatively small increase in heart rate explain why the pressor response rarely causes angina pectoris. Heart rate and blood pressure responses to isometric exercise are attenuated during the early phases of recovery from myocardial infarction.[7] Exercise-induced wall motion abnormalities may activate ventricular baroreceptors. Deformation of these receptors causes bradycardia and vasodilation, which oppose the normal reflex response to isometric exercise and protect against overload.

An early study from our laboratory demonstrated more frequent ventricular ectopic activity during handgrip at 30 percent MVC than during symptom-limited maximal bicycle exercise. However, a majority of the patients in this series had severe left ventricular dysfunction. Subsequent studies[7-9] have failed to support the concept that isometric exercise is arrhythmogenic and therefore dangerous.

Dynamic Arm Exercise

It is well known that at any submaximal workload or level of oxygen uptake, arm exercise produces a higher heart rate and arterial pressure than leg exercise. Maximal oxygen uptake and heart rate are lower than during leg exercise. We have recently examined systematically the relationship between active muscle mass and cardiovascular response during dynamic exercise.[10,11] Four different modes were used: (a) one-arm curl, (b) one-arm, (c) one-leg, and (d) two-leg bicycle exercise. Activity-specific maximal oxygen uptake at modes (a), (b), and (c) averaged 20, 50, and 75 percent of individual two-leg maximal oxygen uptake. Measurements were obtained at relative loads of 25, 50, 75, and 100 percent maximal capacity for each activity. Principal results in 6 young normal subjects are summarized in Figure 2. Car-

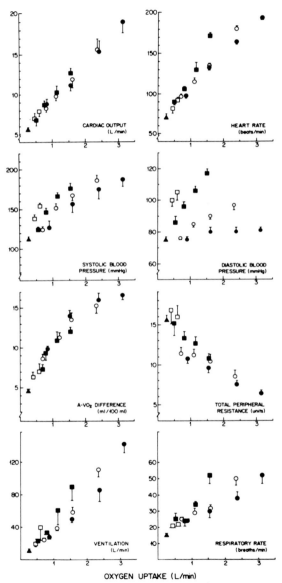

Figure 2. Cardiovascular and respiratory responses to submaximal and maximal exercise as functions of absolute work intensity (plotted as O_2 uptake). ▲, rest; □, 1-arm curl; ■, 1-arm cranking; ○, 1-leg cycling; ●, 2-leg cycling. Data shown are means ± SE; n = 6. (From Lewis, SF, et al,[11] with permission.)

177

Table 1. Effect of active muscle mass on the response to maximal dynamic exercise

Activity Mode	Oxygen Uptake (L/min)	Cardiac Output (L/min)	Heart Rate (beats/min)	Systolic Pressure (mm Hg)	Diastolic Pressure (mm Hg)	Plasma Norepinephrine (ng/ml)
Rest	0.25	5.6	70	112	74	0.08
1–Arm Curl	0.61	7.9	91	154	104	0.32
1–Arm Bicycle	1.55	12.9	172	176	117	0.84
1–Leg Bicycle	2.34	15.6	181	186	97	1.56
2–Leg Bicycle	3.12	18.8	194	188	82	3.75

Data from six young normal men: Blomqvist et al[10] and Lewis et al[11]

diac output and systemic arteriovenous oxygen difference were strongly related to oxygen uptake without significant differences between modes of exercise. The slope of the relationship between heart rate and oxygen uptake was inversely proportional to active muscle mass, that is, the smaller the active muscle mass, the higher the heart rate at any absolute level of oxygen uptake. Arterial pressures (systolic, diastolic, and mean) were even more strongly affected by active muscle mass, with large increases in pressure at low levels of oxygen uptake during exercise involving a small muscle mass. Mean data during maximal exercise are presented in Table 1.

These data show a gradual transition from a dynamic to a static hemodynamic pattern as active muscle mass decreases. Subsequent studies[2] have confirmed that heart rates and blood pressures are virtually identical during static and dynamic handgrip performed with identical small muscle groups to a common end-point of local fatigue. This does not mean that all aspects of the cardiovascular responses are identical. The mode of contraction affects local hemodynamic conditions. There is vasodilation and a markedly increased blood flow to skeletal muscle during dynamic exercise, whereas static exercise causes mechanical obstruction of flow and local ischemia. However, the different local conditions have little impact on systemic hemodynamics so long as the active muscle mass is small. Systemic vascular resistance remains near resting levels and any increase in cardiac output causes a proportional increase in blood pressure. Thus, the pressor response to isometric and dynamic exercise of small muscle groups is linked to a relative absence of metabolic vasodilation. That metabolic vasodilator activity is a principal determinant of systemic hemodynamics is demonstrated by the relationship between plasma norepinephrine levels (which may be viewed as a measure of the strength of neurogenic vasodilator drive) and peripheral resistance. One-arm dynamic and isometric exercises cause only minor changes in norepinephrine levels and peripheral resistance. Norepinephrine increases exponentially with oxygen uptake during exercise and is highest during maximal two-leg dynamic exercise when total peripheral resistance is minimal (Fig. 2 and Table 1). The general relationship between active muscle mass and hemodynamic response is similar in young and middle-aged normal subjects and in angina-free patients with ischemic heart disease (Martin, W, work in progress).

The response to arm exercise in patients with angina pectoris has been examined by several investigators.[12–16] Schwade and associates[15] compared arm and leg bicycle ergometry and included a group of patients who often had chest pain during arm work but rarely during leg work. This subpopulation had responses that were no different from patients who predominantly had their angina during leg work, that is, walking. The maximal workload that can be achieved during two-arm bicycle work varies from less than half to 70 percent of the load during two-leg work. Mechanical efficiency is highly variable but significantly lower during arm work, that is, oxygen uptake is higher at any given workload than during leg work. The lower mechanical efficiency combines with a steeper increase (Fig. 3) in heart rate and systolic blood pressure during arm work to cause a high myocardial oxygen demand relative to workload. However, heart rate-blood pressure products at the onset of myocardial ischemia and the incidence of chest pain and ST segment abnormalities were similar during arm and leg work in the series of 33 patients studied by Schwade and coworkers.[15] Others[14,16] have reported a slightly higher rate-pressure product threshold for angina during arm work. This is consistent with lower filling pressures[17] and, most likely, with lower ventricular volumes during arm work.

Thus, the cost of performing arm work is higher both in terms of myocardial work and systemic energy expenditure. There is little or no correlation between the peak workloads that

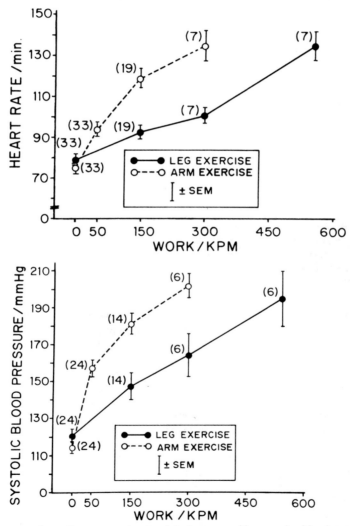

Figure 3. Mean heart rate and systolic pressure at rest and during arm and leg exercise. Numbers within brackets indicate number of patients. Only patients with measurements during both arm and leg exercise at a given load have been included. (From Schwade, J, et al,[15] with permission.)

can be achieved during arm and leg exercise. Arm work is therefore an effective alternate test method if the objective is to document myocardial ischemia, but large interindividual variations in mechanical efficiency and heart rate-blood pressure responses make it impossible to use arm work to derive a valid general estimate of systemic functional capacity.

Combined Static and Dynamic Work

Static and dynamic work are often combined in daily life, for example, when carrying a suitcase. Studies in normal subjects[18] and patients with ischemic heart disease[19] indicate that the pressor response to isometric exercise is superimposed on the response to dynamic exercise at low workload levels. The pressor effects gradually become less prominent as the intensity of dynamic exercise increases. Kerber and coworkers[19] found no significant effect on the incidence of myocardial ischemia, and they suggested that the elevated diastolic pressure during combined exercise actually may improve myocardial perfusion.

EFFECTS OF PHYSICAL TRAINING

We have recently reviewed the cardiovascular effects of physical training in normal subjects and in patients with ischemic heart disease.[20,21] Dynamic exercise training produces adaptations that involve multiple organ systems and functions. The spectrum includes anatomic, metabolic, and regulatory changes. The principal effects are increased maximal oxygen uptake, stroke volume, and cardiac output with relative bradycardia at submaximal levels of work. The increased cardiac pump capacity is due to a combination of cardiac and extracardiac adaptations. There is a modest increase in cardiac dimensions at rest and an increased Starling effect during exercise. An increased blood volume may enhance preload. A relative afterload reduction contributes significantly to the improved pump function. An increased ability to vasodilate enables the trained individual to achieve a higher maximal cardiac output without any increase in arterial pressure. No convincing evidence for training-induced changes in intrinsic contractile performance is available from human studies, and the results of animal experiments are inconclusive.

Many patients with heart disease also improve significantly after physical training. Performance is often enhanced in the absence of any demonstrable changes in cardiac pump function or myocardial blood supply. The improvement has generally been linked to peripheral adaptations, particularly to an increased oxidative capacity of skeletal muscle. However, there is no conclusive experimental support for the concept that metabolic adaptations are the principal mechanism. Recent studies have shown that there are no direct links between maximal oxygen uptake and oxidative capacity. The primary effect of the metabolic adaptations in skeletal muscle is to increase endurance by facilitating the use of fat as fuel and by decreasing the dependence on carbohydrates.[21]

Occupational work often involves more arm work than leg work. The effects of training of small muscle groups differ in many respects from those induced by two-leg dynamic exercise. Hellerstein and Franklin[22] have argued strongly that therapeutic training programs should include arm work, particularly for patients with angina pectoris. The rationale is that training effects tend to be activity-specific.

The extent to which training effects are transferable is a controversial issue. The problem is important from a practical point of view, and a solution will also provide crucial information on the mechanisms that contribute to the cardiovascular training effects. Several investigators have used training programs involving either arm or leg training and compared the effects on the cardiovascular responses to exercise with trained and untrained limbs.[23-25] Others have studied one-leg training.[26,27]

Clausen and colleagues[23] initially concluded that arm training produces a significant reduction in the heart rate during this type of work but has no effect on the response to leg work.

The effect of leg training on the response to arm work was also insignificant. A later study,[24] based on a larger series of subjects, confirmed that arm training does not affect the response to leg exercise but demonstrated that leg training causes a significant reduction in submaximal heart rates during both modes of exercise. Thompson and associates[25] performed a similar study in patients with angina pectoris with similar results. However, the heart rate reduction attributable to a transfer effect is less prominent than that achieved by arm training.

Studies of single leg training[26,27] have shown no transfer of training effects to the untrained limb but a small increase in systemic (or two-leg) maximal oxygen uptake. Further support for the specificity of training effects is derived from a study by Gaffney and coworkers[28] who attempted to achieve a leg training effect at minimal levels of cardiac stress. They used a set of exercises (knee-bend, heel-lift, hip flexion, and hip extension) that were performed separately with each leg. Heart rates during training were less than 125 beats/min and peak oxygen uptake less than one-third of maximal oxygen uptake during two-leg bicycle exercise. Training significantly decreased the heart rate during performance of each exercise but did not affect the response to two-leg bicycle exercise. Leg strength and muscle fiber areas increased but there was no change in the oxidative capacity of skeletal muscle.

Together these studies provide some insight into the mechanisms underlying systemic and local training effects. Systemic or general effects are unlikely to develop if the training program is carried out at low levels of systemic maximal oxygen uptake. Arm training at 70 percent of the capacity for arm work will usually require less than 50 percent of maximal two-leg oxygen uptake. One-leg training[26,27] requires a larger fraction of systemic maximum and produces a small but significant effect on two-leg exercise performance.

Metabolic changes in skeletal muscle are not a prerequisite for a training effect. A significant training-induced relative bradycardia can be achieved in the absence of any changes in oxidative capacity.[28] An increased capacity for vasodilation in working muscle with improved performance may be an important contributor to both local and systemic training effects. Any improvement in maximal systemic oxygen uptake is associated with a decrease in systemic neurogenic vasoconstrictor drive, and local adaptations may include an increased metabolic vasodilator drive.[21,24,27] Training-induced improvements in the ability of working muscle to extract available oxygen from arterial blood have previously been attributed to improved oxidative capacity. However, it is unlikely that this is a causal link. Both bed rest and training increase the A-V O_2 difference across the working leg and lower the O_2 content of femoral vein blood.[21] A training-induced increase in the metabolic vasodilator drive provides a possible alternate explanation.

The mechanisms whereby training alters the function of the autonomic nervous system are still poorly understood. Vagal tone is enhanced by endurance training, and experimental studies have demonstrated changes in the tissue concentrations and metabolism of acetylcholine.[29] There is less compelling evidence for a change in intrinsic sympathetic function.[21,29] The density of beta-adrenergic receptors and the responses to agonists are probably not affected by training. It is possible that the decreased sympathetic activity during exercise in the trained state primarily reflects a reduced afferent impulse traffic.

Skeletal muscle hypertrophy with increased strength may be a major cause of the reduction in heart rate and blood pressure after training, particularly for modes of exercise that can be performed at levels of oxygen uptake well below systemic maximum.[28] Finally, an increase in mechanical efficiency will be manifest as a training effect and go undetected if the evaluation is based on measurements of work capacity and does not include determination of oxygen uptake.

It should be evident from this discussion that there still is a lack of basic knowledge regarding the mechanisms that control the cardiovascular responses to exercise and how they are affected by various forms of physical training. However, in a general sense the physiologic data support the concept[22] that therapeutic exercise programs should not be limited to dynamic leg exercise but should include upper body activities. Exercise specifically designed to improve muscle strength may be beneficial, and the exclusion of all activities requiring predominantly static efforts is not warranted.

REFERENCES

1. SHEPHERD, JT, BLOMQVIST, CG, LIND, AR, ET AL: *Static (isometric) exercise. Retrospection and introspection.* Circ Res 48(Suppl I):179, 1981.

2. LEWIS SF, TAYLOR WF, BASTIAN, BC, ET AL: *Haemodynamic responses to static and dynamic handgrip before and after autonomic blockade.* Clin Sci 64:593, 1983.

3. HASKELL, WL, SAVIN, WM, SCHROEDER, JS, ET AL: *Cardiovascular responses to handgrip isometric exercise in patients following cardiac transplantation.* Circ Res 48(Suppl I):156, 1981.

4. MITCHELL, JH, PAYNE, FC, SALTIN, B, ET AL: *The role of muscle mass in the cardiovascular response to static contractions.* J Physiol 309:45, 1980.

5. PEREZ-GONZALES, JF, SCHILLER, NB, AND PARMLEY, WW: *Direct and non-invasive evaluation of the cardiovascular response to isometric exercise.* Circ Res 48(Suppl I):138, 1981.

6. KRAYENBUEHL, HP, GRIMM, J, TURINA, M, ET AL: *Assessment of left ventricular function in aortic valve disease by isometric exercise.* Circ Res 48(Suppl I):149, 1981.

7. WOHL, AJ, LEWIS, HR, CAMPBELL, W, ET AL: *Cardiovascular function during early recovery from acute myocardial infarction.* Circulation 56:931, 1977.

8. ATKINS, JM, MATTHEWS, OA, BLOMQVIST, CG, ET AL: *Incidence of arrhythmias induced by isometric and dynamic exercise.* Br Heart J 37:465, 1976.

9. DEBUSK, RF, VALDEZ, R, HOUSTON, N, ET AL: *Cardiovascular responses to dynamic and static effort soon after myocardial infarction: Application to occupational work assessment.* Circulation 58:368, 1978.

10. BLOMQVIST, CG, LEWIS, SF, TAYLOR, WF, ET AL: *Similarity of the hemodynamic responses to static and dynamic exercise of small muscle groups.* Circ Res 48(Suppl I):87, 1981.

11. LEWIS, SF, TAYLOR, WF, GRAHAM, RM, ET AL: *Cardiovascular responses to exercise as functions of absolute and relative work load.* J Appl Physiol: Respirat Environ Exercise Physiol 54(5):1314, 1983.

12. WAHREN, J AND BYGDEMAN, S: *Onset of angina pectoris in relation to circulatory adaptation during arm and leg exercise.* Circulation 44:432, 1971.

13. SHAW, DJ, CRAWFORD, MH, KARLINER, JS, ET AL: *Arm-crank ergometry: A new method for the evaluation of coronary artery disease.* Am J Cardiol 33:801, 1974.

14. CLAUSEN, JP AND TRAP-JENSEN, J: *Heart rate and arterial blood pressure during exercise in patients with angina pectoris: Effects of training and nitroglycerin.* Circulation 53:436, 1976.

15. SCHWADE, J, BLOMQVIST, CG, AND SHAPIRO, W: *A comparison of the response to arm and leg work in patients with ischemic heart disease.* Am Heart J 94:203, 1977.

16. LAZARUS, B, CULLINANE, E, AND THOMPSON, PD: *Comparison of the results and reproducibility of arm and leg exercise tests in men with angina pectoris.* Am J Cardiol 47:1075, 1981.

17. BEVEGARD, S, FREYSCHUSS, U, AND STRANDELL, T: *Circulatory adaptation to arm and leg exercise in supine and sitting positions.* J Appl Physiol 21:37, 1966.

18. KILBOM, Å AND PERSSON, J: *Cardiovascular response to combined dynamic and static exercise.* Circ Res 48(Suppl I):93, 1981.

19. KERBER, RE, MILLER, RA, AND NAJJAR, SM: *Myocardial ischemic effects of isometric, dynamic and combined exercise in coronary artery disease.* Chest 67:388, 1975.

20. BLOMQVIST, CG AND LEWIS, SF: *Physiological effects of training: General circulatory adjustments.* In COHEN, LS, MOCK, MB, AND RINGQVIST, I (EDS): *Physical Conditioning and Cardiovascular Rehabilitation.* John Wiley & Sons, New York, 1981, pp 57–76.

21. BLOMQVIST, CG AND SALTIN, B: *Cardiovascular adaptations to physical training.* Ann Rev Physiol 45:169, 1983.

22. HELLERSTEIN, HK AND FRANKLIN, BA: *Exercise testing and prescription.* In WENGER, NK AND HELLERSTEIN, HK (EDS): *Rehabilitation of the Coronary Patient,* ed 2. John Wiley & Sons, New York, 1984, pp 197–284.

23. CLAUSEN, JP, TRAP-JENSEN, J, AND LASSEN, NA: *The effects of training on the heart rate during arm and leg exercise.* Scand J Clin Lab Invest 26:295, 1970.

24. CLAUSEN, JP, KLAUSEN, K, RASMUSSEN, B, ET AL: *Central and peripheral circulatory changes after training of the arms or legs.* Am J Physiol 225:675, 1973.

25. THOMPSON, PD, CULLINANE, E, LAZARUS, B, ET AL: *Effects of exercise training on the untrained limb. Exercise performance of men with angina pectoris.* Am J Cardiol 48:844, 1981.

26. DAVIES, CTM AND SARGEANT, AJ: *Effects of training on the physiological responses to one- and two-leg work.* J Appl Physiol 38:377, 1975.
27. SALTIN, B, NAZAR, K, COSTILL, DL, ET AL: *The nature of the training response: Peripheral and central adaptations to one-legged exericse.* Acta Physiol Scand 96:289, 1976.
28. GAFFNEY, FA, GRIMBY, G, DANNESKIOLD-SAMSØE, B, ET AL: *Adaptation to peripheral muscle training.* Scand J Rehab Med 13:11, 1981.
29. SCHEUER, J AND TIPTON, CM: *Cardiovascular adaptations to physical training.* Ann Rev Physiol 39:221, 1977.

Cardiac Rehabilitation:
Current Status
and Future Possibilities

John Naughton, M.D.

Cardiac rehabilitation is a process of continuing, comprehensive patient care designed to restore a cardiac patient to optimal overall health status and to maintain that status once achieved. The process begins with the identifiable onset of illness or of overt cardiovascular symptoms. By necessity, the process is inter- and multi-disciplinary inasmuch as a successful rehabilitation effort is explicitly defined in terms of vocational and avocational pursuit. To achieve a positive vocational and/or avocational result the process must involve medical, physiologic, psychologic, and sociologic restoration. The level of restoration may be comparable to that enjoyed before the cardiac event, or it may be to a new level compatible with the patient's cardiovascular reserve. In the latter circumstance, the new level may be lower or higher than that which existed before the illness.

Since World War II there have been many significant contributions to the understanding and implementation of cardiac rehabilitation. Each of these contributions has enhanced the ability to define better a patient's potentials and limitations for physical effort. Of all reported advances, three are uniquely identified with the cardiac rehabilitation process. These are patient-spouse education, exercise testing, and physical reconditioning programs. This chapter summarizes the current status of exercise testing and physical conditioning programs and indicates their applications to clinical medicine in the years ahead.

EXERCISE TESTING

General Principles

Graded, multistage exercise testing is currently used to screen patients with probable heart disease, to evaluate cardiac patients' potentials and limitations for work and/or physical activity, and to determine the effectiveness of various therapeutic interventions. A number of methods have been described using instruments such as treadmills, stationary bicycle ergometers, and steps. For the study of cardiac patients it is now accepted that: (1) a testing procedure should have several thresholds of workload; (2) the initial workload should be quite low in terms of an individual's anticipated aerobic threshold; (3) each workload should be maintained for a minimum of two minutes, preferably three; and (4) the testing procedure must be terminated with the onset of definable abnormality, that is, symptoms. significant electrocardiographic changes, inappropriate systolic blood pressure or heart rate response, or life-threatening arrhythmia. Because relatively few cardiac patients can reach the age-predicted peak heart rate (APHR), this end-point must be used with caution, and only for asymptomatic patients with relatively high aerobic thresholds.

Early Testing

In many centers, early testing is now applied to the study and evaluation of selected cardiac patients, especially those recovering from acute episodes of myocardial infarction. This approach is acceptable because the test can be conducted safely and because early testing helps detect patients at high risk for future events or mortality during the first year of recovery. In most centers, early testing is performed when the patient is ready for hospital discharge. Generally, this means that the procedure is performed between the second and third weeks after myocardial infarction.

Table 1 depicts a summary of the results of early exercise testing reported by five groups of clinical investigators.[1-5] The variables reported are listed in the left-hand column, and those with an established statistically significant relationship to the occurrence of future events in each study are indicated in each column by a plus (+). If the variable bore no relationship or was not reported, the appropriate space is represented by a blank, that is, the absence of a plus (+).

It can be appreciated readily that, even though comparable testing methods were employed to study the various patient populations, the variables reported reflected the particular physiologic and clinical interests of the investigating groups. Nevertheless, it is apparent that exercise testing was conducted in a large number of patients after myocardial infarction and that findings indicating further clinical problems following recovery were defined. In general, patients with a low level of physical work capacity, short exercise testing time, low peak heart rate response, low peak systolic blood pressure response, low peak double product, and/or significant ST segment depression on the exercise electrocardiogram have a worse prognosis than those without any of these testing abnormalities.

Because each groups's criteria for an abnormal response differed slightly, it is difficult to assign absolute numbers to each abnormal response. However, in general a low work capacity is defined as one of five METs or lower. A single MET is equivalent to the oxygen consumption of rest adjusted to body weight, that is, 3.5 ml O_2 per kg $\cdot$ min. An aerobic capacity of 5 METs indicates that a patient can work safely to an O_2 consumption of approximately 17.5 ml O_2 per kg $\cdot$ min. This level of work capacity is comparable to a functional cardiovascular status of Class II according to the New York Heart Association (NYHA) classification.[6]

Although it is preferable to define testing outcome in terms of work capacity or oxygen consumption, some methods only report exercising time. It is apparent that a shorter duration of exercise tolerance is usually associated with a reduced cardiovascular reserve and a poorer clinical course.

Interest has been directed toward defining the value of peak heart rate, peak systolic blood pressure, and peak double product responses during exercise in predicting prognosis. Because these variables indirectly reflect the adequacy of myocardial contractility and overall cardiovascular integrity, they should provide additional information regarding the patient's clinical

Table 1. Relationship of exercise testing results early after myocardial infarction to subsequent clinical events

	Investigators				
Finding	DeBusk et al[1]	Starling et al[2]	Swartz et al[3]	Theroux et al[4]	Fuller et al[5]
No. Patients	300	72	48	210	40
Low Work Capacity	+	+	+		
Short Exercise Time		+	+		
Low Peak Heart Rate		+			
Low Double Product	+	+			
Marked ST Segment Depression	+	+	+	+	+

status. The data depicted in Table 1 tend to confirm their importance. There is general agreement that a low peak response of one or more of these variables carries with it a poor prognosis and the likelihood of more cardiac events in the future. Of the three variables, it appears that a peak systolic blood pressure below 140 mm Hg is the most significant predictor of subsequent events, and a low peak heart rate response the next most important. Some investigators question the use of the double product (systolic blood pressure) (heart rate) (10^{-2}), because a low peak value could be related independently to a low peak systolic blood pressure or low peak heart rate response, or to both. Thus, with only the double product to evaluate, it is not possible to make as critical an analysis of the underlying cause of the abnormal adaptation to exercise.

It is apparent that a relatively large number of selected cardiac patients can be tested during the early phases of convalescence and recovery and that the results will help identify patients at relatively high or low risk for subsequent events. Thus, early exercise testing will probably be used with increased frequency in the years ahead, particularly as new interventions designed to enhance prognosis and patient well-being are developed and applied to the future care of cardiac patients.

Late Testing

In current terms, a late exercise test is one that is performed following recovery from an acute event. For patients following myocardial infarction, this late testing may be done as early as two months post-event or many months later. During the early development of cardiac rehabilitation, exercise testing was routinely performed late. However, very few reports on the value of late exercise testing in determining its prognostic value have been reported. One study, the National Exercise and Heart Disease Project (NEHDP),[7] provided such an opportunity. In this study, 651 patients who had recovered from one or more episodes of myocardial infarction performed a graded exercise test prior to their randomized assignment to an exercise training (treatment) or to a nonexercise (control) group. The patients were studied from as early as 8 weeks to as late as 156 weeks after infarction.

The NEHDP investigators evaluated variables comparable to those listed in Table 1 for the investigators who employed early testing procedures. The NEHDP patients were followed for three years. The results are tabulated in Table 2. Among the NEHDP patients, a low

Table 2. Relationship of three-year mortality to outcomes of baseline exercise test in the National Exercise and Heart Disease Project

Outcome	Total Patients	No. With Finding	No. Deaths	%	Relative Risk	p
Work Capacity	651					
METs						
<6		199	26	13.0	3.3	.0001
≥7		452	13	3.9		
Peak Systolic Pressure	641					
mm Hg						
<140		123	16	13.0	3.2	.0001
≥140		518	21	4.0		
Peak Heart Rate	651					
% APHR						
<85		301	24	7.9	1.9	.05
≥85		350	15	4.2		
ST Segment Depression	439					
Microvolts						
≥1.0		85	10	10.2	2.1	.05
<1.0		354	17	4.8		

Table 3. Relationship of mortality over three years to baseline work capacity and peak heart rate responses in the National Exercise and Heart Disease Project

	Work Capacity (METs)			
	<6		≥7	
	Peak Heart Rate (% APHR)			
	<85	>85	<85	≥85
No. With Finding	148	51	153	299
No. Deaths	18	8	6	7
% Deaths	12.1	15.1	3.9	2.4
% Deaths/Year	4.3	5.3	1.3	0.8
p	NS		NS	

level of work capacity, low peak systolic blood pressure response, low peak heart rate level, and significant ST segment depression on the electrocardiogram were each associated with statistically significant higher mortality rates. These findings indicate not only that each of these abnormal variables carries with it a higher relative risk for future mortality, but that regardless of the timing of an exercise test to the recurrence of a myocardial infarction, it is possible to identify high- and low-risk patients.

Inasmuch as a low work capacity carried with it the highest relative risk for mortality among the four outcomes studied and a peak heart rate response the lowest relative risk, the relationship of low to high work capacity and of each to peak heart rate levels was determined. The data are tabulated in Table 3. The findings indicate clearly that of the two outcome variables, that is, work capacity and heart rate, work capacity is of most significance. For patients with a work capacity in excess of 7 METs, the level of peak heart rate achieved had little influence on mortality. In those patients whose work capacity was 6 METs or less, the overall mortality was statistically significantly higher than those with work capacity of 7 METs or higher, regardless of peak heart rate response. In fact, for patients with a reduced level of work capacity there was an excess mortality, although statistically insignificant, in patients with a high compared with a low peak heart rate response. Clinically, this finding should not be surprising inasmuch as at low workloads the heart rate should normally be low and at such workloads a higher than expected heart rate response might signal the presence of latent left ventricular dysfunction.

PHYSICAL CONDITIONING PROGRAMS

Many clinical investigators have confirmed that regular physical activity performed by cardiac patients can lead to an increased level of physical working capacity, a reduction of systolic blood pressure and of heart rate at submaximal levels of work, and a reduction in myocardial oxygen requirements at rest and during the performance of submaximal work. These changes in physiologic adaptation are believed to be not only desirable but beneficial. Other effects of regular physical activity have been reported sporadically and with less consistency. Included are a reduction of serum and/or plasma lipids, especially cholesterol and triglycerides, an increase in high density lipoproteins (HDL), changes in well-being characterized by reductions in anxiety and depression and an increase in ego strength, and changes in other aspects of life-style.

As with exercise testing, there have been few large scale randomized studies performed that were designed to determine the effects of physical activity per se on selected rehabilitation outcomes. The NEHDP was designed to determine the effects of medically prescribed

Table 4. Factors studied for the effect of physical activity over one year in the National Exercise and Heart Disease Project

	Exercise Group	Control Group	p
A. Factors Affected Positively			
Resting Diastolic Blood Pressure	Decreased	Unchanged	<.03
Plasma Triglycerides	Decreased	Increased	<.04
Work Capacity	Increased	Decreased	<.0001
Body Fat	Decreased	Increased	<.0005
B. Unaffected Factors			
Resting Systolic Blood Pressure	Increased	Increased	N.S.
Plasma Cholesterol	Increased	Increased	N.S.
Plasma LDL	Increased	Increased	N.S.
Plasma HDL	Increased	Unchanged	N.S.
Smoking Cigarettes	Increased	Increased	N.S.

and supervised physical activity on a number of outcomes. Although the project followed each patient for three years, it limited its analysis of intervention effects on physiologic and metabolic outcomes to the first year of study because adherence and compliance were higher during this phase than during years two and three. The results are summarized in Table 4. The findings indicate that the exercise treatment group experienced statistically significant decreases of resting diastolic blood pressure, plasma triglycerides and body fat, and a statistically significant increase in work capacity. These outcomes are in keeping with the expected outcomes of a physical conditioning program and serve to confirm the positive effects of regularly performed exercise by patients after myocardial infarction. However, in the NEHDP the levels of resting systolic blood pressure, plasma cholesterol, plasma LDL, and plasma HDL were apparently not affected by the intervention. Over the year of study both groups of patients reported a slight increase in the number of cigarettes smoked, a finding which suggests that regular physical activity does not influence this important cardiovascular risk factor.

The effect of regular physical activity on three cardiovascular risk factors—cigarette smoking, hyperlipidemia, and a history of hypertension—and on three baseline exercise test variables related to subsequent mortality—ST segment depression, peak systolic blood pressure response, and work capacity—were also evaluated in the NEHDP.[8] Mortality was lower in patients without antecedent cardiovascular risk factors and in those with normal exercise test responses, regardless of their randomized group assignment. Mortality was lower for the exercise training patients with the three cardiovascular risk factors and two of the three exercise test abnormalities than that observed in the control patients. These findings suggest that exercise was beneficial in these subgroups. There was a slightly higher mortality rate in the physically active patients with a low peak systolic blood pressure response than in the control patients with this finding.

The effect of physical activity on subsequent mortality and morbidity is a public health issue that still awaits clarification. The effect can be determined only by a well-conducted clinical trial. During the past decade, five exercise clinical trials have been reported. Their results are summarized in Table 5. Three of the five trials reported a substantial degree of effectiveness favoring physical activity. Mortality in these three trials was reduced 37, 31, and 28 percent in patients undergoing exercise training. In one trial no differences between regular physical activity and a control group were reported. In the Ontario Heart Study, only data on fatal myocardial infarction events were reported, and the trial actually compared two levels of medically prescribed physical activity rather than contrasting physical activity with a control group. Although the differences between the two subject groups were very small, a

Table 5. Comparative effectiveness of regular physical activity in reducing mortality and nonfatal recurrent myocardial infarction among five clinical trials

| | | | Percent Effectiveness | |
Exercise Trial	No. Patients	Study Duration (mos.)	Mortality	Recurrent Infarction
NEHDP[8]	651	36	−37	+39
Sweden[9]	315	48	−31	−12
Finland[10]	370	30	−28	+62
Finland[11]	158	21	0	+50
Ontario[12]	733	48	−7.9	+5.9

− = reduced
+ = increased

slightly higher mortality was observed in the high intensity exercise patients than in the low intensity group.

Although it appears that regular physical activity might effect a major reduction in mortality and therefore prolong life following myocardial infarction, only one trial reported statistically significant differences. That trial was conducted in Finland by Kallio and coworkers[10] and used multifactorial intervention rather than exercise alone. Regular physical activity may have influenced the outcome, but there is no way to decide its value with certainty. It was of interest, however, that in this Finnish trial there was no evidence that a physical conditioning effect occurred among the patients assigned to the treatment group.

The data in Table 5 indicate that the effectiveness of regular physical activity as a therapeutic intervention apparently differs. Whereas mortality rates are generally and substantially lowered, the incidence of nonfatal myocardial infarction events is not affected. In fact, in four of the five exercise clinical trials the recurrence rate was higher in the training than in the control patients. Again the differences did not reach statistical significance. The need to better define the role of physical activity on fatal and nonfatal outcomes requires further careful study, and cardiologists must assume a moderate-to-conservative attitude when recommending physical activity as a means of reducing morbid events or of prolonging life. However, its effectiveness as an adjunct to improving physiologic performance is well established.

FUTURE POSSIBILITIES

Cardiac rehabilitation has progressed rapidly during the past generation. Cardiologists and members of the health care team have come to appreciate the importance of patient-spouse education, early ambulation, improved noninvasive assessment of a patient's limitations and potential for physical work, and of performance of regular physical activity. It is clear that each contribution applied to the comprehensive care of cardiac patients has resulted in an improved quality of life and care and demonstrated physiologic and psychologic benefits. It is less clear whether the underlying disease process or the natural history of coronary heart disease is affected significantly by the performance of regular activity throughout the remainder of a patient's lifetime.

Given the current state-of-the-art it seems warranted to encourage the continued application of exercise testing to the noninvasive evaluation of cardiac patients. These procedures can be performed safely, relatively inexpensively, and in ambulatory settings, within either a hospital or clinic. Regardless of the timing of a testing procedure to the onset of a cardiac event, meaningful information regarding a patient's current status and relative prognosis can be readily obtained. Patients at high risk for major complications or death can be identified, and appropriate diagnostic and therapeutic interventions can be prescribed more readily and rationally. In the years ahead there is a need to refine exercise testing procedures further so that more detailed information about cardiovascular adaptation to graded exercise and more accurate assessments of coronary blood flow and myocardial contractility can be made.

Although there is every reason to encourage the further development and application of exercise testing procedures, there is a need to proceed more cautiously with the expansion of physical conditioning programs. It seems reasonable and prudent to provide selected patients with the needed counseling for performing physical activity regularly and safely and to encourage every major medical center to conduct a well-organized and structured program. However, given the current state of knowledge, these programs should be presented with a very objective set of goals, and formal supervised participation should be limited to the reconditioning phase. This program will usually range from a minimum of 8 to a maximum of 16 weeks. Thereafter patients should be counselled to exercise at home and given regimens as inexpensive yet safe as possible. Clearly, an unmet challenge to today's clinical investigator is to demonstrate the value of regular physical activity in reducing the severity of coronary heart disease and in prolonging life.

ACKNOWLEDGMENTS

This manuscript includes, in part, data from the National Exercise and Heart Disease Project. The author is grateful to the collaborating investigators: University of Alabama in Birmingham: Albert Oberman, M.D., Stephen Barton, M.D., Glenda Barnes, R.N., and Del Eggert, M. Ed.; Case-Western Reserve University: Herman K. Hellerstein, M.D., Jorge Insua, M.D., Chaim Yoran, M.D., Paul Fardy, Ph.D., Barry A. Franklin, Ph.D., and Krishna P. Kaimal, M.D.; Emory University: Charles Gilbert, M.D., Daniel L. Blessing, M.D., and Barbara Johnson, R.N.; George Washington University: Patrick Gorman, M.D., Margie LaVille, R.N., and Marcia Everette, M.S.; Lankenau Hospital: Alan Barry, Ph.D., James Daly, M.D., John Satinsky, M.D., and William Marley, Ph.D.; Coordinating Center: Lawrence Shaw, A.M., Patricia Cleary, M.S., Jorge Rios, M.D., Melvin Stern, M.D., Donald Paup, Ph.D., Dan Bogaty, Patti Kavanaugh, Sara Schlesselman, M.S., John C. LaRosa, M.D., and John Naughton, M.D.

REFERENCES

1. DeBusk, RF and Haskell, W: *Symptom-limited versus heart rate limited exercise testing after myocardial infarction.* Circulation 61:738, 1980.
2. Starling, MR, Crawford, MH, Kennedy, GT, et al: *Treadmill exercise tests predischarge and six weeks post-myocardial infarction to detect abnormalities of known prognostic value.* Ann Intern Med 94:221, 1981.
3. Schwartz, KM, Turner, JD, Sheffield, LT, et al: *Limited exercise testing soon after myocardial infarction.* Ann Intern Med 94:727, 1981.
4. Theroux, P, Waters, DD, Halphen, C, et al: *Prognostic value of exercise testing soon after myocardial infarction.* N Engl J Med 301:341, 1979.
5. Fuller, CM, Raizner, AE, Verani, MS, et al: *Early post-myocardial infarction treadmill stress testing.* Ann Intern Med 94:734, 1981.
6. The Criteria Committee of the New York Heart Association, Inc: *Diseases of the Heart and Blood Vessels: Nomenclature and Criteria for Diagnosis,* ed 6. Little, Brown & Company, Boston, 1964.
7. Shaw, LW (for the Project Staff): *The National Exercise and Heart Disease Project: Effects of a prescribed supervised exercise program on mortality and cardiovascular morbidity in patients after a myocardial infarction.* Am J Cardiol 48:39, 1981.
8. Oberman, A, Cleary, P, LaRosa, JC, et al: *Changes in risk factors among participants in a long-term exercise rehabilitation program.* Adv Cardiol 31:168, 1982.

9. WILHELMSEN, L, SANNE, H, ELMFELDT, D, ET AL: *A controlled trial of physical training after myocardial infarction.* Prev Med 4:491, 1975.

10. KALLIO, V, HAMALAINEN, H, HAKKILA, J, ET AL: *Reduction in sudden death by a multifactorial intervention programme after acute myocardial infarction.* Lancet 2:1091, 1979.

11. KENTALA, E: *Physical Fitness and Feasibility of Physical Rehabilitation after Myocardial Infarction in Men of Working Age.* Ann Clin Res Suppl. 9, 1972.

12. RECHNITZER, PA, CUNNINGHAM, DA, ANDREW, GM, ET AL: *Relation of exercise to the recurrence rate of myocardial infarction in men. Ontario Exercise-Heart Collaborative Study.* Am J Cardiol 51:65, 1983.

Supervised Versus Nonsupervised Exercise Rehabilitation of Coronary Patients

Henry S. Miller, Jr., M.D.

The value of physical conditioning in patients with heart disease is not a new concept. Heberden[1] in the early 19th century and Stokes,[2] some 50 years later, discussed physical conditioning and its beneficial effect in these patients. Increased functional capacity associated with physical activity programs in middle and older aged adults, and also in patients with coronary disease, has been described by our group and many others.[3,4] Since the mid 1950s cardiologists have promoted early activity and encouraged progressive exercise following myocardial infarction and cardiovascular surgery. Hospitalization for myocardial infarction has been shortened to approximately 10 days, and for coronary artery bypass grafting to 6 to 7 days. Patients are now out of bed in the first few hospital days and caring for themselves in the hospital by 5 to 7 days. They are observed and at times monitored during personal care and other home activity routines (stair climbing and so on) during the last 2 to 3 days in the hospital. Following coronary artery bypass and valvular surgery, patients perform upper and lower extremity exercise by walking, using wall pulleys, bicycling, and doing arm cranking activities to mobilize the incisional areas and to reassure them that these exercises are safe and helpful.

These Phase I, or in-hospital, rehabilitation programs are now available in most hospitals. These programs are designed to counteract the disability associated with bed rest and to promote control of risk factors by dietary and psychologic counselling in addition to the usual medical treatment. Physicians caring for patients with cardiac disease under these circumstances began to seek ways and later to develop programs in which these patients can continue the comprehensive rehabilitation therapy begun in the hospital. These outpatient community programs gradually became more plentiful in the United States but are not available in all areas. Even though it is believed that the effectiveness of exercise and dietary and psychologic intervention is better in a supervised, comprehensive rehabilitation program, frequently the physician is asked to prescribe a safe, effective exercise program for patients in an unsupervised setting. The decision as to which patients can be safely and effectively rehabilitated in an unsupervised program, when a supervised rehabilitation program is also available, will be addressed more specifically.

In the last few years, cardiologists and other physicians treating patients with ischemic heart disease commonly have been evaluating their patients for the extent of the residual cardiac problems 10 days to 4 weeks following the event. The screening procedures have been designed primarily to identify myocardial ischemia, left ventricular dysfunction, and arrhythmias. Studies have shown that the presence of ST segment depression and angina during treadmill exercise testing is related to an increased incidence of myocardial infarction and sudden death during the first year after infarction.[5] Patients with arrhythmias that occur late in the hospital course and those who have complex ventricular ectopy are also at higher risk.[6] Exercise tolerance of 4 METs or less, a decrease or plateau in blood pressure with exercise of less than 9 METs, and inability to develop a systolic blood pressure greater than 120 mm Hg with exercise are also associated with a higher risk of myocardial infarction and sudden death in one year, as noted both in our patient population and by others.[7] Congestive failure, as evidenced by the presence of an S_3 gallop, rales, edema, and cardiomegaly on physical examination, suggests significant myocardial damage associated with infarction. Schwartz and Wolfe suggested that prolongation of QT interval is a predictor of sudden death following myocardial infarction.[8] Electrocardiographic findings of conduction defects, particularly trifascicular block, necessitate careful evaluation of medications and possibly the use of a pacemaker to prevent sudden cardiac events.

Simple evaluative procedures can detect the majority of these problems and allow the physician to determine which patients will be more likely to experience sudden death or coronary occlusive events within the year. Observation of the patient while doing daily living activities, with telemetry monitoring, treadmill exercise testing, echocardiography, Holter monitoring, and radioisotopic studies with and without exercise, has provided the information necessary to determine the need for invasive studies. From all these investigations, the need for early intervention with surgical and/or medical therapy can be decided.

SUPERVISED VERSUS UNSUPERVISED PROGRAMS: PATIENT EVALUATION

Following this initial evaluation, which is designed for therapeutic intervention, all subjects entering a cardiac rehabilitation program need a more comprehensive evaluation to determine their total rehabilitative needs. The aforementioned screening procedures include an exercise test on which an exercise prescription can be based. Dietary therapy is based on the lipid profile, height and weight, percent body fat, and a 7-day food diary and food preference chart. With these data, the nutritionist can instruct the patient and the patient's spouse in proper eating and nutritional habits and in the foods to be used to produce the proper weight and lipid control. Psychologic testing also is important to determine the patient's daily stresses. Identifying and discussing the psychologic problems have improved the patient's and family's understanding of the importance of these factors in coronary artery disease control. The association of psychologic stress with syncope and sudden death is seemingly rare but has been described.[9] Even for patients who refuse psychologic therapy for their specific problems, recognizing the fact that they are present has helped to structure their rehabilitation program. Having the patient associate with other patients who are not depressed or not anxious, if that happens to be the patient's problem, and with those who will give them encouragement and psychologic support is frequently of great benefit.

The decision as to whether a patient should be in a supervised or unsupervised exercise program must include the need for all phases of rehabilitation. Physical activities are the means used to improve functional capacity. Patients are very encouraged as they see improvement in their activity level, decrease in amount of angina with daily activities, and a slower heart rate after climbing stairs. However, the need for weight loss in the obese cardiac patient, the need for group support for patients with psychologic problems, the need for group therapy in a stop smoking program, and the need for group encouragement to increase the compliance in the exercise phase of the program should all be considered.

It is essential to provide explicit instruction for a specific aerobic activity program including exercise tehniques, proper warm-up and cool-down activities, and stretching. The ability of patients to monitor their pulse rate and to perceive exertional signs and symptoms, such as a feeling of fatigue or shortness of breath or angina that occurs at a safe or therapeutic activity level, is needed to maximize the safety of their exercise routine. The exercise intensity level, duration of each exercise session, frequency as to times per day and days per week, have to be assessed individually. To evaluate the patient's personal exercise prescription, having them exercise under supervision for four or five sessions allows modification of the routine if necessary. During this time, the patients can become familiar with the intensities and duration of different activities that will produce and maintain the proper heart rate.

In our unsupervised program, patients attend six supervised sessions following their testing and evaluation. During this time, their exercise prescription is appropriately established and modified, if necessary. They appear very comfortable about their ability to control activity levels within the heart rate range prescribed. They return once each month for three months and then every two months for one year. Unfortunately, only two of twenty patients appropriately adhered to the program for more than three months, even though attempts were made to have them record their heart rates, exercise time, exercise distances, and frequency. The two patients that did comply, however, improved their maximum capacity and other physiologic changes similar to those in a supervised program. In a compliant group of patients who have the ability to exercise at a moderate level without undue fear of cardiac events that might hamper their exercise routine, the physiologic improvement should be equally good in a supervised or an unsupervised program.

Regulation of the intensity of exercise in patients with ischemic heart disease can frequently be a problem. In patients who seem to deny that they have had a myocardial infarction because of lack of pain or limitation, it is more difficult to control the intensity of exercise. In contrast, patients who are depressed and are concerned about sudden events that may cause reinfarction or death are very hard to motivate to a level of activity that is adequate. Both types of patients probably should be in a supervised program at least longer than the initial training period. A minimum of three to six months is usually needed to educate them to the intensity level they can safely accomplish and to give them and the physician an adequate opportunity to determine whether proper intensity, duration, and frequency are practiced and improvement is accomplished. This approach encourages underachievers to exercise a bit harder in order to accomplish what they wish to accomplish. It also proves to overachievers that improvement can be made in physical capacity without an all-out pace from the beginning. The attention required by the staff in our program to these two types of patients is about equal, possibly more with those who tend to believe we are unnecessarily restricting their activity, even when the exercise heart rate restrictions are established by worrisome ischemic electrocardiographic changes. Again, psychologic testing has proved to be very valuable in identifying these patients if they are not obvious from general observation.

SUPERVISED VERSUS UNSUPERVISED PROGRAMS: RELATIVE SAFETY

As has been noted by others,[10,11] the frequency of cardiac arrest in supervised cardiac rehabilitation programs has been relatively small. The reports to date have noted that those patients who have cardiac arrest in the supervised programs are almost always successfully resuscitated. We have had four such events from the spring of 1975 to the fall of 1983, with approximately 150 patients in attendance at each session during the last five years; and all four have been resuscitated. All have returned to the program following recovery from their event. One subsequently died from a sudden arrhythmia, some five months later. The other three have continued in the Cardiac Fitness Program, a maintenance program that is available beyond the Phase III Rehabilitation Program. All had been in the program more than one year after a myocardial infarction, except for one who was at five months. This information is in keeping with data reported by Haskell in which 84 percent of patients who arrested were resuscitated successfully.[11] The number of arrests per patient hour of exercise was 1 per 32,000 in his study, which compares with approximately 1 per 33,500 patient hours in our program. In contrast, eight other patients died during the time they were enrolled in our cardiac rehabilitation program or cardiac fitness program. Two were identified as having new infarctions, and both died in cardiogenic shock. The other six were unobserved deaths, but none of the patients was apparently engaged in physical activity when the infarction or death occurred. The circumstances under which they were found led us to believe that the deaths were probably due to sudden arrhythmias.

Except for the four patients we resuscitated, it is difficult to know whether there would have been any difference in the number of sudden deaths occurring during supervised or unsupervised exercise. However, supervision has provided us with recognition of arrhythmias, change in blood pressure associated with exercise, and change in degree of angina, dyspnea, and fatigue with specific activity levels. This recognition has allowed investigation of these problems with appropriate studies to determine changes in the myocardial function or coronary anatomy. It is difficult to say whether instruction to the patients prior to entering an unsupervised program could account for the same recognition of symptoms and signs. Intensive screening of patients before discharge from the hospital or in the early postdischarge period following myocardial infarction would seem to be the best mechanism to detect those individuals who are more prone to sudden death. Careful evaluation of the patients throughout the rehabilitation program, whether supervised or unsupervised, is essential. In our supervised program, the patients are re-evaluated at 3, 6, and 12 months. At those times, many problems are suspected, if not accurately diagnosed. Further diagnostic studies can then be accomplished and corrective therapy begun. The same frequency of testing should obviously be available in an unsupervised program.

SUPERVISED VERSUS UNSUPERVISED PROGRAMS: COST OF COMMUNITY PROGRAMS

As noted, supervised rehabilitation programs, whether monitored in a hospital or supervised by personnel in a university, college, YMCA, Jewish Community Center, private dedicated facility, health club facility, and so on, are not available in all areas. In North Carolina, a system of comprehensive multiphasic rehabilitation programs applicable to towns of modest-to-large size has been developed. Obviously, these programs are not located in every town, but they are operational in 16 cities in the state at present. None has continuous telemetry or hardwire monitoring of patients. Most meet once a day, before the work day begins, on a 3 day per week schedule. Patients are referred to the program by their physicians at 3 to 6 weeks following myocardial infarction or coronary artery bypass surgery. The physicians send a hospital summary and appropriate laboratory and office records. The average stay of patients in the program is 6 to 12 months. Patient evaluation includes exercise testing, the usual blood screening tests including lipid profile, anthropometric measurements to determine body fat, and nutritional and psychologic evaluations as noted previously. The vocational counselor consults with the patient and evaluates the patient's job as to physical work requirements, assessing his ability to return to the same job, with or without modifications. The cost of the program varies throughout the state, but rehabilitation therapy sessions range from $1000 to $1500 for patients attending three exercise sessions per week for one year. Except for membership dues and activity charges at an exercise facility, there should be no other cost for an unsupervised program after the evaluation and instruction period. The cost of this instruction period depends on the degree of rehabilitative evaluation and therapy. The laboratory tests including resting and exercise electrocardiograms with oxygen uptake measurements, pulmonary function studies, routine blood tests including lipid profile, nutritional evaluation and therapy, and psychologic evaluation and advice, plus five or six orientation sessions in our cardiac rehabilitation program, cost approximately $450. The graded exercise test with oxygen uptake and exercise prescription instruction costs about $200, and $240 if laboratory studies are included. These costs are the same in either program.

Followup evaluation should be established in the unsupervised programs. Seeing the patient for the purpose of encouragement, preferably in an area where the exercise routine can be carried out with supervision every 4 to 6 weeks, is helpful in maintaining the proper exercise intensity. If necessary, the warm-up and cool-down activities can be improved, body weight assessed, and blood collected for lipid evaluation. In our initial experience with such programs 6 years ago, compliance was not good. Perhaps 6 years later, the national physical fitness trend will have changed the attitude of the unsupervised patient to one of increased compliance.

The cost seems insignificant if the patient has an increased risk of sudden death and needs supervision to detect changes in arrhythmia patterns, ischemic symptoms, and left ventricular functional status that could modify therapy and prevent sudden events. Is the cost truly measurable if one includes not only the safety but the overall benefit of the program? How much does the camaraderie and the assurance of a supervising staff add to a person's psychologic security and reduce stress concerning the disease? How much does the constant instruction and reminders from a nutritionist improve one's dietary habits and weight control? Is the patient likely to return to work as quickly in the unsupervised setting as with encouragement from a vocational counselor, ending the sick leave much sooner? These questions are unanswerable generally but frequently can be answered for an individual patient. The degree of disease, risk of sudden events, nutritional and psychologic problems all determine the justification of cost. The prevention of a hospitalization for a patient with known heart disease will more than offset the cost of all evaluation and therapy sessions for one year in many locations in the United States.

A less expensive mechanism has been established for patients to remain under partial supervision for an extended period of time after they have completed our cardiac rehabilitation program. This maintenance program, labeled the Cardiac Fitness Program, is one in which patients can be placed following 6 to 12 months in a cardiac rehabilitation program if they elect to do so. Patients in the rehabilitation program who are hospitalized for coronary artery bypass surgery or myocardial infarction are placed in the Cardiac Fitness Program 3 months after returning to the rehabilitation program. With their previous instruction, this has been an adequate period to evaluate and re-establish the exercise and other therapeutic needs and to minimize the overall cost. Most patients can afford the charge of $300 to $350 a year for approximately 140 exercise sessions. In this setting, exercise personnel and emergency equipment are available. The patients exercise at the same time in an adjacent location or with the more advanced cardiac rehabilitation patients. This program serves as a constant reminder that coronary artery disease does not disappear with coronary artery bypass surgery or when pain ceases following an infarction and that one must continue to modify life-style if the improvement attained with rehabilitation is to continue. This type of exercise can also be done in an unsupervised setting and is the case for 60 to 65 percent of our patients. Upon completion of the rehabilitation program, precise compliance to exercise routines and other rehabilitative needs in this group is unknown; but it is hoped that they are interested enough to continue with all they have learned. Perhaps if the patient has not been influenced to practice secondary prevention in a one-year period, he or she will not be likely to do so.

SUPERVISED VERSUS UNSUPERVISED PROGRAMS: GUIDELINES

As we found in 1981,[12] it was difficult to formulate definite recommendations for patients who could safely exercise in an unsupervised setting. Rehabilitative needs other than physical deconditioning must be considered when determining whether a patient can obtain all appropriate care without supervision.

The types of patients that are presently being referred to cardiac rehabilitation programs have changed as these programs have proven their value and safety to physicians who care for patients with ischemic and valvular heart disease. We now see many patients who have inoperable coronary artery occlusive disease and/or poor left ventricular function and also patients who have done poorly after surgery or who have had graft closure owing to ongoing disease in the coronary arteries following grafting. The potential risk and problems associated with improving the physical status in these patients are greater than those we experienced between 1975 and 1979. Most of the patients have had post-event evaluations and medical and surgical therapeutic interventions that seemed appropriate. Many have been therapeutic failures because of the complications of ischemic coronary disease, and this has increased the number of patients that are not suitable for unsupervised rehabilitative programs.

Perhaps the patients with uncomplicated myocardial infarction are being selected out by their personal physicians and instructed in unsupervised home programs. In patients following myocardial infarction, Savin and coworkers[13] noted improvement in aerobic activity from resuming daily activities in the absence of a prescribed exercise program. If these patients are tested at 3 months after myocardial infarction, their improvement is significant and the need for physical rehabilitation may not be apparent. The attending physician often disregards the need for other rehabilitative needs and does not refer the patient for additional care. Nonetheless, one should assess the patients in a comprehensive manner to determine their rehabilitative needs and the ability to respond in an unsupervised setting.

Patients should exercise in a medically supervised setting if they have one or more of the conditions listed below. In most situations, the length of time they remain in a supervised program will be determined by their rehabilitative needs and their ability to properly monitor their exercise heart rate and rhythm and control their symptoms.

A. Abnormal hemodynamic response to exercise and left ventricular dysfunction.
   1. Decrease or inappropriate rise in blood pressure with increased exercise.
   2. Inability to attain a blood pressure of greater than 120 mm Hg systolic.
   3. Presence of an ejection fraction of less than 40 percent.
   4. Cardiomegaly and/or the presence of an S_3 gallop and other signs of heart failure.
B. Presence of angina pectoris or evidence of myocardial ischemia (ST segment depression greater than 2 mm) at a workload of less than 7 METs.
C. Electrocardiographic changes.
   1. Development of complex ventricular arrhythmias of Class III or greater: multifocal PVCs; couplets, triplets, or salvos of PVCs; ventricular tachycardia; early cycle PVCs (R-on-T phenomenon).
   2. Evidence of multiple premature atrial beats or supraventricular tachyarrhythmia with exercise.
   3. QT intervals greater than 440 msec corrected for heart rate.
   4. Development of AV block and/or bundle branch block during exercise.
D. Maximal functional capacity of less than 5 METs with or without other aforementioned conditions.
E. Historical findings.
   1. Previous episodes of ventricular or supraventricular tachyarrhythmias and survival after previous episodes of ventricular fibrillation in the absence of acute myocardial infarction at the time of or following the event.
   2. History of syncopal episodes in the presence of known ischemic heart disease.
   3. Patients with pacemakers who have an inappropriate or fixed heart rate with activity.
F. Noncardiac conditions.
   1. Uncontrolled hypertension with exercise.
   2. Psychologic problems that make compliance unlikely, for example, anxiety, depression, and denial.
   3. Arthritic or other orthopedic problems necessitating special exercise requirements.
   4. Need for temporary supervision until condition is adequately managed.
      a. Inability to self-monitor heart rate, degree of fatigue, dyspnea, or angina during exercise.
      b. Hyperlipidemia and/or obesity.
      c. Diabetes mellitus.

This list is not all-inclusive but should serve as a guideline for recommendations for patients entering a rehabilitation program. Those that are free of these problems during testing and have the appropriate personality and motivation to be compliant with recommendations for exercise and diet can maintain a good rehabilitation program without supervision. As noted, re-evaluation of their program and testing at 3, 6, and 12 months, as is practiced in many supervised programs, should ensure better safety and compliance of the patient.

Unfortunately, many high-risk patients do not have a supervised rehabilitation program available. These patients need careful screening for obvious problems that will lead to greater likelihood of disabling angina, re-infarction, or sudden death during the first year following their event. The exercise prescription in these individuals should be very carefully calculated, considering not only the pulse rate and rhythm, blood pressure, and ischemic response to exercise testing, but the presence or absence of left ventricular failure, even if manifested only by the development of an S_3 sound or minimal lung rales with exercise.

In all exercise programs, the first 4 to 8 weeks should be slowly progressive without an attempt to maintain a calculated exercise heart rate of 60 to 85 percent. Peripheral deconditioning in this group will usually not allow the patient to tolerate this exercise intensity, even when the heart has minimal functional impairment. Even a lower percentage of the calculated symptom-limited heart rate for the high-risk patient will increase safety, decrease overall fatigue, and encourage the patient to be more compliant in the initial exercise program. To avoid undue fatigue in patients at high risk, it may be necessary to modify the usual activity program, beginning with 10-minute exercise periods 2 to 3 times a day for the first week, and increasing to 15 minutes twice a day for a week before the patient returns to work. The regimen is then changed to 20 minutes of exercise once daily, 5 days per week. Thereafter, 5 minutes is added to each exercise period each week or two, until approximately 30 to 40 minutes of sustained exercise can be tolerated 3 to 4 days a week. The patient should always be instructed in warm-up and cool-down activities and stretching exercises to minimize muscle soreness and joint stiffness. All programs have to be individualized. Whether the intensity and duration are too great can be observed by exercising with the patients and/or monitoring their cardiovascular and symptomatic responses during and after exercise. The frequency of exercise required depends on the intensity and duration plus other factors, such as musculoskeletal status and available time.

The less the intensity, the more frequent the exercise should be performed to attain a training effect, unless a prolonged duration of effort is tolerated. In an unsupervised home program, intermittent exercise, suggested by many exercise physiologists, is a method to reduce undue fatigue in an extremely deconditioned patient. Repetitions interrupted by rest, for example, two minutes of exercise, one minute of rest, or five minutes of exercise, two minutes of rest, and so on, can be better tolerated than sustained exercise in these patients.

Controlled studies are necessary to determine which patients should be supervised, when they should progress from a supervised to an unsupervised program, by whom and how they should be supervised, or even if supervision is required. We currently believe that supervised rehabilitation is generally appropriate and we use those previously cited conditions to make a decision regarding unsupervised exercise. The medical condition and all rehabilitative needs of the patient should be the primary determinants used to answer the question—to supervise or not to supervise?

REFERENCES

1. HEBERDEN, W: *Commentaries on the History and Cure of Diseases.* T. Payne, London, 1802.
2. STOKES, W: *Diseases of the Heart and Aorta.* Hodges and Smith, Dublin, 1854.
3. CLAUSEN, JP: *Circulatory adjustments to dynamic exercise and effect of physical training in normal subjects and in patients with coronary artery disease.* Prog Cardiovasc Dis 18:459, 1976.

4. REDWOOD, DR, ROSING, DR, AND EPSTEIN, SE: *Circulatory and symptomatic effects of physical training in patients with coronary artery disease and angina pectoris.* N Engl J Med 286:959, 1972.

5. THEROUX, P, WATERS, DD, HALPHEN, C, ET AL: *Prognostic value of exercise testing soon after myocardial infarction.* N Engl J Med 301:341, 1979.

6. VISMARA, LA, ANDERSON, EA, AND MASON, DT: *Relation of ventricular arrhythmias in the late hospital phase of acute myocardial infarction to sudden death after hospital discharge.* Am J Med 59:6, 1975.

7. BRUCE, RA, DE ROUEN, T, PETERSON, DR, ET AL: *Non-invasive predictors of sudden cardiac death in men with coronary heart disease: Predictive value of maximal stress testing.* Am J Cardiol 39:833, 1977.

8. SCHWARTZ, PJ AND WOLFE, S: *QT interval prolongation as predictor of sudden death in patients with myocardial infarction.* Circulation 57:1074, 1978.

9. ENGEL, GL: *Psychologic stress, vasodepressor (vasovagal) syncope, and sudden death.* Ann Intern Med 89:403, 1978.

10. MEAD, WF, PYFER, HR, TROMBOLD, JC, ET AL: *Successful resuscitation of two near simultaneous cases of cardiac arrest with a review of fifteen cases occurring during supervised exercise.* Circulation 53:187, 1976.

11. HASKELL, WL: *Cardiovascular complications during exercise training of cardiac patients.* Circulation 57:920, 1978.

12. WILLIAMS, RS, MILLER, HS, KOISCH, FP, ET AL: *Guidelines for unsupervised exercise in patients with ischemic heart disease.* J Car Rehab 1,3:213, 1981.

13. SAVIN, WM, DE BUSK, RF, HOUSTON, N, ET AL: *Spontaneous improvement in aerobic capacity between 3 and 11 weeks after myocardial infarction.* Am J Cardiol 45:391, 1980.

Exercise Testing and Training of the Elderly Patient

Ronald J. Landin, M.D., Thomas J. Linnemeier, M.D., Donald A. Rothbaum, M.D., Jane Chappelear, B.S., and R. Joe Noble, M.D.

Aging is a complex phenomenon, and the mechanism of the diminished effort tolerance attendant with the aging process has proven elusive. Is loss of function the result of a sedentary lifestyle, an incipient disease, or an effect of aging per se?[1,2]

That the first factor—inactivity—is of paramount importance is suggested by anecdotal accounts of supreme effort expenditure in well-conditioned elderly people. For instance, in the recent Senior Classic held in Indianapolis, 514 individuals over the age of 55 competed in track and field events, bicycling, swimming, and other sports. Figure 1 captures an 81-year-old man winning at hurdles, with a time of 19.79 seconds. A 67-year-old woman set a new world record at high jump for her age group; and an 81-year-old man set a new record of 35.34 seconds for the 200 meter dash. Less extreme examples of excellent mental and physical conditioning are common in aged individuals.

Perhaps even more supportive of the role of inactivity in explaining some of the loss of effort tolerance in the elderly has been the experience of rehabilitation programs for the very inactive, institutionalized elderly population. Figure 2 illustrates a calisthenic and stretching exercise program that has been initiated in a nursing home in our city; and Figure 3 depicts a 92-year-old patient with known coronary artery disease and prior myocardial infarction, complicated by chronic atrial fibrillation with a slow ventricular response, who is now active, alert, completely functional, and contributing importantly to the society of the elderly in our city—related in large part to an exercise program.

Controlled analyses of physical rehabilitation efforts in institutionalized patients indicate improved cardiovascular performance, strength, and overall activity and self care, as a result of participation in exercise programs of light to moderate intensity.[3,4]

Though anecdotal, there are enough examples of happy, functional, active, exercising senior citizens to suggest that the medical profession should have much more intense interest in exercise testing and training of elderly patients.

This chapter will review the effects of aging on the musculoskeletal, respiratory, and cardiovascular systems. Several objective analyses of the effect of exercise in impeding deterioration in these organ system functions in the elderly are now available, and these studies will be reviewed as well. Certainly much scientific work remains to be accomplished, yet must we await this information before encouraging our elderly patients to be more physically active? We think not. Enough information is currently available to encourage our healthy, elderly patients to be much more physically active. In this chapter we will also present examples of exercise programs prescribed for the elderly.

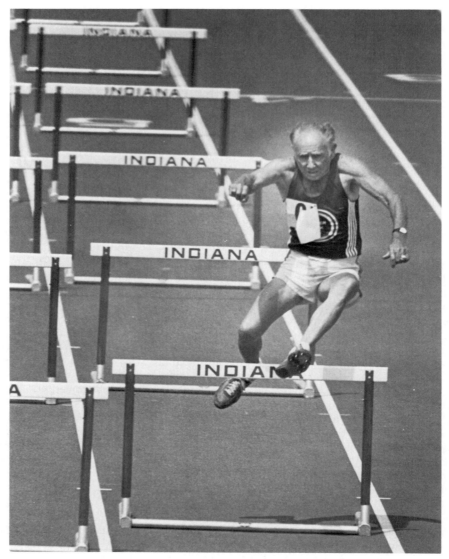

Figure 1. Participant in Senior Classic, Indianapolis, Indiana. See text for additional information. (Photograph kindly provided by Mr. Gregory J. Griffo, Indianapolis Star and News, Indianapolis, Indiana.)

EFFECTS OF AGING ON PHYSIOLOGIC FUNCTION

Biogerontologists have long known that, after maturity, function declines with advancing age. Specifically, the functional capacity of most organ systems declines at a rate of approximately 0.75 to 1.0 percent per year from a peak in function at approximately age 30.[5]

Thus, overall work capacity declines approximately 30 percent over the 40-year interval from age 30 to age 70.[6,7] Muscle strength and muscle mass decrease to the same degree.[6,8,9]

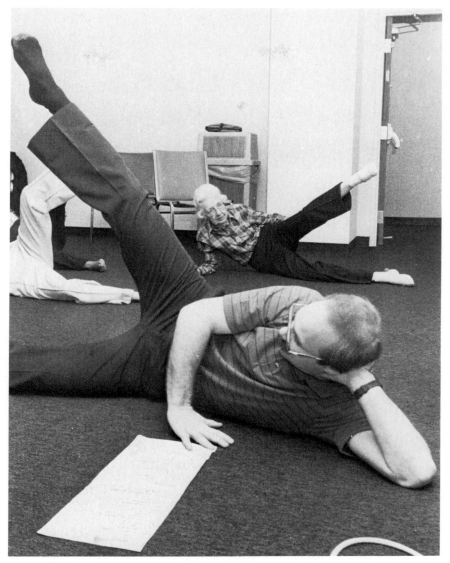

Figure 2. Exercise program for residents of a nursing home. (Photograph kindly provided by Mr. William Oates, Indianapolis Star and News, Indianapolis, Indiana.)

Cardiac output, maximum heart rate, and respiratory vital capacity show a similar trend.[6,10-14] Females have lost 30 percent of their bone mass by age 70, whereas males lose approximately half that amount.[6,15] Joint flexibility is reduced 25 to 30 percent.[16] The decrement in renal and liver function is of the same order of magnitude.[6,17]

Perhaps 50 percent of this diminished function can be attributed to disuse, and conceivably this portion of the functional decline could be prevented by physical activity.[18,19] Before exploring that potential, however, it is important to review the effects of aging on the cardiovascular, respiratory, and musculoskeletal systems.

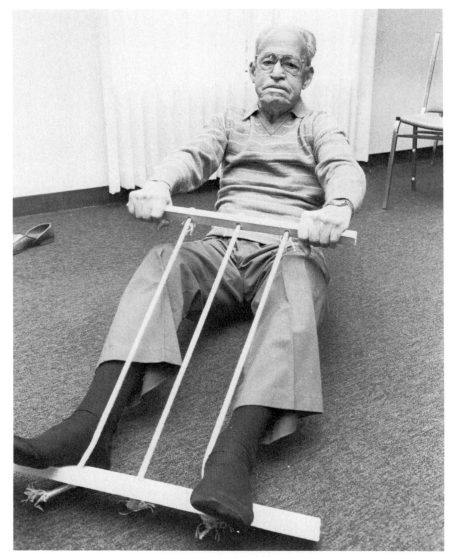

Figure 3. Elderly patient with heart disease has been helped through an exercise program. (Photograph kindly provided by Mr. William Oates, Indianapolis Star and News, Indianapolis, Indiana.)

Cardiovascular System

The cardiovascular system, more than any other organ system, illustrates the difficulty in distinguishing between the aging process, disease, and disuse in explaining declining function. From a clinical standpoint, the incidence of cardiac disease is markedly increased in the elderly population. One half of subjects aged 65 to 74 percent have evidence of heart disease.[20] Therefore, the question of cardiovascular dysfunction is of major importance in the elderly patient.

The term presbycardia has often been used to denote changes in cardiac function caused by aging. If aging changes per se are defined as those responsible for symptoms of heart failure at rest, then presbycardia is an extremely rare entity or may not actually exist at all. On the other hand, if this term is used to describe an inability to respond to imposed stress, then the term does have meaning.[21]

Structural Changes

From an anatomic standpoint, several changes occur in the heart with aging; these changes are microscopic, not macroscopic.[22] Thus, cardiomegaly is secondary to such disease processes as hypertension or coronary artery disease, rather than aging per se.

Histologically, collagen and fat deposition is increased, particularly in the interventricular septum and atrium.[22] Deposition of lipofuscin appears to be a true manifestation of myocardial aging; however, there is no correlation between lipofuscin deposition (brown atrophy) and cardiomegaly or heart failure. Although lipofuscin has no functional significance, it has been hypothesized that lipofuscin may be composed of mitochondrial fragments and that decreased cardiac efficiency with aging may indicate mitochondrial damage.[23]

Another age-associated phenomenon is myofibrilar degeneration. No functional significance has yet been attributed to this degenerative process.[24]

Anatomic changes in the endocardium, including thickening and proliferation of elastic fibers and collagen, are believed to be caused primarily by mechanical factors related to aging.[25] Cardiac valves demonstrate local endocardial thickening at the closure lines, which is believed to be mechanically induced.

The same disease processes that affect younger patients also affect older patients, but with a greater frequency in the older population. Myocardial infarction is found at necropsy in 30 percent of elderly patients, even in the absence of symptoms of ischemia; in patients with heart failure, the incidence of myocardial infarction exceeds 50 percent.[22] Cardiomyopathies, both hypertrophic and congestive, are common in the elderly.[26-28]

Two forms of cardiac pathology are relatively specific to the elderly. One is senile cardiac amyloidosis. Rare before the age of 70, the prevalence of amyloidosis increases sharply after this age.[29] Ventricular involvement is encountered in only 17 percent of patients. Cardiac dysfunction is directly related to the amount of amyloid deposition and is manifested either as atrial arrhythmias, especially atrial fibrillation, or congestive heart failure. The etiology of amyloidosis is unknown.

A second type of cardiac pathology unique to the elderly is mechanical damage to the cardiac valves, particularly the left-sided valves. The degenerative process begins as fibrosis and progresses to calcium deposition. Aortic valve abnormalities range from mild, asymptomatic sclerosis to severe stenosis with sufficient calcium deposition to immobilize the cusps. In fact, calcific aortic stenosis on a tricuspid aortic valve is the most common cause of isolated aortic stenosis after the age of 75.[30]

Mitral valvular calcification is uncommon before the age of 70, yet the frequency increases markedly after this age.[31] The calcification initially involves the annulus, and the process may result in hemodynamically significant mitral regurgitation or, very rarely, mitral stenosis owing to immobilization of valve cusps by large calcium deposits.

Calcification extending into the conducting system may cause bundle branch block or complete heart block with resultant syncope.

Functional Changes

In the absence of cardiac disease, a correlation between physiologic changes and the aforementioned histologic alterations of aging has proven difficult.[32] There is a slight decrease in the resting heart rate with aging; yet there is a greater decrease in the intrinsic heart rate, that is, the heart rate after pharmacologic denervation or after elimination of vagal and adrenergic tone.[33] Of greater functional significance is the fact that the maximal heart rate with exercise decreases with age.[32] The cause of this phenomenon is unknown, although it has been hypothesized that decreased sensitivity to catecholamine stimulation is responsible.[34] Cardiac output decreases steadily with age, by approximately one percent per year.[35] Also, the increase in cardiac output for any level of oxygen uptake or workload is less in elderly than in young individuals.[36] Maximal oxygen consumption and maximal stroke volume also decrease with age.[12,37] The decrease in stroke volume is the result of several factors—diminished contractility, increased afterload, and perhaps reduced compliance.[32]

At rest, there appears to be a slowing of diastolic filling of the ventricle owing to decreased compliance. This alteration may be the result of delayed relaxation of the myofibrils owing to decreased calcium accumulation by the sarcoplasmic reticulum.[38] Impaired diastolic left ventricular filling would be expected to result in an increase in left ventricular diastolic pressure, particularly in response to exercise or any other stress that increases the heart rate. An elevated left ventricular diastolic pressure would explain the symptom of exertional dyspnea in the elderly. The fact that the pulmonary capillary wedge pressure is higher during exercise in the elderly than in young patients supports this contention.[39]

Of equal importance to the diastolic changes are systolic alterations in left ventricular function. Impedance to left ventricular ejection is increased owing both to decreased compliance of the large arterial vessels, especially the aorta, causing an increased systolic blood pressure, and also to increased peripheral vascular resistance.[32] The rise in blood pressure at any level of exertion is greater in the older than in the younger patient. Increased impedance causes an increased afterload on the myocardium and therefore impairs left ventricular performance. Finally, myocardial contractility may be reduced in the elderly, in part as a result of decreased cardiac responsiveness to catecholamines.[40]

Although it is difficult to demonstrate significant changes in cardiac performance at rest in the elderly, these changes are more obvious when function is measured in response to stress. Under these circumstances, the combination of a blunted heart rate response to exercise, increased preload and afterload, and decreased contractility probably combine to produce the lesser increase in stroke volume, cardiac output, and maximum oxygen consumption encountered in the elderly in response to stress.[32]

The aforementioned anatomic changes related to presbycardia are rarely of functional significance. When elderly patients experience symptoms of cardiac dysfunction, they invariably have evidence of structural disease, whether ischemic, hypertensive, or degenerative calcific disease. Multiple cardiac morphologic abnormalities correlate significantly with congestive heart failure, in that at least two or more abnormal morphologic processes are found in 65 percent of elderly patients who present with clinical evidence of heart failure.[22]

On the other hand, less significant alterations in function commonly accompany the aging process, independent of disease processes. Unequivocal physiologic alterations of cardiovascular function—that is, the decrease in maximum oxygen consumption, the decrease in maximum heart rate with exercise, and the decrease in exercise stroke volume, with a resultant decrease in exercise cardiac output—occur in the elderly, in the absence of cardiovascular disease.[21,32] Inasmuch as a portion of this functional decline can be reversed or prevented by exercise training, it is possible that inactivity has contributed to the functional decline.[41]

Respiratory System

Respiratory function deteriorates with aging, as do all other organ system functions.[42] A type of emphysema develops with aging, characterized histologically by abnormalities in the alveolar membrane, with consequent increase in size of the alveoli and an overall decrease in lung tissue.[43,44] As a consequence, the actual alveolar surface area diminishes with age, resulting in a reduction in pulmonary diffusion capacity.[42]

Overall pulmonary compliance is reduced. Because of kyphoscoliosis and changes within the bony thorax, the chest wall becomes less compliant. In contrast, the lung is even more compliant, probably as a result of loss of lung tissue. Inasmuch as the chest wall compliance decreases more than the lung compliance increases, the overall compliance of the lung and thorax is reduced. As a result, older individuals must expend more work than younger patients to overcome chest wall compliance at the same level of ventilation.[45]

Total lung capacity changes little with age. The residual volume, however, more than doubles from youth to old age owing to an increase in airway resistance; therefore, vital capacity decreases.[13,46] As the patient exchanges air at high volumes (near the total lung capacity), the maximal expiratory flow is determined by the patient's physical effort.[42] Hence, maximal respiratory flow rate ($FEV_{1.0}$) and the maximal voluntary level of ventilation (MVV) are reduced with age.[47,48]

Arterial oxygen tension (P_{a02}) declines with age, probably related to a ventilation:perfusion imbalance which, in turn, may be the result of diminished ventilation of distal alveoli.[49] The expected inhomogeneity of ventilation and perfusion in different regions of the lung is augmented in old age.[50]

In summary, when one compares the respiratory capabilities of old versus young healthy subjects, the following changes are found to occur with aging: the vital capacity decreases as the residual volume increases and total lung capacity is unchanged. Overall thoracic compliance is reduced, that is, the chest is stiff. The elderly patient expends more effort in moving air for a given amount of work. Respiratory minute volume is greater, and oxygen consumption per unit of body work is less. Respiratory frequency increases and tidal volume declines.[42]

With exercise, oxygen transport in the elderly individual is limited by these alterations in chest wall compliance, ventilation:perfusion inequality, and alterations in lung volumes. The maximal oxygen intake is reduced with advanced age. The ventilatory response to exercise in older patients consists of an increase in the tidal volume. Inasmuch as dyspnea develops when the tidal volume exceeds 55 to 60 percent of the vital capacity, and because the vital capacity is reduced in the elderly, dyspnea often limits the exercise potential of older individuals.[42] Much of the dyspnea in the elderly individual probably results also from muscle weakness of the chest wall and conceivably of the diaphragm.

Musculoskeletal System

Muscles

With aging, muscles tend to lose their strength and mass and thus their effectiveness to do work. Major structural and functional changes occur at the neuromuscular junction, leading to a gradual reduction in synaptic contact and in hormonal influence. During this process, both the size and the total number of fibers recruited decrease, with a significant loss in the fast twitch, type II fibers, which are the red oxidative fibers; thus, the absolute senile muscle size is reduced by 50 percent in comparison with young adult muscle.[51] Together with the decreased recruitment of motor units, there is a reduction in strength and contractile properties of aged muscle. For instance, the muscle fibers of the proximal lower limb show a great amount of atrophy and loss of strength with advanced age.[52,53]

Because there is a loss of muscle mass with age, a loss of muscle strength follows. There is also a decrease in the intramuscular concentration of substances rich in energy. As a result, muscles lose their ability to work at maximum strength, power, and endurance. This loss of strength translates specifically into diminished isometric and dynamic strength, with a lesser loss in speed of movement. Endurance, defined as the ability to continue an activity at a given workload, decreases.

Joints

The joint is the primary anatomic determinant of the flexibility of an individual. The aging process brings a loss of stability and mobility to this structure. The four major components of a human joint are the cartilage, tendons, ligaments, and synovial fluid. Several functional and structural changes occur simultaneously in these tissues with aging.[16] Collagen fibers tighten and the membrane separating the connective tissue from other tissues thickens. As a result, the aged tissue is less responsive to mechanical stress and is less compliant.[16,54]

Enzymatic activity, cell count, and certain metabolic substrates are reduced in aged cartilage. As a consequence of these age-related changes, total joint space is reduced and the range of motion of joints inhibited, especially that of the hips and knees.[55]

The range of motion for each joint of the body is specific to that joint and its unique structure and is also relative to the amount of activity performed by that joint. Younger joints are more flexible than aged joints; athletes tend to increase flexibility in the joints specific to their sport. Furthermore, the longer an individual uses the same posture, the more one encounters a loss in the flexibility of certain joints. Joints stiffen and their range of motion decreases as a result of the wear and tear of surfaces, thickening of the joint capsule itself, waste accumulation in the joint, and the growth of osteocytes. Furthermore, the range of motion in joints is reduced after a period of inactivity.[56,57]

Bones

Bone atrophy or osteoporosis is the result of bone loss and is characterized by decreased mineral mass and an oversized medullary cavity. Bone loss progresses at a rate of about 0.75 to 1.0 percent per year for women, starting at age 30 to 35; the process begins for men at age 50 to 55.[58] For about five years after the menopause, the rate of bone mineral loss increases to about two or three percent. At this rate of progression, women can lose about 30 percent of their bone mass by age 70.

Bone strength is directly related to bone mineral mass, and decreased bone mineral density results in an increased risk of fracture in the elderly.[59,60]

Certainly several factors contribute to osteoporosis, including genetic, hormonal, nutritional, and mechanical forces. Recently, the involvement of mechanical stress on bone mineral composition has been emphasized: mechanical forces may prevent bone loss. Immobilization, weightlessness, or loss of muscle function results in bone loss. With prolonged bed rest, for instance, negative calcium balance occurs, with as much as a 39 percent mineral loss documented in a 26-week period of bed rest.[61] The reduced gravitational and muscular forces acting on bones cause a reduction in the mineral content of that bone.[62] Bone mineral composition seems to be locally controlled; and hypertrophy can occur in response to a specific mechanical stress.

EFFECTS OF EXERCISE ON REVERSING PHYSIOLOGIC DETERIORATION IN THE ELDERLY

In the preceding section we restated and detailed the conclusions of biogerontologists that function declines at a rate of approximately 0.75 percent per year after the age of 30. Perhaps 50 percent of this diminished function can be attributed to disuse; and conceivably this half of the functional decline could be prevented by physical activity.[18,19] Two lines of reasoning support the protective role of exercise in impeding the decline of function in the elderly: (1) the physiologic effect of inactivity in the normal population, and (2) the physiologic effects of exercise training on cardiovascular, respiratory, and musculoskeletal structure and function in the elderly.

Physiologic Effects of Bed Rest

Several investigators have studied the effects of bed rest on body composition and function, but by far the most comprehensive analysis is that provided by Saltin and coworkers in 1968.[63]

The cardiopulmonary function of five healthy college students was studied longitudinally, first in the control state, second, following a three-week period of absolute bed rest, and finally, after a 55-day period of intensive physical training.

With bed rest, maximal oxygen uptake fell by 20 to 46 percent (mean, 28 percent). Lung volumes and ventilatory mechanics changed little at rest, but ventilatory volume during maximal work declined significantly as a result of bed rest. A ventilation-perfusion mismatch indicated that pulmonary blood flow was less uniform. With exercise, the maximum heart rate increased and cardiac output decreased as a result of bed rest, with a decrease in stroke volume of approximately 30 percent. Peripheral resistance did not change substantially.

After the period of physical training, there was no effect on lung volumes nor ventilatory mechanics, although pulmonary blood flow was more homogeneous with respect to ventilation. Maximal oxygen uptake increased by about one third. With submaximal work, the stroke volume was higher and heart rate lower after training.

Recall the previously mentioned, separate study of bone mineralization in young men, in which six months of bed rest resulted in a 39 percent decrease in mineralization.[61]

It is of considerable interest that the deterioration in cardiopulmonary and probably musculoskeletal function and structure experienced by young, healthy men as a result of three weeks of bed rest parallels that experienced by older individuals in the process of aging 30 or 40 years.[64] The fact that these deteriorations in function can be remedied by training in the young raises the fascinating question as to whether exercise training might reverse the disuse atrophy and function of the inactive elderly.

Effects of Training on the Cardiovascular System

Studies of the effects of strenuous physical training in the elderly have shown somewhat conflicting results. At rest, heart rate, cardiac output, and blood pressure are altered little, if at all, by a training program. At submaximal levels of exercise, these parameters also change only insignificantly. However, the exercise heart rate does decelerate toward the control state more quickly after submaximal exercise in the trained, elderly subject.[7] When measured at levels of maximal exercise, short-term exercise results in little increase in exercise capacity. Prolonged training, on the other hand, has resulted in a 10 to 15 percent increase in maximal oxygen consumption, stroke volume, and cardiac output.[66-70] Interestingly, this increment in cardiac function consequent to training accounts for about one half of the 30 percent decrement anticipated with aging. The improved cardiac output results more from an increase in stroke volume than in heart rate.

In studies of the elderly athlete, the rate of decline of maximal oxygen consumption is the same as for sedentary individuals: 0.6 to 0.7 ml/kg min per year.[71] However, the initial and maximal values of oxygen consumption are higher for athletes than nonathletes. Indeed, the maximal oxygen consumption of a trained 65-year-old athlete approximates that of a sedentary 25-year-old subject.[7] The systemic blood pressure is only minimally lower for athletes than nonathletes, both at rest and with exercise, and the differences are not significant. Of importance, however, the exaggerated increase in systolic blood pressure with exercise in the elderly appears to be blunted considerably with training.

Activity performance, endurance, and ability to tolerate stress, all of which are characteristically impaired in the elderly subject, may be improved with physical training. Even training as brief as 10 weeks can result in improvement in these parameters, with an increase in aerobic capacity to a level comparable to that of subjects 10 to 20 years younger.[67]

Endurance exercise training appears to increase maximal oxygen consumption in sedentary elderly subjects, even though it does not seem to benefit previously well-conditioned elderly subjects. The improvement ranges from 0 to 38 percent, with the largest improvement measured in those patients who were sedentary at the initiation of training.[72]

Effects of Training on the Respiratory System

Inasmuch as oxygen transport depends more on cardiovascular than respiratory function, the influence of exercise training on lung volumes and flow is probably not of great importance in determining the effort tolerance of older individuals.[42,73] Studies of the response of respiratory function to exercise training in the elderly have been contradictory. No consistent responses, in terms of lung volumes, flow rates, and gas exchange have been demonstrated, although deVries observed a significant, training-induced increase in vital capacity and minute volume in elderly men.[74] In short, even though physical training may not improve respiratory function substantially, such an improvement is probably not essential to improved effort tolerance in elderly subjects.

Effects of Training on the Musculoskeletal System

There are at least two approaches to answering the question: does exercise improve muscle strength and function in the elderly? The first is to compare the muscle strength of young and old individuals involved in equivalent levels of physical exertion; the second is to evaluate any exercise-induced gains in muscle strength and function in the deconditioned elderly. Both approaches indicate that the implementation of an exercise program retards the expected deconditioning of the elderly.

For example, the strength and endurance of men approaching age 65 did not differ from that of men as young as age 22, when they were involved in equivalent work activities.[75]

DeVries found nearly a 12 percent increase in arm strength in elderly subjects involved in a 42-week exercise regimen consisting of a walk-run program with stretching exercises, but no isometric arm exertion.[74] Moritani noted an equivalent increase in muscle strength in older subjects after eight weeks of isotonic training.[9] In both of these studies, muscle girth increased little, suggesting that increased neural activation may play a more important part than muscle hypertrophy in improving strength in the older subjects. The oxygen delivered to working muscles is increased by regular exercise; and oxidative enzyme levels increase as well, to account for the greater aerobic capacity observed in older, exercising subjects.[76]

Thus, muscle strength increases in elderly persons involved in a regular exercise program related to at least two factors: an increased recruitment of motor units, approaching maximal levels in the working muscle group, and structural and metabolic changes in the muscle tissue per se.[9]

Not only does muscle strength improve as a result of exercise, but several studies indicate that a regular training program will enhance flexibility as well. For instance, Munns engaged 40 subjects whose age exceeded 65 years in a dance exercise session of one hour, three times a week, for 12 weeks and measured a significant improvement in flexion/extension of the neck, wrist, hip, knee, ankle, and lower back, and in abduction/adduction of the shoulder.[77] Similar results have been described by other investigators, whether the exercise program involved a single joint or multiple joints.[78-80] The improvement in joint flexibility as a result of a properly designed exercise program probably contributes more to the patient's sense of improved function and well-being than does the observed increase in muscle strength.

Exercise does not prevent osteoporosis. However, just as it is obvious that inactivity and disuse lead to bone demineralization, it is also apparent that physical activity and the resultant stress imposed on the bone improves bone mineralization.[81] Smith and associates[62] studied the mineralization of the midshaft of the radius in 30 elderly women, approximately half of whom participated in a chair exercise program for three years. Bone mineralization decreased in the control group but increased in the exercising subjects. The mechanism of the enhanced bone growth probably involves improved circulation in the bone and increased gravitational and muscular stress that influences the bones' cellular activity.[81]

EXERCISE PRESCRIPTION

Evaluation

Principally because of the high frequency of occult cardiac disease in the elderly, a careful cardiovascular evaluation is a prerequisite to the initiation of an exercise program. The exercise prescription will be based on a careful history, a meticulous cardiovascular examination, an electrocardiogram, and an exercise test.[82] With these modes of evaluation the physician is interested in excluding evidence of ischemic heart disease; significant rhythm disturbances, whether tachyarrhythmias or bradyarrhythmias; aortic, and to a lesser extent, mitral valve disease; significant hypertension; and myocardial disease manifested by heart failure.[83] Demonstration of any of these abnormalities either precludes an exercise program or at least dictates a substantial modification in the exercise prescription.[41]

Exercise testing may be undertaken with either a bicycle ergometer or treadmill, whichever is available and consistent with the patient's capabilities. Because a walking program will probably be included in the exercise prescription, the treadmill test seems preferable. However, if the elderly patient is incapable of performing adequately on a treadmill, the physician may improvise by recording a standard electrocardiogram during and immediately following a simple walking exercise, or even after chair exercises.

Several different protocols of exercise testing have been recommended, from which the target heart rates or MET levels may be calculated. Actually, it seems that the specific protocol is relatively unimportant, inasmuch as the objective of the test is to determine the patient's effort tolerance and the heart rate that can be achieved without cardiovascular or musculoskeletal deterioration.[84] The individual should exercise on the treadmill until 80 to 85 percent of predicted maximal heart rate is achieved, in order to document that this level of exertion can be tolerated. The patient's maximum heart rate may be calculated by the formula 220 minus age; he or she is then exercised until 80 to 85 percent of this value is achieved. However, it must be borne in mind that the maximum heart rate that an elderly person can attain may be considerably less than that calculated, because the older individual is more likely to display sinus node or autonomic dysfunction. If the patient tolerates this level of exertion, he or she would be exercised in a training program at a level designed to achieve a somewhat lesser rate.

With the exercise test, should the patient experience angina or inappropriate dyspnea or develop impressive repolarization changes on the electrocardiogram, or significant rhythm disturbances such as heart block or a complex ventricular rhythm disturbance, or should the systolic blood pressure fall more than 20 to 30 mm Hg, then an unsupervised exercise program is clearly contraindicated.[82] Instead, a more intensive evaluation of the patient's cardiovascular status is required.

Principles of Exercise

Certain modifications of an exercise program are essential for the elderly subject. An increased warm-up period is necessary, both from a cardiovascular and a musculoskeletal standpoint. Also, the time for the heart rate to return to normal after exercise is longer in the elderly than in a younger counterpart. Therefore, there should be a longer period of low-level activity or a longer rest period between exercise sessions in the elderly. Another factor that limits exercise capacity in the elderly is the decreased ability to sweat efficiently, which may lead to heat intolerance. Decreased perspiration may be the result of decreased skin blood flow (which also lowers the skin temperature in the elderly) and of atrophy of the sweat glands. Therefore, high-level physical activity may be hazardous in the elderly, although moderate exercise is extremely beneficial. Physical activity should be limited or avoided in hot or humid weather.[41]

To improve cardiovascular fitness, the exercise program should be devised to achieve a heart rate of approximately 60 to 75 percent of the maximum heart rate predicted for that age individual.[84] Also, for an effective training response, the elderly individual should exercise for at least 30 minutes three times a week, with no more than two days separating each exercise period. As the intensity of the exercise diminishes, the duration should increase; it may be necessary for the patient to divide the exercise program into two or more periods each day. A five- to ten-minute warm-up period of calisthenics or slow walking should precede the more vigorous activity. A five- to ten-minute cool-down period should follow the exercise period in order to avoid lightheadedness, syncope, or other cardiovascular complications of the exercise period. The individuals must learn to count their own pulse rate and should record the pulse rate periodically on at least one occasion during the warm-up period, on at least one occasion during the cool-down period, and every 10 to 15 minutes during the exercise period. The exercise period per se is otherwise uninterrupted and should persist for at least 20 to 30 minutes.[82,84]

Specific Prescription

The exercise prescription should be quite specific. The interested physician should refer to detailed exercise programs such as those described by deVries, Smith, and Leslie and McLure; and the physician may want to consult with a physical therapist or exercise physiologist in recommending a program for the individual patient.[6,85-87] DeVries' program consists of three exercise periods per week of a walk-jog program, preceded by stretching calisthenics. Illustrations of the warm-up stretching calisthenics are reproduced in Figures 4 and 5. Assuming that the rate of repetition is not excessive, most healthy, elderly subjects tolerate

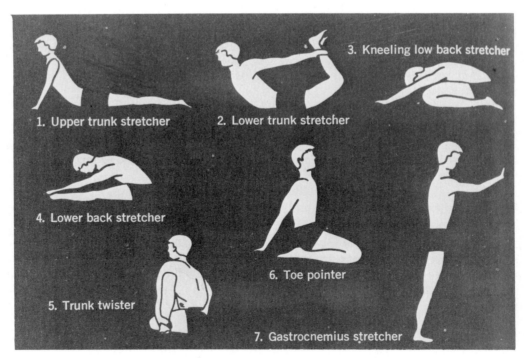

Figure 4. Stretching calisthenics for warm-up. (From deVries, HA.: Prescription of exercise for older men from telemetered exercise heart rate data. Geriatrics 26:102, 1971, with permission.)

212

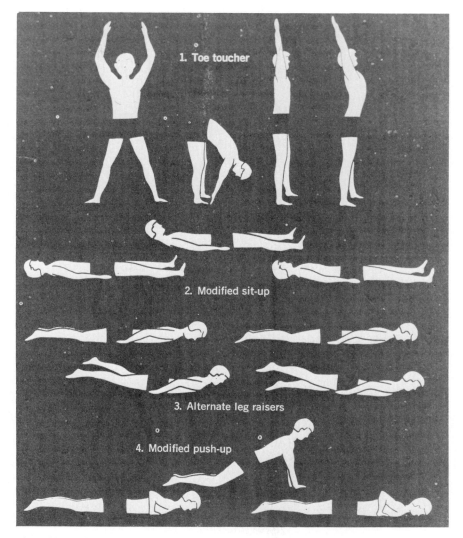

Figure 5. Stretching calisthenics for warm-up. (From deVries, H.A.: Prescription of exercise for older men from telemetered exercise heart rate data. Geriatrics 26:102, 1971, with permission.)

these exercises, which are adequate to prevent muscle stiffness and to improve flexibility. An example of the walk-jog program characterized by increments in the number of steps jogged, corresponding to decrements in number of steps walked, is reproduced in Figure 6. Such a program may prove too vigorous for some elderly patients; deVries noted an inappropriate tachycardia or actually diminished effort tolerance in a limited number of elderly subjects exercising at this level.[74]

Swimming, bicycling, and other aerobic activities, such as square dancing, may achieve precisely the same results. Because they avoid joint trauma, these activities are preferred for selected patients. Walking at 3.0 to 3.5 miles per hour may prove just as effective as jogging for an overall conditioning effect in the elderly, without the orthopedic complications associated with jogging.[62]

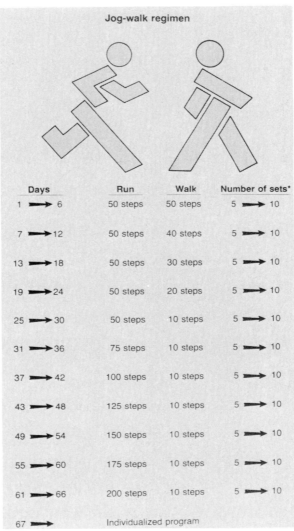

Jog-walk regimen

Days		Run	Walk	Number of sets*	
1 → 6		50 steps	50 steps	5 → 10	
7 → 12		50 steps	40 steps	5 → 10	
13 → 18		50 steps	30 steps	5 → 10	
19 → 24		50 steps	20 steps	5 → 10	
25 → 30		50 steps	10 steps	5 → 10	
31 → 36		75 steps	10 steps	5 → 10	
37 → 42		100 steps	10 steps	5 → 10	
43 → 48		125 steps	10 steps	5 → 10	
49 → 54		150 steps	10 steps	5 → 10	
55 → 60		175 steps	10 steps	5 → 10	
61 → 66		200 steps	10 steps	5 → 10	
67 →		Individualized program			

Figure 6. Jog-walk regimen (See text for discussion.) (From deVries, H.A.: Tips on prescribing exercise regimen for your older patient. Geriatrics 34:75, 1979, with permission.)

Whichever program is selected, it must be acceptable to the patient and must satisfy the aforementioned criteria of sufficient intensity to achieve 60 to 75 percent of the maximum predicted heart rate for age, and must be of sufficient duration to result in a positive training effect; it must be preceded by and followed by appropriate warm-up and cool-down periods; and it must be monitored by the patient with intermittent heart rate checks.

Finally, the elderly patient should be re-evaluated periodically by the physician to ascertain progress and determine tolerance of the prescribed program. A repeat evaluation, including an exercise test, is advisable to determine the efficacy and safety of training.

SUMMARY

As an invariable accompaniment of the aging process, cardiac function declines, that is, cardiac output, stroke volume, heart rate, and maximum oxygen consumption all decrease.

The vital capacity declines as residual volume increases, and ventilation-perfusion imbalance increases. Muscles atrophy and weaken, joints stiffen, and bones are demineralized.

Certainly the aging process per se explains a portion of this functional deterioration. Disease states also account for some deterioration. However, inasmuch as approximately one half of the deterioration in function can be prevented or reversed by an exercise training program, it would seem that disuse or inactivity is responsible for at least a portion of the functional decline characteristic of aging.

Special considerations in prescribing exercise training for the elderly include careful cardiovascular assessment; evaluation of orthopedic problems; consideration of heat intolerance; and careful attention to motivation.

The exercise prescription should be specific and tailored to the subject's individual cardiovascular status, musculoskeletal limitations, and personal goals. Walking, stretching calisthenics, and other aerobic activities, if of reasonable intensity and duration, and when preceded and followed by an appropriate warm-up and cool-down period, respectively, can result in a substantial, positive training effect in the elderly.

In response to such a training program, elderly subjects demonstrate an increase in stroke volume, cardiac output, and maximum heart rate. Respiratory function changes little, yet maximal oxygen consumption is increased. Fat may be replaced by lean muscle mass as muscle strength and endurance improve. Flexibility is improved and bone demineralization retarded or even reversed. Exercise has a tranquilizing effect on elderly subjects so that anxiety and depression may be prevented.[88] The subject develops self-respect as effort tolerance improves.

An excessively conservative attitude on the part of physicians, families, and elderly subjects has resulted in inappropriate activity limitations with a consequent decrement in effort tolerance. Elderly individuals can maintain a reasonable level of effort tolerance or can be rehabilitated to this level of activity with an appropriate exercise program. The decline in overall function expected with age can be substantially retarded. Consequently, physicians, families, and the subjects themselves should consider the potential advantages of an exercise program.

ACKNOWLEDGMENTS

The authors gratefully acknowledge the advice provided by Herbert A. deVries, Ph.D., Director, Exercise/Fitness Laboratory, Andrus Gerontology Center, University of Southern California, and Everett L. Smith, Ph.D., Directory of Biogerontology Laboratory, Department of Preventive Medicine, University of Wisconsin, Madison, Wisconsin, in the preparation of this manuscript.

REFERENCES

1. deVRIES, HA: *Physiology of exercise and aging.* In WOODRUFF, DS AND BIRREN, JE (EDS): *Scientific Perspectives and Social Issues.* Van Nostrand, New York, 1975.

2. NOBLE, RJ AND ROTHBAUM, DA: *Prologue.* In NOBLE, RJ AND ROTHBAUM, DA (EDS): *Geriatric Cardiology.* FA Davis, Philadelphia, 1981.

3. CLARK, BA, WADE, MG, MASSEY, BH, ET AL: *Response of institutionalized geriatric mental patients to a twelve-week program of regular physical activity.* J Gerontol 30:565, 1975.

4. STAMFORD, BA: *Physiological effects of training upon institutionalized geriatric men.* J Gerontol 27:451, 1972.

5. SMITH, EL: *The interaction of nature and nurture.* In SMITH, EL AND SERFASS, RC (EDS): *Exercise and Aging: The Scientific Basis.* Enslow Publishers, Hillside, New Jersey, 1981, pp 11–17.

6. SMITH, EL AND GILLIGAN, C: *Physical activity prescription for the older adult.* Sports Med 11:83, 1983.

7. SIDNEY, KH: *Cardiovascular benefits of physical activity in the exercising aged.* In SMITH, EL AND SERFASS, RC (EDS): *Exercise and Aging: The Scientific Basis.* Enslow Publishers, Hillside, New Jersey, 1981, pp 131–147.

8. FITTS, RH: *Aging and skeletal muscle.* In SMITH, EL AND SERFASS, RC (EDS): *Exercise and Aging: The Scientific Basis.* Enslow Publishers, Hillside, New Jersey, 1981, pp 31–44.

9. MORITANI, T: *Training adaptations in the muscles of older men.* In SMITH, EL AND SERFASS, RC (EDS): *Exercise and Aging: The Scientific Basis.* Enslow Publishers, Hillside, New Jersey, 1981, pp 149–166.

10. BECKLAKE, MR, FRANK, H, DAGENAIS, GR, ET AL: *Influence of age and sex on exercise cardiac output.* J Appl Physiol 20:938, 1965.

11. HARRIS, R: *The Management of Geriatric Cardiovascular Disease.* JB Lippincott, Philadelphia, 1970.

12. ASTRAND, I: *Aerobic work capacity in men and women with special reference to age.* Acta Physiol Scand 49:1, 1960.

13. JONES, RL, OVERTON, T, HAMMERLINDEL, D, ET AL: *Effects of age in regional residual volume.* J Appl Physiol: Respirat Envirn Exer Physiol 44:195, 1978.

14. NIINIMAA, V AND SHEPHARD, RJ: *Training and oxygen conductance in the elderly. I. The respiratory system.* J Gerontol 33:354, 1978.

15. SMITH, DM, KHAIRI, MRA, NORTON, J, ET AL: *Age and activity effects on rate of bone mineral loss.* J Clin Invest 58:176, 1976.

16. ADRIAN, MJ: *Flexibility in the aging adult.* In SMITH, EL AND SERFASS, RC (EDS): *Exercise and Aging: The Scientific Basis.* Enslow Publishers, Hillside, New Jersey, 1981, pp 45–57.

17. ROWE, JW, SHOCK, NW, AND DE FRONZO, RA: *The influence of age on the renal response to water deprivation in man.* Nephron 17:270, 1976.

18. DEVRIES, HA AND ADAMS, GM: *Comparison of exercise responses in old and young men. II. Ventilatory mechanics.* J Gerontol 27:349, 1972.

19. SMITH, EL: *Physical activity: The foundation of youth in aging. A synopsis of the National Conference on Fitness and Aging.* September 10–11, 1981.

20. KENNEDY, RD, ANDREWS, GR, AND CAIRD, FI: *Ischaemic heart disease in the elderly.* Br Heart J 39:1121, 1977.

21. GERSTENBLITH, G: *Congestive heart failure.* In NOBLE, RJ AND ROTHBAUM, DA (EDS): *Geriatric Cardiology.* FA Davis, Philadelphia, 1981, pp 131–144.

22. POMERANCE, A: *Cardiac pathology in the elderly.* In NOBLE, RJ AND ROTHBAUM, DA (EDS): *Geriatric Cardiology.* FA Davis, Philadelphia, 1981, pp 9–54.

23. KOOBS, DH, SCHULTZ, RL, AND JUTZY, RV: *The origin of lipofuscin and possible consequences to the myocardium.* Arch Pathol Lab Med 102:66, 1978.

24. HAUST, MD, ROWLANDS, DT, GARANCIS, JC, ET AL: *Histochemical studies on cardiac 'colloid'.* Am J Pathol 40:185, 1962.

25. MC MILLAN, JB AND LEV, M: *The aging heart. I. Endocardium.* J Gerontol 14:268, 1959.

26. BERGER, M, RETHY, C, AND GOLDBERG, E: *Unsuspected hypertrophic subaortic stenosis in the elderly diagnosed by echocardiography.* J Am Geriat Soc 27:178, 1979.

27. PENTHER, P, COUSTEAU, JP, AND GAY, J: *Some peculiar aspects of obstructive cardiomyopathy of subjects over 55 years of age (with reference to 14 cases).* Arch Mal Coeur 63:1230, 1970.

28. WHITING, RB, POWELL, WJ, DINSMORE, RE, ET AL: *Idiopathic hypertrophic subaortic stenosis in the elderly.* N Engl J Med 285:196, 1971.

29. HODKINSON, HM AND POMERANCE, A: *The clinical significance of senile cardiac amyloidosis: A prospective clinocopathological study.* Q J Med 46:381, 1977.

30. POMERANCE, A: *The pathogenesis of aortic stenosis and its relation to age.* Br Heart J 34:569, 1971.

31. POMERANCE, A, DARBY, AJ, AND HODKINSON, HM: *Valvular calcification in the elderly: Possible pathogenic factors.* J Gerontol 33:672, 1978.

32. KENNEDY, RD AND CAIRD, FI: *Physiology of aging of the heart.* In NOBLE, RJ AND ROTHBAUM, DA (EDS): *Geriatric Cardiology.* FA Davis, Philadelphia, 1981, pp 1–8.

33. JOSE, AD AND COLLISON, DL: *The normal range and determinants of the intrinsic heart rate in man.* Cardiovasc Res 4:160, 1970.

34. ROBINSON, S: Quoted by Strandell, T. In CARID, FI, DALL, JLC, AND KENNEDY, RD (EDS): *Cardiology in Old Age.* Plenum Press, New York, 1976.

35. BRANDFONBRENER, M, LANDOWNE, M, AND SHOCK, NW: *Changes in cardiac output with age.* Circulation 12:557, 1955.

36. STRANDELL, T: *Cardiac output in old age.* In CARID, FI, DALL, JLC, AND KENNEDY, RD (EDS): *Cardiology in Old Age.* Plenum Press, New York, 1976.

37. ASTRAND, PO: *Physical performance as a function of age.* JAMA 205:729, 1968.

38. FROEHLICH, JP, LAKATTA, EG, BEARD, E, ET AL: *Studies of sarcoplasmic reticulum function and contraction duration in young adult and aged rat myocardium.* J Mol Cell Cardiol 10:427, 1978.

39. GRANATH, A, JONSSON, B, AND STRANDELL, T: *Circulation in healthy old men studied by right heart catheterization at rest and during exercise in supine and sitting position.* Acta Med Scand 176:425, 1964.

40. LAKATTA, EG, GERSTENBLITH, G, ANGELL, CS, ET AL: *Diminished inotropic response of aged myocardium to catecholamines.* Circ Res 36:262, 1975.

41. WENGER, NK: *Rehabilitation of the elderly cardiac patient.* In NOBLE, RJ AND ROTHBAUM, DA (EDS): *Geriatric Cardiology.* FA Davis, Philadelphia, 1981, pp 221–230.

42. REDDAN, WG: *Respiratory system and aging.* In SMITH, EL AND SERFASS, RC (EDS): *Exercise and Aging: The Scientific Basis.* Enslow Publishers, Hillside, New Jersey, 1981, pp 89–107.

43. LIEBOW, AA: *Biochemical and structural changes in the aging lung.* In CANDER, L AND MOYER, JH (EDS): *Aging of the Lung.* Grune & Stratton, New York, 1964, pp 97–104.

44. PUMP, KK: *The aged lung.* Chest 60:571, 1971.

45. TURNER, JM, MEAD, J, AND WOHL, ME: *Elasticity of human lungs in relation to age.* J Appl Physiol 35:664, 1968.

46. STANESCU, S: *Investigations into changes of pulmonary function in the aged.* Bull Europ Physiopath Resp 15:171, 1979.

47. MORRIS, JF, KOSKI, A, AND JOHNSON, LC: *Spirometric standards for healthy non-smoking adults.* Am Rev Resp Dis 103:57, 1971.

48. STORNSTEIN, O AND VOLL, A: *New prediction formulas of ventilatory measurements: A study of normal individuals in the age group 20–59 years.* Scand J Clin Lab Invest 14:633, 1962.

49. NEUFELD, O, SMITH, J, AND GOLDMAN, S: *Arterial oxygen tension in relation to age in hospital subjects.* J Am Ger Soc 21:4, 1973.

50. WAGNER, P, LARAVUSO, R, UHL, R, ET AL: *Continuous contributions of ventilation-perfusion ratios in normal subjects breathing air and 100% O_2.* J Clin Invest 54:54, 1974.

51. CAMPBELL, JM, MC COMAS, AJ, AND PETTITO, F: *Physiological changes in aging muscles.* J Neurol Neurosurg Psychiatry 36:174, 1973.

52. FROLKIS, VV, MARTZNENKO, OA, AND ZAMOSTYAN, VP: *Aging of the neuromuscular apparatus.* Gerontology 22:244, 1976.

53. GUTMANN, E, HANZLIKOVA, V, AND VYSKOCEL, F: *Age changes in cross striated muscle of the rat.* J Physiol 216:331, 1971.

54. HALL, DA: *The Aging of Connective Tissue.* Academic Press, London, 1976.

55. BALAZS, EA: *Intercellular matrix of connective tissue.* In *Handbook of Biology of Aging.* New York, 1977, pp 222–240.

56. BUTLER, DL, GROOD, ES, NOVES, FR, ET AL: *Biomechanics of ligaments and tendons.* In *Exercise and Sport Sciences Reviews.* Philadelphia, 1979, pp 125–282.

57. TIPTON, CM, MATTHES, RD, MAYNARD, JA, ET AL: *The influence of physical activity on ligaments and tendons.* Med Sci Sports 7:165, 1975.

58. SMITH, EL, SEMPOS, CT, AND PURVIS, RW: *Bone mass and strength decline with age.* In SMITH, EL AND SERFASS, RC (EDS): *Exercise and Aging: A Scientific Basis.* Enslow Publishers, Hillside, New Jersey, 1973, pp 59–75.

59. SMITH, EL: *Exercise for prevention of osteoporosis: A review.* Physician and Sports Medicine, 1982, 72–83.

60. BASSETT, CA AND BECKER, RO: *Generation of elective potentials by bone in response to mechanical stress.* Science 137:1063, 1962.

61. DONALDSON, C, HALLEY, SB, VOGE, JM, ET AL: *Effect of prolonged bedrest on bone mineral.* Metabolism 19:1071, 1970.

62. SMITH, EL, REDDAN, W, AND SMITH, PE: *Physical activity and calcium modalities for bone mineral in aged women.* Med Sci Sports Ex 13:60, 1981.

63. SALTIN, B, BLOMQVIST, G, MITCHELL, JH, ET AL: *Response to exercise after bed rest and after training.* Circulation 37-38:VII-l, 1968.

64. DEVRIES, HA: *Functional Fitness for Older Americans. A Synopsis of the National Conference on Fitness and Aging.* September 10–11, 1981.

65. BENESTAD, AM: *Trainability of old men.* Acta Med Scand 178:321, 1965.

66. GRANATH, A AND STRANDELL, T: *Relationships between cardiac output, stroke volume, and intracardiac pressures at rest and during exercise in supine position and some anthropometric data in healthy old men.* Acta Med Scand 176:447, 1964.

67. ADAMS, GM AND DE VRIES, HA: *Physiological effects of an exercise training regimen upon women aged 52 to 79.* J Gerontol 28:50, 1973.

68. Rost, R, Dreisbach, W, and Hollmann, WL: *Hemodynamic changes in 50- to 70-year-old men due to endurance training.* In Landry, F and Orban, WAR (eds): *Sports Medicine, Vol. 5.* Symposia Specialists, Miami, 1978, pp 121–124.

69. Dehn, MM and Bruce, RA: *Effects of physical training on exertional ST segment depression in coronary heart disease.* Circulation 44:390, 1971.

70. Hollman, W: *Diminution of cardiopulmonary capacity in the course of life and its prevention by participation in sports.* In Kato, K (ed): *Proceedings of International Congress of Sports Sciences.* Japanese Union of Sport Sciences, Tokyo, 1966, pp 91–93.

71. Sheuer, J and Tipton, CM: *Cardiovascular adaptations to physical training.* Ann Rev Physiol 39:221, 1977.

72. Barry, AJ, Daly, JW, Pruett, EDR, et al: *The effects of physical conditioning on older individuals. I. Work capacity, circulatory-respiratory function, and electrocardiogram.* J Gerontol 21:182, 1966.

73. Shephard, RJ (ed): *Physical Activity and Aging.* Year Book Medical Publishers, Chicago, 1978.

74. deVries, HA: *Physiological effects of an exercise training regimen upon men aged 52–88.* J Gerontol 25:325, 1970.

75. Petrofsky, JS and Lind, AR: *Aging, isometric strength and endurance, and cardiovascular responses to static effort.* J Appl Physiol 39:91, 1975.

76. Suominen, H, Heikkinen, E, and Parkatti, T: *Effect of eight weeks' physical training on muscle and connective tissue of the m. vastus lateralis in 69-year-old men and women.* J Gerontol 32:33, 1977.

77. Munns, K: *Effects of exercise on the range of joint motion in elderly subjects.* In Smith, EL and Serfass, RC (eds): *Exercise and Aging: The Scientific Basis.* Enslow Publishers, Hillside, New Jersey, 1981, pp 167–177.

78. Chapman, EA, deVries, HA, and Swezey, R: *Joint stiffness: Effects of exercise on young and old men.* J Gerontol 27:218, 1972.

79. Leslie, DK and Frekany, GA: *Effects of an exercise program on selected flexibility measures of senior citizens.* The Gerontologist 4:182, 1978.

80. Lesser, M: *The effects of rhythmic exercise on the range of motion in older adults.* Am Correct Ther J 32:118, 1978.

81. Smith, EL: *Bone changes in the exercising older adult.* In Smith, EL and Serfass, RC (eds): *Exercise and Aging: The Scientific Basis.* Enslow Publishers, Hillside, New Jersey, 1981, pp 179–186.

82. American Heart Association, Committee on Exercise: *Exercise Testing and Training of Apparently Healthy Individuals: A Handbook for Physicians.* AMA, New York City, 1972.

83. Noble, RJ, and Rothbaum, DA: *History and physical examination.* In Noble, RJ and Rothbaum, DA (eds): *Geriatric Cardiology.* FA Davis, Philadelphia, 1981, pp 55–64.

84. Pollock, ML, Wilmore, JH, and Fox, SM, III: *Health and Fitness Through Physical Activity.* John Wiley & Sons, New York, 1978, pp 130–131.

85. deVries, HA: *Prescription of exercise for older men from telemetered exercise heart rate data.* Geriatrics 26:102, 1971.

86. deVries, HA: *Tips on prescribing exercise regimens for your older patients.* Geriatrics 34:75, 1979.

87. Leslie, DK and Mc Lure, JW: *Exercises for the elderly.* University of Iowa Press, Iowa City, 1975.

88. deVries, HA, Wiswell, RA, Bulbulian, R, et al: *Tranquilizer effect of exercise: Acute effects of moderate aerobic exercise on spinal reflex activation level.* Am J Phys Med 60:57, 1981.

Exercise Training of Patients with Ventricular Dysfunction and Heart Failure

R. Sanders Williams, M.D.

THE RATIONALE FOR CONSIDERING EXERCISE TRAINING OF PATIENTS WITH VENTRICULAR DYSFUNCTION

The systolic and diastolic performance of the left ventricle can be impaired by a variety of pathologic processes including primary valvular heart disease, long-standing systemic hypertension, exposure to environmental toxins, viral or parasitic infection, endocrinopathies, or unknown causes. However, the most common cause of chronic ventricular dysfunction in industrialized nations is myocardial infarction secondary to atherosclerotic coronary artery disease.* Patients with ventricular dysfunction related to coronary artery disease often present difficult therapeutic problems to the practicing clinician. First, such patients are at high risk for sudden death[1] presumably due to ventricular dysrhythmias, and as yet no form of therapy has been clearly demonstrated to reduce mortality in such patients. Second, patients with severe ventricular dysfunction have a high operative mortality[2] and are often excluded as candidates for surgical revascularization procedures, even in the presence of disabling angina pectoris that is not well controlled by pharmacologic therapy. Third, even the impressive recent advances in the drug therapy of symptomatic congestive heart failure including the availability of potent vasodilator compounds that reduce ventricular afterload[3] do not always produce consistent long-term results, in part related to the development of drug tolerance.[4,5] And finally, regardless of the degree of physical disability, subjects with severe ventricular dysfunction may experience greater psychologic and emotional distress than other persons who have survived a myocardial infarction.[6]

These four factors suggest that persons with severe ventricular dysfunction constitute a group of individuals particularly in need of intensive rehabilitative efforts and of vigilant medical followup. However, somewhat paradoxically, subjects with severe ventricular dysfunction have often been excluded from formal cardiac rehabilitation programs,[7] which have generally focused their efforts on patients with less complicated illnesses. For example, the unexpectedly

---

*Because of the lesser prevalence of other forms of cardiomyopathy, and because most of the available studies of physical training in patients with ventricular dysfunction are limited to subjects with coronary disease, this review will focus largely upon this latter population. Although some patients with other etiologies for ventricular dysfunction may exhibit similar physiologic adaptations to acute exercise and to exercise training as those described here, the validity of extrapolating these data to patients with nonischemic cardiomyopathies cannot be assumed a priori, and until other research data are available, patients with ventricular dysfunction related to etiologies other than coronary artery disease should be considered as candidates for exercise training only with extreme caution and after informed consent, including a frank discussion of the uncertain benefits and potential risks that may ensue from this form of therapy.

low mortality in the randomized control population of the recent National Exercise and Heart Disease Project[8] may have reflected a conscious or unconscious bias toward excluding subjects with poor ventricular function from entry into the study, even though ventricular dysfunction was not a stated exclusion criterion.

The rationale for excluding patients with ventricular dysfunction from cardiac rehabilitation programs has been based largely on the legitimate concern that such patients are at excessive risk for adverse events during even controlled exertion, or that exertion might adversely affect the natural history of ventricular dysfunction, precipitating or accelerating decompensation of the left ventricle. Indeed, avoidance of exertion has been a time-honored principle of therapy for congestive heart failure. However, these concerns have not been supported by quantitative evidence for adverse effects of exertion in coronary patients with ventricular dysfunction, and several basic principles of exercise physiology suggest that physiologic adaptations to habitual exercise (physical conditioning) could be beneficial rather than harmful. Dynamic or isotonic exercise involving major muscle groups is associated with a profound decrease in peripheral vascular resistance owing to local vasodilation in exercising muscle groups;[9] the resulting fall in ventricular afterload would be expected to allow some subjects with abnormal ventricles to increase their cardiac output and comfortably support some level of exertion, even in the face of a minimal or absent inotropic reserve of the ventricle.

The important role of biochemical and morphologic adaptations in skeletal muscle (increased capillary density and mitochondrial oxidative capacity) in mediating cardiovascular adaptations to habitual exercise[10] suggests that even subjects with markedly abnormal hearts may be able to increase their maximal oxygen consumption and work capacity by means of exercise training. Furthermore, the ability to perform any given submaximal activity at a lower heart rate and mean arterial blood pressure following physical conditioning, a characteristic response in normal persons and in coronary patients without ventricular dysfunction,[11] could be expected to offer physiologic advantages to persons with ventricular dysfunction, particularly those with residual areas of viable myocardium that become ischemic during exercise.

This line of reasoning—that exercise training may be safe and produce favorable hemodynamic changes in subjects with abnormal ventricles—has led several groups of investigators to study the physiology of acute exercise and of physical conditioning in such subjects, and this review will summarize the results of these investigations. Additional rationale for including such patients in physical conditioning programs has been provided by suggestive evidence from animal models or from preliminary human studies that exercise training may reduce vulnerability to ventricular fibrillation,[12] that training may enhance mechanical performance of the heart under ischemic conditions,[13] that participation in group rehabilitation programs together with exercise training may have psychologic benefits,[14] and that the extremely close surveillance of patients available in the context of a formal rehabilitation program (for example, frequent determination of antiarrhythmic drug levels[15]) may have therapeutic benefits.

LIMITATIONS TO ACUTE EXERTION IN PATIENTS WITH VENTRICULAR DYSFUNCTION

To understand the abnormalities in exercise peformance that may accompany ventricular dysfunction, we should first review the physiologic factors that limit exercise capacity in healthy persons. During dynamic exertion with major muscle groups in the upright position (cycling, walking, running), the maximal level of exercise that can be performed is limited by two dominant factors:[16] the ability of the cardiovascular system to deliver oxygen (and other substrates) to the exercising skeletal muscle (cardiac output × oxygen content of the blood); and the ability of the exercising muscle to extract oxygen from the blood for use as fuel for muscular work (arteriovenous oxygen difference).* When the intensity of muscular work produces energy demands that exceed the capability of the cardiovascular system to deliver (central component) or of the skeletal muscle to use (peripheral component) oxygen, then exercise cannot be maintained for more than a few minutes owing to a rapid consumption of available substrate for anaerobic glycolysis, a progressive accumulation of lactic acid and fall in pH, and a fall in high energy phosphate concentrations,[17] all of which limit continued muscular work.

To reiterate, in normal individuals maximal oxygen consumption ($\dot{V}O_{2\ max}$), and therefore maximal exercise capacity, is determined both by the ability to increase cardiac output during exercise and by the ability to extract oxygen from the blood, as reflected by the maximal arteriovenous oxygen difference. Most normal persons can achieve an oxygen consumption at maximal exercise that is 5 to 12 times greater than resting levels, and they accomplish this by a two- to fourfold increase in cardiac output, and by a two- to fourfold increase in arteriovenous oxygen difference. Highly conditioned athletes may increase $\dot{V}O_{2\ max}$ by twentyfold over resting values, achieved by four- to fivefold increases in both cardiac output and arteriovenous oxygen difference.[16,18]

The increase in cardiac output occurring with acute exercise is attributable both to an increase in stroke volume, as well as to an increase in heart rate. The augmented stroke volume is usually produced by an increase, compared with resting values, of both the ejection fraction (that is, the percent of blood ejected from the left ventricle with each contraction) and of the end-diastolic volume of the heart. Of these three variables—heart rate, ejection fraction, and end-diastolic volume, the product of which equals cardiac output—the heart rate is quantitatively the most important, increasing by 100 to 200 percent above resting values, as compared with only 10 to 20 percent increases in ejection fraction, and 0 to 15 percent increases in end-diastolic volume in most normal individuals. Notably, the enhancement of cardiac output and of end-diastolic volume that occurs during acute exercise in normal persons is accompanied by only slight increases in the filling pressure (left ventricular end-diastolic pressure or pulmonary capillary wedge pressure) of the left ventricle.[19]

What about the patient with ventricular dysfunction? The most striking finding that emerges when persons with abnormal ventricles are submitted to symptom-limited exercise tests is the marked heterogeneity of exercise capacity that exists among subjects with similar degrees of ventricular dysfunction (as defined by the left ventricular ejection fraction). Although studies from several investigators give identical results,[20,21] data from Duke University are representative[22] (Fig. 1) and reveal how some patients retain normal exercise capacity despite a markedly abnormal ejection fraction.

The absence of a strong relationship between left ventricular performance, assessed by the ejection fraction, and exercise capacity, assessed by the $\dot{V}O_{2\ max}$, is surprising to many physicians and cardiologists but is not so unexpected when viewed in light of the relatively minor contribution of increases in stroke volume in comparison with increases in heart rate and arteriovenous oxygen difference, in determining $\dot{V}O_{2\ max}$ in normal individuals.

If the left ventricular ejection fraction—the most readily quantifiable single variable available for assessing ventricular performance—is not an important determinant of exercise capacity in patients with diseased hearts, then what are the factors that limit exercise capacity in patients with ventricular dysfunction?

There is little question that some patients with abnormal ventricles develop dramatic increases in pulmonary capillary wedge pressure during exercise and that their exercise

---

*Although it has been traditional to segregate the factors limiting exercise into central and peripheral components, as described in the text, it should be recognized that these two components are intricately intertwined, and that this segregation is, to some degree, an artificial one. For example, increased vascularity of skeletal muscle produced by physical conditioning may reduce vascular resistance during exercise and contribute to an augmented cardiac output. This adaptation to physical conditioning would generally be classified as a central adaptation, although its morphologic basis is in the skeletal muscle and not in the heart.

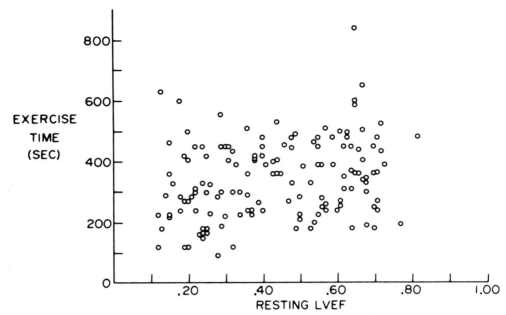

Figure 1. Relationship between symptom-limited exercise duration on a standard bicycle exercise protocol and left ventricular ejection fraction. (From Port et al,[22] with permission.)

capacity may be limited by dyspnea produced by pulmonary vascular congestion. Figure 2 illustrates the response of the pulmonary capillary wedge pressure and pulmonary artery pressures of two such patients, one of whom had an idiopathic congestive cardiomyopathy, and the other of whom had ventricular dysfunction caused by extensive prior myocardial infarction. Such patients may have greater abnormalities of diastolic relaxation of the ventricle than other patients with comparable reductions of systolic function as assessed by the LVEF. On the other hand, as Figure 2 also demonstrates, other subjects with ventricular dysfunction and clinical heart failure reach the point of fatigue during graded exercise testing without any increase in pulmonary capillary wedge pressure above resting values. Recent studies by other investigators, as well as preliminary data from our laboratory, suggest that most subjects with NYHA Class II or III congestive heart failure are limited by the onset of anaerobic metabolism in exercising skeletal muscle, rather than by dyspnea and pulmonary congestion.[23]

Higgenbotham and coworkers have compared the relative importance of a series of hemodynamic variables as determinants of maximal oxygen consumption during bicycle exercise in a group of 17 ambulatory patients with symptomatic congestive heart failure (NYHA Class II or III) and in a group of 9 normal sedentary adults of similar age.[24] There was a wide range of exercise capacities within each group (Table 1), despite marked differences between the two groups and no overlap in left ventricular ejection fraction either at rest or during exertion. The major determinants of exercise capacity, assessed by stepwise multivariable and multiple regression analyses, were identical in the two groups, and included primarily the increment of heart rate and of arteriovenous oxygen difference at maximal exertion over resting values. Neither the absolute value nor the change from rest to exercise of ejection fraction, end-diastolic volume, or stroke volume correlated significantly with maximal oxygen consumption in patients with abnormal ventricles. Figure 3 demonstrates the significant correlation between maximal oxygen consumption (expressed as METs, or multiples of resting oxygen consumption) and the ability to widen the arteriovenous oxygen difference during exertion, and the ability to increase heart rate during exertion, but this study corroborated

222

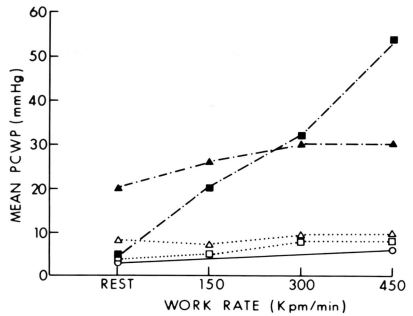

Figure 2. Mean pulmonary capillary wedge pressure (PCWP) during upright bicycle exercise. Mean values from 24 asymptomatic volunteers (mean age 35 years) are shown as open circles. The remaining symbols depict data from four patients with abnormal LVEF (18–34 percent) and NYHA Class II or III congestive heart failure who had identical maximal exercise capacities of 450 kpm/min. Despite identical degrees of functional impairment, marked heterogeneity of the PCWP during exertion is evident.

earlier results (see Fig. 1) in revealing the absence of a correlation between maximal exercise capacity and resting ejection fraction.

These experimental observations are consistent with the theoretical considerations presented earlier and indicate the primacy of hemodynamic factors other than ejection fraction and stroke volume as determinants of exercise capacity in subjects with abnormal ventricular function. The pathophysiologic basis of subnormal elevations of heart rate during exercise in this population remains unknown and is under further investigation in our laboratory. The apparently important role of maximal arteriovenous oxygen difference in determining exercise

Table 1. Hemodynamic and gas exchange variables in 9 normal sedentary subjects and 17 patients with cardiac failure

	Normal Subjects	*Patients*
Exercise capacity	5.5*	3.9
(METs)	(2.9–8.5)	(2.3–5.7)
Resting ejection fraction	60	23
(%)	(50–68)	(9–37)
Exercise ejection fraction	76	23
(%)	(63–87)	(8–33)
$\dot{V}O_{2\ max}$ (ml/kg/min)	23.5 ± 7.6±†	14.8 ± 4.3
Maximal exercise heart rate (bpm)	158 ± 17	132 ± 17
Respiratory quotient at peak exertion	1.12 ± .08	1.16 ± .12

*Mean value (range in parenthesis)
†Mean value ± 1 standard deviation

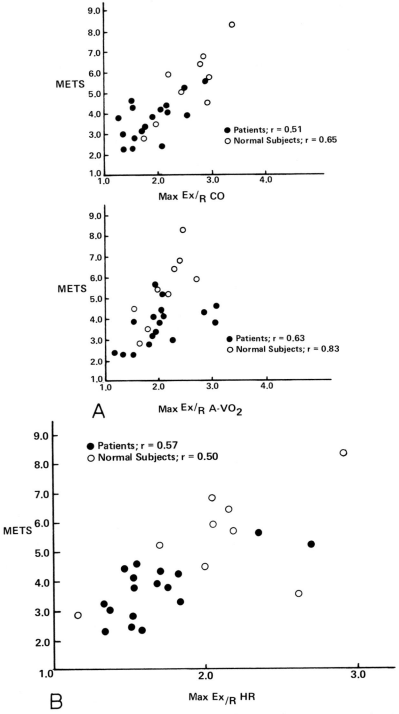

Figure 3. Relationships between maximum exercise capacity (METS) and the ability to increase cardiac output (CO) and arteriovenous oxygen difference (A-VO$_2$) (Panel A) or heart rate (HR) (Panel B) in 9 normal subjects and in 17 patients with cardiac failure. (From Higginbotham et al,[24] with permission.)

performance in such patients is of particular interest, inasmuch as this variable is known to be increased by physical conditioning in normal subjects and in subjects with coronary artery disease.[25] Furthermore, because the physiologic basis of an increased maximal arteriovenous oxygen difference in conditioned subjects is primarily related to biochemical and morphologic adaptations in skeletal muscle, this response to exercise training would be expected to occur even in patients with severely damaged ventricles, who may not develop the adaptations in intrinsic cardiac performance observed in normal hearts in response to habitual exercise.

EXERCISE TRAINING OF PATIENTS WITH VENTRICULAR DYSFUNCTION AND HEART FAILURE

Studies from several institutions appear to confirm the hypothesis that selected patients with severely abnormal ventricular function can perform habitual exercise to a level sufficient to induce favorable physiologic adaptations, without experiencing a high frequency of adverse events during exercise, and without apparent adverse effects on subsequent cardiovascular mortality.

Lee and associates[26] performed symptom-limited exercise testing before and after 12 to 42 months of exercise training in 18 patients wtih LVEF of 40 percent or less. Exercise duration on a standard treadmill protocol (Bruce) increased in 10 of 15 patients (mean change 6.4 to 7.4 min; p = 0.03), and the maximal bicycle workload achieved increased in each of 3 subjects who had orthopedic limitations precluding treadmill testing (mean change 733 to 917 kpm/min). These increases in work capacity occurred in the absence of significant changes in heart rate or blood pressure at peak exertion, and in the absence of changes in resting LVEF, left ventricular end-diastolic pressure, or left ventricular end-diastolic volume quantitated by serial cardiac catheterization. There were significant changes in resting heart rate (71 to 63 bpm; p = 0.01) and in heart rate at a standard submaximal workload (117 to 109 bpm; p = 0.05). No adverse events occurred during exercise testing or training sessions. One patient experienced sudden death unrelated to exertion 21 months after beginning physical conditioning.

Letac and colleagues[27] evaluated the effects of 2 months of exercise training in 8 patients with ejection fractions less than 45 percent and observed similar improvements in exercise capacity and reductions in heart rate during submaximal exercise, without adverse events, and in the absence of changes in resting LVEF.

In an initial publication from our laboratory, Conn and coworkers[28] reported our experience with exercise training of 10 patients with severely impaired ventricular function (LVEF < 27 percent), 6 of whom had clinical congestive heart failure. With a followup duration of 4 to 37 (mean 13) months, 7 of these subjects demonstrated improved work performance during treadmill exercise testing, with significant changes in the group mean values for METs (7.0 to 8.5; p = 0.05) or oxygen pulse (12.8 to 15.7 ml/beat; p = 0.01), the time course of which is depicted in Figure 4. All 10 subjects, regardless of changes in maximum work capacity, demonstrated a reduction in heart rate during submaximal exercise at a standard work rate. No adverse effects occurred during exercise testing or training sessions, although 2 patients died suddenly during the period of observation.

We have proceeded to evaluate the effects of exercise training in a larger number of patients with ventricular dysfunction related to coronary artery disease and to compare these results with those observed in coronary patients with normal resting ventricular function[29] (Fig. 5), with results consistent with all of these earlier investigations. Patients with severe (LVEF < 27 percent) or moderate (LVEF 28 to 49 percent) ventricular dysfunction achieved increments in aerobic work performance similar to those in subjects with normal resting LVEF. In this series of patients, representing 11,000 patient-hours of exercise training in the groups with abnormal ventricular function, no adverse events related to exercise were noted. One episode of ventricular fibrillation occurred during a training session in a subject with a normal ventricle, who was successfully resuscitated. Annualized mortality across this popu-

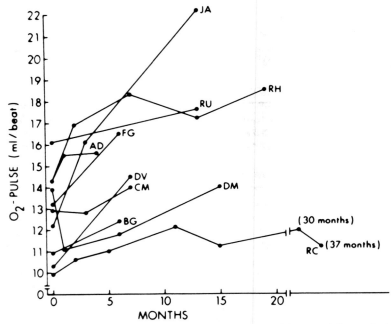

Figure 4. Time course of improvements in aerobic capacity in patients with severe left ventricular dysfunction undergoing exercise conditioning. (Oxygen pulse, the ratio of $\dot{V}O_{2\,max}$/maximal exercise heart rate, is a variable assessing aerobic fitness that is relatively independent of changes in body weight or motivation during serial exercise testing). (From Conn, et al,[28] with permission.)

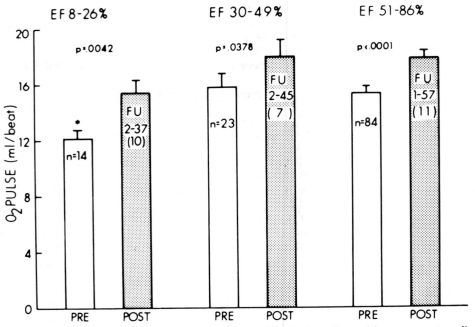

Figure 5. Changes in aerobic capacity following exercise conditioning in patients with coronary artery disease stratified on the basis of resting left ventricular ejection fraction. The numbers of subjects in each stratum are identified (n), as well as the range and median (parenthesis) of the followup (FU) period in months. Patients in all three categories demonstrated similar increments in aerobic capacity.

lation was 16 percent in patients with severe ventricular dysfunction, 4 percent in subjects with moderate ventricular dysfunction, and 1 percent in subjects with normal resting LVEF. For the purposes of comparison, in 95 other subjects with coronary artery disease who had undergone cardiac catheterization at Duke and were found to have an LVEF of 27 percent or less, and who were matched by age to our exercising subjects, annualized mortality was 35 percent.

We are in the process of performing serial radionuclide angiography in subjects with severe ventricular dysfunction undergoing exercise training in order to assess the effects of physical conditioning not only upon work capacity but upon ventricular function as well. This study has not yet been completed, but preliminary results suggest that LVEF at rest or during exertion is either unchanged or shows small improvements following 6 to 12 months of exercise training.

These data indicate that selected patients with severe ventricular dysfunction, including some patients with compensated congestive heart failure, can achieve measurable improvements in exercise capacity following physical conditioning. Although the number of subjects who have been studied remains relatively small and randomized controlled studies have not yet been performed, it appears that these improvements in work performance can be achieved without an unusually high incidence of adverse events during exercise training sessions, without deleterious effects on ventricular function, and without evidence for increased mortality. Although survival curves for patients with poor ventricular function participating in exercise training programs appear to be more favorable than for other patients in our institution with comparable degrees of ventricular dysfunction, the numbers of subjects we have followed are too small, and the possibility of selection bias in favor of the exercise training program is too great to allow firm conclusions regarding longevity in exercising subjects with ventricular dysfunction.

It is also of interest that Franciosa and associates[30] observed improved maximal exercise capacity and a widened arteriovenous oxygen difference during exercise after 3 months of chronic vasodilator therapy of congestive heart failure with disosorbide dinitrate, despite the absence of acute effects of this drug on maximal exercise capacity. One potential explanation for this response is that favorable hemodynamic changes ensuing from acute administration of vasodilators allowed these subjects to pursue more vigorous day-to-day activities, and that, in these severely impaired persons, this augmented activity was sufficient to induce a physical training effect comparable to that described in the studies cited above.

Recommendations for Clinicians

The available evidence suggests that physical training, when conducted under carefully controlled conditions, represents a therapeutic modality that may improve exercise capacity in subjects with ventricular dysfunction related to coronary artery disease, including some subjects with clinical congestive heart failure. Furthermore, irrespective of the physiologic effects of physical conditioning, patients may derive psychologic benefits from participation in cardiac rehabilitation programs and may benefit from the close medical surveillance available in the context of a formal rehabilitation program. It remains uncertain whether patients with other forms of cardiomyopathy will exhibit similar favorable effects of exercise training, and it remains uncertain whether exercise training can be safely recommended to subjects with ventricular dysfunction related to coronary artery disease outside of a carefully supervised medical environment.

In considering patients with ventricular dysfunction for an exercise training program or in making recommendations about occupational or leisure time activities for such patients, a careful physiologic assessment of each patient is mandatory. In our center we recommend that no patient should perform activities that produce demonstrable myocardial ischemia, that produce or increase pulmonary vascular congestion, that produce exertional hypotension, or that produce sustained ventricular dysrhythmias. Patients with overt cardiac decompensation manifested by significant pulmonary vascular congestion at rest that cannot be controlled by pharmacologic therapy are not candidates for exercise training. Among other patients, our primary criterion for determining the suitability of patients with ventricular dysfunction for exercise training can be defined with a single question: Can the patient perform any level of exertion, however low, for several minutes without subjective dyspnea or excessive fatigue and without adverse hemodynamic effects, dysrhythmias, or evidence of myocardial ischemia?

We evaluate patients by a variety of laboratory tests, in addition to a complete medical history and physical examination. All subjects being considered for exercise training undergo graded treadmill or bicycle exercise testing with electrocardiographic monitoring and with frequent determinations of the blood pressure by cuff sphygmomanometry. Subjects suspected of having severe ventricular dysfunction or who have a history of congestive heart failure also undergo radionuclide ventriculography either by the first-pass or multigated technique at rest, and during several stages of exercise on a stationary bicycle. Subjects with extremely low functional work capacity (less than 4 METs), or subjects who are otherwise judged to be more severely ill, generally undergo treadmill or bicycle exercise in conjunction with expired gas analysis and direct measurements of oxygen consumption and carbon dioxide production. And finally, some subjects will undergo invasive testing with direct measurement of pulmonary artery and pulmonary capillary wedge pressures during several stages of work on a stationary bicycle. The goal of all of these studies is to quantitatively determine the maximal level of activity that each person can tolerate without hemodynamic or metabolic effects that might render exertion unpleasant or unsafe. The results of the physiologic testing are used to develop an exercise prescription for use in an exercise training program and for making rational recommendations to the patient about physical activity during daily living.

Although serious adverse events during controlled exercise in patients with severe ventricular dysfunction appear to be rare, definitive data regarding the risks of habitual exercise in such patients are not yet available. Therefore, it is still reasonable to assume that these patients have a higher risk than apparently healthy adults, or than other less severely impaired persons with coronary artery disease. For this reason we recommend that particular caution and a high level of supervision be employed during exercise training of these patients. Currently we recommend that exercise training of patients with severe ventricular dysfunction be limited, at least for an initial period, to settings in which emergency medical assistance, including a portable defibrillator, is immediately at hand, and in which personnel trained in cardiopulmonary resuscitation are present. Perhaps even more important, in an effort to prevent life-threatening complications of exercise therapy in these patients, the personnel assisting patients with ventricular dysfunction in a physical conditioning program should be experienced in the recognition of subtle signs and symptoms suggesting cardiac decompensation, as well as in basic principles of exercise training for coronary patients.

We prescribe exercise for patients with severe ventricular dysfunction by essentially the same methods employed for other persons with coronary disease, relying heavily upon the concept of a training range of heart rates during exercise. For patients who can exercise to fatigue without adverse hemodynamic effects or symptoms, we calculate the training range as 60 to 80 percent of the increment between the resting heart rate and the maximal heart rate attained, added back to the resting heart rate. For patients who develop angina, a fall in LVEF, an elevation of pulmonary capillary wedge pressure, or a fall in systemic arterial pressure during exertion, we attempt to quantitate the heart rate at which such adverse effects first occur and prescribe the upper limit of subsequent exercise at a level 10 bpm below the heart rate at which such evidence for hemodynamic compromise occurs. For practical purposes we round off these heart rate values to the nearest multiple of 6, such that patients may count their pulse rate during exertion for 10 seconds and multiply by 6 to estimate their exercising heart rate. For example, a patient with a resting LVEF of 17 percent who exercises to heart rate of 150 bpm and is limited by fatigue without abnormal changes in blood pressure, LVEF, or the exercise electrocardiogram would have exercise prescribed in a heart rate range of 114 to 132 bpm. Another patient with a resting LVEF of 28 percent who develops dyspnea and a rise in pulmonary capillary wedge pressure from 16 to 24 mm Hg at a heart rate of 102 bpm, but who can exercise comfortably without a rise in wedge pressure at 90 bpm, will have exercise prescribed in a range of 78 to 90 bpm.

We attempt to perform the physiologic testing used to quantify the training range while the patients are receiving the same medication regimen that they are to receive during the subsequent exercise training program. Medication changes and clinical observation of the patients during the exercise sessions will sometimes necessitate changes in the training range. For exercise performed outside of direct medical supervision, essentially any occupational or recreational activity, including sexual intercourse, we think it prudent to recommend a lesser intensity of effort (heart rates 12 to 18 bpm lower) than that permitted during supervised exercise sessions. Our patients are taught to determine their own pulse rates during exertion, to recognize irregularities of heart rhythms, and to recognize warning symptoms that may render a particular activity inadvisable. They are also taught that certain situations (for example, exercise in a cold environment or isometric work) may present stresses to the cardiovascular systems that are not accurately reflected by the heart rate.

Exercise training sessions at Duke University Medical Center for patients with ventricular dysfunction usually involve some combination of bicycle ergometry, light calisthenics and flexibility exercises, walking on a flat track, and stair climbing. Severely impaired patients may begin with as little as five minutes of walking. At the other end of the spectrum, some extraordinary patients with resting LVEF less than 25 percent, after months of training, have been able to bicycle at work loads in excess of 900 kpm/min for 15 minutes and jog continuously for 30 minutes as a daily exercise regimen. Within a few weeks of beginning a training program, most patients will perform bicycle ergometry for 15 minutes and track activities (walking mixed with jogging) for 30 minutes at an intensity sufficient to elevate their heart rate to the desired training range three to five times weekly, supplemented with flexibility exercises and stair climbing.

We determine body weight, resting heart rate, and resting blood pressure in these patients on a daily basis before the exercise sessions, and the patients are questioned concerning any unusual symptoms occurring since the previous session. Individuals with new or increasing symptoms, rapid weight fluctuations, or changes in vital signs do not exercise until clearance from a physician has been obtained.

Our patients with ventricular dysfunction participating in exercise training generally undergo followup exercise testing after 6 to 12 weeks, 6 months, and 1 year. Invasive studies are not repeated except as part of specific research protocols or for evaluation of new symptoms.

It is important to emphasize that exercise training of patients with severe ventricular dysfunction does not necessarily involve levels of effort that normal individuals would regard as strenuous. For a person with congestive heart failure whose activities have been limited to sitting in a chair and walking to the bathroom, walking continuously for 15 minutes at 1.5 to 2.0 mph may represent a level of exertion sufficient to induce favorable physiologic adaptations and therefore constitute physical conditioning. Some physicians may be deterred from advising exercise training for severely impaired cardiac patients by making an incorrect association between exercise training and jogging or other forms of strenuous effort that are clearly inappropriate for most individuals with serious ventricular dysfunction. Somewhat surprisingly for many clinicians, the potential for achieving gratifying improvements in the quality of life through participation in an exercise training program may actually be greater in cardiac patients who are severely impaired than in relatively uncomplicated patients. An individual whose functional work capacity improves from 3 to 5 METs will experience a dramatic change in his or her ability to perform routine activities of daily living, whereas the same absolute improvement of 2 METs in a person with a baseline work capacity of 10 METs would be imperceptible unless the individual is customarily engaged in fairly strenuous activities.

CONCLUSION

Exercise training appears to be a therapeutic modality that should be considered for patients with ventricular dysfunction related to coronary artery disease. When patients are carefully selected and when exercise training sessions are conducted under close supervision, life-threatening complications of exercise training are infrequent, and favorable physiologic adaptations, most prominently an increase in functional work capacity, occur in most patients. Although only limited data are available, increased levels of physical activity do not appear to have adverse effects on subsequent cardiac mortality or on ventricular function in patients with ventricular dysfunction. In addition, these patients may derive psychologic benefits from participation in exercise training, and the close medical surveillance available in the context of a supervised exercise program may facilitate better clinical decisions concerning pharmacologic therapy, interpretation of symptoms, or the necessity for and timing of operative procedures.

REFERENCES

1. Harris, PJ, Harrell, FE, Lee, RL, et al: *Survival in medically treated coronary artery diseases.* Circulation 60:1259, 1979.
2. Kennedy JW, Kaiser, GC, Fisher, LD, et al: *Clinical and angiographic predictors of operative mortality from the collaborative study in coronary artery surgery (CASS).* Circulation 63:793, 1981.
3. Cohn, JN and Franciosa, JA: *Vasodilator therapy of cardiac failure.* N Engl J Med 297:254, 1977.
4. Arnold, SB, Williams, RL, Ports, TA, et al: *Attenuation of prazosin effect on cardiac output in chronic heart failure.* Ann Intern Med 91:345, 1979.
5. Packer, M, Meller, J, Medina, N, et al: *Hemodynamic characterization of tolerance to long-term hydralazine therapy in severe chronic heart failure.* N Engl J Med 306:57, 1982.
6. Blumenthal, JA, Williams, RS, Wallace, AG, et al: *Physiological and psychological variables predict adherence to prescribed medical therapy in patients recovering from myocardial infarction.* Psychosom Med 44:519, 1982.
7. McHenry, MM: *Medical screening of patients with coronary artery disease: Criteria for entry into exercise conditioning programs.* Am J Cardiol 33:752, 1974.
8. Shaw, LW: *Effects of a prescribed supervised exercise program on mortality and cardiovascular morbidity in patients after a myocardial infarction: The National Exercise and Heart Disease Project.* Am J Cardiol 48:39, 1981.
9. Clausen, JP: *Circulatory adjustments of dynamic exercise and effects of physical training in normal subjects and in patients with coronary artery disease.* Prog Cardiovasc Dis 19:91, 1976.
10. Holloszy, JO: *Adaptations of muscular tissue to training.* Prog Cardiovasc Dis 18:445, 1976.
11. Scheuer, J and Tipton, CM: *Cardiovascular adaptations to physical training.* Annu Rev Physiol 39:221, 1977.
12. Noakes, TD, Higginson, L, and Opie, LH: *Physical training increases ventricular fibrillation thresholds of isolated rat hearts during normoxia, hypoxia, and regional ischemia.* Circulation 67:24, 1983.
13. Bersohn, MM and Scheuer, J: *Effects of ischemia on the performance of hearts from physically trained rats.* Am J Physiol 234:H215, 1970.
14. Hackett, TP and Cassem, NH: *Psychological factors related to exercise.* In Wenger, NK (ed): *Exercise and the Heart.* FA Davis, Philadelphia, 1978.
15. Myerburg, RJ, Conde, C, Sheps, DS, et al: *Antiarrhythmic drug therapy in survivors of prehospital cardiac arrest: Comparison of effects on chronic ventricular arrhythmias and recurrent cardiac arrest.* Circulation 59:855, 1979.
16. Wasserman, K and Whipp, BJ: *Exercise physiology in health and disease.* Am Rev Resp Dis 112:219, 1975.
17. Karlsson, J and Saltin, B: *Lactate, ATP, and CP in working muscles during exhausive exercise in man.* J Appl Physiol 29:598, 1970.

18. EPSTEIN, SE, BEISER, GD, STAMPFER, M, ET AL: *Characterization of the circulatory response to maximal upright exercise in normal subjects and patients with heart disease.* Circulation 35:1049, 1967.

19. HIGGINBOTHAM, MB, MORRIS, KG, WILLIAMS, RS, ET AL: *Hemodynamic responses during upright bicycle exercise in normal men: Relation to exercise performance and age* (submitted for publication).

20. LITCHFIELD, RL, KERBER, BE, BENGE, JW, ET AL: *Normal exercise capacity in patients with severe left ventricular dysfunction: Compensatory mechanisms.* Circulation 66:129, 1982.

21. FRANCIOSA, JA, PARK, M, AND LEVINE, B: *Lack of correlation between exercise capacity and indices of resting left ventricular performance in heart failure.* Am J Cardiol 47:33, 1981.

22. PORT, S, MCEWAN, P, COBB, FR, ET AL: *Influence of resting left ventricular response to exercise in patients with coronary artery disease.* Circulation 63:856, 1981.

23. WILSON, JR AND FERRARO, N: *Exercise intolerance in patients with chronic left heart failure: Relation to oxygen transport and ventilatory abnormalities.* Am J Cardiol 51:1358, 1983.

24. HIGGENBOTHAM, MB, MORRIS, KG, CONN, EH, ET AL: *Determinants of variable exercise performance among patients with severe left ventricular dysfunction.* Am J Cardiol 51:52, 1983.

25. DETRY, JMR, ROUSSEAU, M, VANDERBRONCHE, G, ET AL: *Increased arteriovenous oxygen difference after physical training in coronary heart disease.* Circulation 44:109, 1971.

26. LEE, AP, ICE, R, BLESSEY, RPT, ET AL: *Long-term effects of physical training on coronary patients with impaired ventricular function.* Circulation 60:1519, 1979.

27. LETAC, B, CRIBIER, A, AND DESPLANCHES, JF: *A study of left ventricular function in coronary patients before and after physical training.* Circulation 56:375, 1977.

28. CONN, EH, WILLIAMS, RS, AND WALLACE, AG: *Exercise responses before and after physical conditioning in patients with severely depressed left ventricular function.* Am J Cardiol 49:296, 1982.

29. WILLIAMS, RS, CONN, EH, AND WALLACE, AG: *Enhanced exercise performance following physical training in coronary patients stratified by left ventricular ejection fraction.* Circulation 64:IV-186, 1981.

30. FRANCIOSA, JA, GOLDSMITH, SR, AND COHN, JN: *Contrasting immediate and long-term effects of isosorbide dinitrate on exercise capacity in congestive heart failure.* Am J Med 69:559, 1980.

Use of Exercise Testing in Noncoronary Heart Disease

Jerre F. Lutz, M.D. and Nanette K. Wenger, M.D.

In 1978 Gilbert and Schlant[1] listed as the major uses of exercise testing: (1) diagnostic aid in the detection of coronary artery disease and (2) determination of functional capacity or exercise tolerance in patients with a variety of known or suspected heart diseases. Indications for exercise testing have significantly broadened in recent years; additionally, the current emphasis is on specific questions being asked for each disease process. Rather than a universal approach to all patients, exercise testing is used to answer a series of questions that depend on the disease either known or suspected to exist.

The designation *noncoronary heart disease* encompasses a wide gamut of diagnoses. During exercise testing of the patient with noncoronary heart disease, a variety of aspects are currently evaluated. Perhaps most important is the physical work capacity or functional capacity, as determined by the duration of exercise and/or the maximal oxygen uptake. Oxygen uptake, either during bicycle exercise or walking on a treadmill, is proportionate to the workload at submaximal levels of effort. Aerobic capacity or maximal oxygen uptake is defined as the level of oxygen uptake at which an increase in workload produces no further increase in oxygen uptake. Maximal cardiac output of the systemic circulation is the main determinant of maximal oxygen uptake.[2] A number of exercise testing protocols are available; however, the most frequently used are the Bruce[3] and the Naughton[4] protocols (Fig. 1). The determination of oxygen uptake allows comparison among different forms of exercise testing.

Also of importance are the heart rate and the blood pressure responses to activity. Symptoms to be assessed during exercise testing include the development of dyspnea, fatigue, palpitations, chest pain, weakness, dizziness, and/or claudication. A change in cardiac murmurs and heart sounds during exercise testing (particularly the development of a third heart sound) or the appearance of abnormal precordial impulses derserves specific identification. Finally, the exercise electrocardiogram should be scrutinized for evidence of dysrhythmia or repolarization (ST segment) changes. Objective end-points for terminating a maximal or symptom-limited exercise test are listed in Table I.

The addition of radionuclide-based procedures to assess ventricular function has greatly increased our knowledge of the sensitivity and specificity of routine measurements made during exercise testing and has significantly modified the standard evaluation of the patient with noncoronary heart disease. This chapter emphasizes the role of exercise testing in patients with valvular heart disease. Recent information about exercise testing in primary cardiac muscle diseases (predominantly hypertrophic and congestive cardiomyopathy) will also be discussed. Data about the effect of exercise on disturbances of cardiac rhythm, congenital heart diseases, and other selected cardiovascular disorders such as systemic arterial hypertension will be presented.

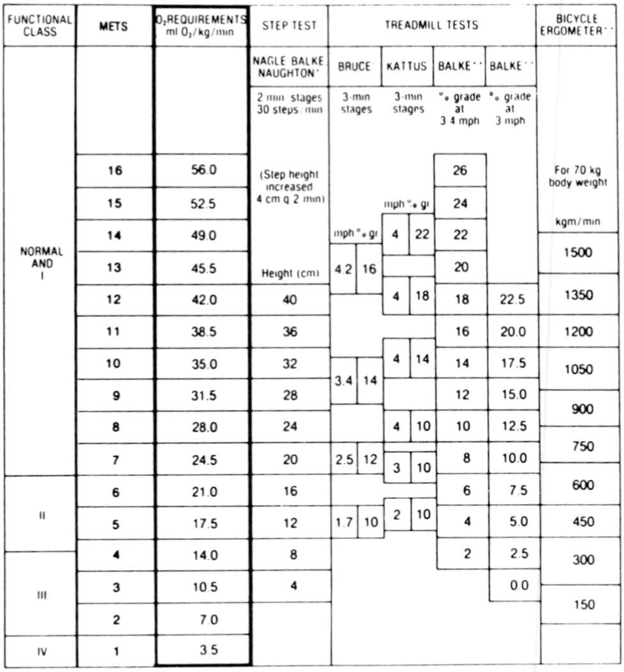

FUNCTIONAL CLASS	METS	O₂ REQUIREMENTS ml O₂/kg/min	STEP TEST NAGLE BALKE NAUGHTON* 2 min stages 30 steps/min	TREADMILL TESTS BRUCE 3-min stages	KATTUS 3-min stages	BALKE** % grade at 3.4 mph	BALKE** % grade at 3 mph	BICYCLE ERGOMETER**
NORMAL AND I	16	56.0	(Step height increased 4 cm q 2 min)			26		For 70 kg body weight
	15	52.5			mph %gr	24		
	14	49.0		mph %gr	4 22	22		kgm/min
	13	45.5	Height (cm)	4.2 16		20		1500
	12	42.0	40		4 18	18	22.5	1350
	11	38.5	36			16	20.0	1200
	10	35.0	32	3.4 14	4 14	14	17.5	1050
	9	31.5	28			12	15.0	900
	8	28.0	24		4 10	10	12.5	750
	7	24.5	20	2.5 12	3 10	8	10.0	
II	6	21.0	16			6	7.5	600
	5	17.5	12	1.7 10	2 10	4	5.0	450
	4	14.0	8			2	2.5	300
III	3	10.5	4				0.0	150
	2	7.0						
IV	1	3.5						

†Bruce RA. Multi-stage treadmill test of submaximal and maximal exercise Appendix B, this publication

‡Kattus AA, Jorgensen CR, Worden RE, Alvaro AB. S-T-segement depression with near-maximal exercise in detection of preclinical coronary heart disease Circulation 41 585-595, 1971

*Nagle FS, Balke B, Naughton JP. Gradational step tests for assessing work capacity. J Appl Physiol 20 745-748, 1965

**Fox SM, Naughton JP, Haskell WL. Physical activity and the prevention of coronary heart disease. Ann Clin Res 3 404, 1971

Figure 1. Oxygen requirements increase with workloads from bottom of chart to top in various exercise tests of the step, treadmill, and bicycle ergometer types. (From American Heart Association, with permisson.)

Selection of a patient for exercise testing must follow the tenet that the benefit of the procedure must substantially outweigh the risk; and acceptability of testing must consider the entire clinical picture defining the importance of the information to be derived from testing and its relationship to data derived from other evaluative procedures. Contraindications to exercise testing in patients with noncoronary heart disease include (1) evidence of overt congestive heart failure; (2) any recent acute illness such as a respiratory infection, gastrointestinal bleeding, and so forth; (3) resting blood pressure greater than 180 mm Hg systolic or 100 mm Hg diastolic; (4) orthostatic hypotension, especially if symptomatic; (5) orthopedic

Table 1. Objective end-points for maximal or symptom-limited exercise testing*

1. Marked ST segment elevation or depression (2 mm from baseline), with or without chest pain
2. Sustained supraventricular tachycardia other than sinus tachycardia
3. Frequent premature beats that significantly decrease cardiac output or fail to disappear with a brief continuation of exercise
4. Ventricular tachycardia (three or more ventricular ectopic complexes in a row)
5. Drop in systolic arterial blood pressure during exercise[7]
6. Excessive elevation of arterial blood pressure with exercise (260/120 mm Hg)
7. Signs of cerebral hypoxemia (ataxia, failure to answer questions or obey commands)
8. Signs of peripheral circulatory insufficiency (pallor, development of cyanosis, clammy skin)

*Adapted from Gilbert and Schlant,[1] with permission.

problems making exercise testing potentially hazardous or unlikely to yield adequate information; (6) recognition of a recent change in frequency or severity of anginal episodes and/or new electrocardiographic changes compatible with myocardial infarction or injury (these changes should persuade the clinician to defer exercise testing until an adequate evaluation and treatment of this concomitant process has been accomplished); (7) presence of significant anemia that could confuse the results of testing; (8) recognition of an electrolyte disturbance that could confound interpretation of test results or make exercise potentially dangerous; (9) failure to sign an informed consent form.

The decision *not* to exercise the patient for these reasons or other reasons often indicates the seriousness or severity of the disease process and should suggest that more intensive evaluation and management may be indicated.

EXERCISE TESTING IN VALVULAR HEART DISEASE

Mitral Stenosis

The decrease in exercise performance associated with progressively severe mitral stenosis has been well established.[5] In general, there is good correlation between the severity of the valvular obstruction and the decline in exercise tolerance. A notable exception may occur when atrial fibrillation develops in a patient with mitral stenosis, leading to a precipitous decline in exercise tolerance related both to the tachycardia, which limits ventricular filling, and to loss of the atrial kick, which further decreases the stroke output. Additionally, patients with controlled atrial fibrillation reach maximal heart rates at low to moderate workloads and may then, with an increase in workload, have no further increase in heart rate.[2]

Patients with significant mitral stenosis are unable to maintain their stroke volume during exercise.[2] Left atrial pressure rises progressively with exercise, whereas the cardiac output tends to remain fixed or even may decline.[6] Thus, both symptoms (predominantly fatigue, weakness, and exertional dyspnea) and the duration of exercise correlate well with the severity of mitral valvular obstruction.

As the patient with mitral stenosis adapts to these limitations by diminishing the work effort, serial exercise testing may document progressive severity of mitral valvular obstruction in the individual who is unaware of the progressive disability because work intensity has been gradually and progressively decreased, or in the stoic individual who refuses to acknowledge any impairment of function. Conversely, an exercise test that documents a normal or near normal treadmill duration time and/or maximal oxygen uptake for sedentary normal persons or Class I cardiac patients should indicate that the mitral valvular obstruction is not severe and that cardiac catheterization to assess the need for surgery should probably be deferred.

Almendral and associates[7] found a significant correlation between the duration of exercise and the extent of mitral valvular obstruction; however, there was poor correlation between the mitral valve area at cardiac catheterization and the development of exercise-induced hypotension. They found that the inability to reach Stage III of a Bruce protocol was associated with critical mitral stenosis in patients with isolated mitral valve disease.

Postoperative exercise testing[8,9] tends to point out the disparity between symptomatic results, which are typically excellent, and improvement in exercise performance as determined by exercise testing which, although improved, is generally significantly lower than that of sex and age matched sedentary control subjects. The extent to which this reflects decreased fitness prior to surgery is problematic.

Mitral Regurgitation

In patients with mitral regurgitation, as with mitral stenosis, there is generally a good correlation between the degree of valvular regurgitation and the duration of treadmill exercise. However, Borer and coworkers[10] demonstrated that radionuclide ventriculography in patients with mitral regurgitation helped to unmask left ventricular dysfunction, which correlated poorly with or anteceded the development of symptoms. The left ventricular ejection fraction was normal at rest in 18 of 20 patients tested, but fell with exercise in 10 of the 20 patients. At present, rest and exercise radionuclide ventriculography studies are performed in an effort to detect early those patients with exercise-induced left ventricular dysfunction who may benefit from medical or surgical intervention prior to their development of symptoms.

Mitral Valve Prolapse

The clinician is often in a predicament trying to differentiate patients with isolated mitral valve prolapse from those with concomitant coronary heart disease because of (1) the high frequency of both typical angina pectoris and atypical chest pain in patients with mitral valve prolapse; (2) the frequency of abnormal exercise electrocardiograms with this disorder; and (3) the clinical association of the two entities.[11] The resting electrocardiogram in patients with isolated mitral valve prolapse frequently reveals ventricular ectopy; however, 70 percent of patients have ventricular ectopy during exercise. The development of ST segment depression also occurs frequently during exercise in patients with isolated mitral valve prolapse.

Exercise myocardial perfusion scintigraphy using thallium 201 has correctly differentiated patients with isolated mitral valve prolapse (normal exercise thallium) from those with significant associated atherosclerotic coronary artery disease (myocardial perfusion defect with exercise) with a high degree of accuracy.[12,13] Routine exercise testing may help detect arrhythmias in patients with mitral valve prolapse and may be useful in assessing the response of these patients to pharmacologic interventions.

Aortic Stenosis

Exercise testing is contraindicated in the patient suspected to have severe aortic stenosis, inasmuch as exercise-induced syncope and/or sudden cardiac death may occur secondary to an inability to increase the stroke volume and an actual or relative decrease in cardiac output with exercise.

However, in the patient documented to have only modest aortic stenosis, serial exercise testing may help identify the progression of its severity and define the need for surgery. Such testing is particularly important in the patient with congenital aortic stenosis, in which the significance of the obstruction often increases with age and the growth of the patient.

In patients with modest aortic stenosis, the compensatory mechanisms for an increased ventricular pressure load may enable normal exercise performance. However, with progressive severity of the aortic obstruction, repolarization (ST segment) changes on the electrocardiogram in response to exercise may identify unmet myocardial oxygen needs. Another abormal feature that may be encountered at exercise testing is an inadequate increase in the systolic blood pressure in response to exercise. Almendral and colleagues[7] found that, unlike the poor correlations in patients with mitral stenosis, exertional hypotension was characteristic of patients with the most severe grades of aortic valve obstruction.

Because many patients with moderate or severe aortic stenosis describe chest pain, the question has been raised as to whether exercise radionuclide (thallium) myocardial perfusion studies can differentiate the patient with isolated aortic stenosis from the individual with both aortic stenosis and significant atherosclerotic coronary artery obstruction.[14] Unfortunately, this differentiation is not possible, as both groups of patients may develop myocardial ischemia and therefore may exhibit thallium perfusion abnormalities with exercise which resolve with rest.

Exercise thallium studies can be used, however, to assess the efficacy of surgical correction of aortic stenosis; a decrease in or absence of exercise-induced ischemia on a thallium myocardial perfusion study indicates a good surgical result. Conversely, identification of a new defect at rest on a radionuclide (thallium) myocardial perfusion study suggests that the patient may have sustained a perioperative myocardial infarction.

Aortic Regurgitation

Evidence of impaired exercise tolerance, elicited either on the basis of symptoms described in the clinical history or at exercise testing, occurs late in the natural history of chronic aortic regurgitation. Exercise tolerance is often normal with moderate or severe aortic regurgitation, and even in the presence of an elevated left ventricular end-diastolic pressure and/or a diminished left ventricular ejection fraction.[15] The exercise-related decrease in peripheral vascular resistance that favors forward flow and the decrease in diastolic time during which the aortic regurgitation can occur are potential explanations for this disparity.

Symptoms of congestive heart failure and, less commonly, chest pain and syncope also occur late in the clinical course of patients with chronic aortic regurgitation.

After aortic valve replacement in a patient with significant left ventricular enlargement, left ventricular function typically improves either slowly or not at all, suggesting that earlier intervention might have been associated with a better operative result.[16,17] Radionuclide assessment of the left ventricular ejection fraction at rest and after exercise testing appears to represent an advance in earlier definition of those patients with developing left ventricular dysfunction who might benefit from early therapeutic intervention.[18,19] The response of the pulmonary capillary wedge pressure (and therefore the left ventricular diastolic pressure) during exercise in patients with aortic regurgitation has been variable. Absolute rest and exercise ejection fractions, as well as maximum levels of exercise, correlate with the pulmonary capillary wedge pressure, but the change in ejection fraction with exercise does not.[15]

EXERCISE TESTING IN CONGENITAL HEART DISEASE

Particularly during the last decade, exercise testing has become a valuable adjunctive procedure in the evaluation of children or adolescents with cardiac disorders. Freed's[20] survey of members of the Cardiology Section of the American Academy of Pediatrics determined that 38 percent of those responding used exercise testing, predominantly isotonic treadmill or bicycle testing, in the evaluation of these patients. Complications of testing were infrequent (1.7 percent) and no deaths were attributed to exercise testing in 6722 tests reported for 1979.

Normal exercise responses in children and adolescents have been established for both a bicycle protocol[21] and a Bruce treadmill protocol.[22] James and associates[21] described an 8.9 percent incidence of 1 to 2 mm ST segment depression on the exercise electrocardiogram among normal males and a 16.9 percent incidence among normal females within the pediatric age group. Godfrey[23] found that the maximum capacity for exercise as well as the maximum exercise heart rate increased with height in the pediatric age group. Peak heart rate increased to about 210 beats per minute at age 10 and reached a plateau thereafter. As in adults, the heart rate was the major contributor to cardiac output, as stroke volume reached its maximum value at a lower level of exercise.

Important data are available regarding exercise testing in the following subsets of congenital heart disease.

Large Atrial Septal Defect

A disproportionately large number of patients have a very low functional capacity,[22] both prior to and even after closure of a large atrial septal defect. A proposed mechanism is the decrease in left ventricular stroke work. Exercise training may be considered after surgery as a means to improve left ventricular performance.

Ventricular Septal Defect

Cumming[22] described a significant number of patients with moderate-sized or large ventricular septal defects who had a low functional capacity at exercise testing. Postoperatively, some patients with corrected ventricular septal defects elevate their pulmonary artery pressure in response to exercise; others have decreased exercise cardiac outputs, both with and without elevation of their pulmonary artery pressures. These findings raise the question as to whether earlier closure of the ventricular septal defect might obviate this problem.

Congenital Aortic Stenosis

The indications and results for exercise testing in children with congenital aortic stenosis are similar to those in adults with aortic stenosis of various etiologies, as previously discussed. One significant difference may be the greater reliance on exercise-induced ST segment and T wave changes on the electrocardiogram in the pediatric population as indications of borderline myocardial ischemia, thereby identifying patients in need of careful surveillance or intervention.[24]

Coarctation of the Aorta

Despite adequate surgical correction of coarctation of the aorta, some patients have significant exercise-induced hypertension, particularly if the coarctation is corrected at an older age. Exercise testing may document this response, identify the need for therapy, and serve to assess the adequacy of antihypertensive medication.

Conner[25] described the use of treadmill exercise prior to and after corrective surgery to evaluate the success of operation in patients with coarctation of the aorta. Two of 13 patients studied were found to have residual aortic coarctation on the basis of a post-exercise systolic blood pressure difference between the upper and lower extremities that was not appreciated on the routine postoperative physical examination at rest. A post-exercise arm-to-leg systolic gradient of greater than 35 mm Hg is recommended to be an indication for recatheterization.

Tetralogy of Fallot

As is the case with other cyanotic congenital cardiac lesions, Cumming[22] described the inability of any cyanotic patients with tetralogy of Fallot to attain greater than 50 percent of their age-predicted exercise capacity prior to corrective surgery. A significant number of patients continue to exhibit low exercise capacities even after corrective surgery. One explanation is that time and possibly exercise training are required for the left ventricle to fully develop. James and coworkers[26] described an inverse relationship between the maximum physical work capacity and the age at surgery in both males and females, suggesting that earlier surgical repair may be preferable.

Additionally, exercise testing after correction of tetralogy of Fallot may help identify postoperative arrhythmias requiring therapy. James and associates[26] described premature atrial or ventricular contractions in 10 of 43 patients who had undergone correction of tetralogy of Fallot. Five of the 10 had multiform premature ventricular contractions (PVCs) and four had uniform PVCs. Among the 5 with multiform PVCs, ventricular tachycardia occurred in 2, PVC pairs in 1, and ventricular bigeminy in 2.

EXERCISE TESTING IN PATIENTS WITH RHYTHM OR CONDUCTION DISTURBANCES

Sinus Node Dysfunction

Patients with sinus node dysfunction may develop a wide variety of exercise-induced rhythm disburbances: tachyarrhythmias, both ventricular and supraventricular; bradycardias due to increased vagal tone; or progressive atrioventricular block. Latent heart failure may become evident in patients with underlying myocardial dysfunction.[27] Exercise testing in patients with sinus node dysfunction may elucidate the etiology of exercise-related symptoms (before or after pacemaker insertion) and may help to establish the need either for antiarrhythmic therapy or for permanent cardiac pacing.

Supraventricular Tachyarrhythmias

Some patients experience exercise-induced tachyarrhythmias, predominantly atrial fibrillation, atrial flutter, or re-entrant tachycardias. Exercise testing may be used to document the type of tachycardia, as well as the efficacy of therapy, particularly the use of beta blocking drugs that blunt the chronotropic effects of exercise.

Atrioventricular (AV) Block

Both patients and apparently healthy individuals, especially endurance-trained athletes, may exhibit AV block at rest as evidence of increased vagal tone, usually first or second degree AV block. When exercise overcomes the vagal tone, the patient may demonstrate a normal functional capacity, with 1:1 AV conduction occurring at sinus rates up to 200 beats per minute.

Exercise testing in patients with congenital complete AV block permits assessment of the linear increase in atrial and ventricular rates in response to exercise; these data serve as a basis for establishing or guiding activity recommendations and/or ascertaining the need for pacemaker insertion.

Ventricular Ectopy

Although in general not as sensitive as the ambulatory electrocardiogram in detecting ventricular ectopy, exercise testing more effectively detects exercise-induced arrhythmias and may have diagnostic and therapeutic usefulness in some patients.

Nevertheless, exercise testing is far from ideal if the evaluation of the patient for heart disease is based on the appearance of ventricular ectopy; this is true for several reasons. First, ventricular ectopy is frequently present in normal patients, and this occurrence increases with age.[28] Although frequent PVCs, multiform PVCs, and ventricular tachycardia occur with cardiovascular disease, they may also occur in persons without evidence of a cardiovascular problem. Therefore, even exercise-induced complex ventricular ectopy has limited predictive value as an indicator of the presence of latent heart disease. Furthermore, Faris and associates[29] demonstrated that the reproducibility of the occurrence of exercise-induced ventricular arrhythmias at two consecutive exercise tests was only slightly greater than the reproducibility expected by chance alone.

EXERCISE TESTING IN MISCELLANEOUS CARDIOVASCULAR DISORDERS

Hypertrophic Cardiomyopathy

Patients with hypertrophic cardiomyopathy (either obstructive or nonobstructive) may experience exercise-induced hypotension or arrhythmias, which often indicate the need for medical or surgical intervention. Serial exercise testing allows delineation of the presence and severity of these exercise-induced arrhythmias and can help document the efficacy of therapy.

Severely Depressed Left Ventricular Function

Conn and coworkers[30] demonstrated the ability of 10 patients who had sustained a myocardial infarction and who had a residual left ventricular ejection fraction of less than 27 percent both to safely undertake a closely supervised program of physical training and to attain the benefits of the training effect. Thus, patients with substantial left ventricular dysfunction need not automatically be excluded from supervised exercise training programs but may require exercise testing for precise exercise prescription.

Although these patients with severely depressed ventricular function were not randomly selected, the principle of the potential trainability of patients with severely depressed left ventricular function is important. Whether this approach applies to other groups of patients with significant left ventricular dysfunction, including congestive cardiomyopathy, remains to be ascertained.

Myocarditis

Although contraindicated in the acute phase of myocarditis, exercise testing during recovery may reveal unsuspected residual functional impairment, arrhythmias requiring treatment, and so forth.

Systemic Arterial Hypertension

In patients with borderline hypertension, multilevel exercise testing produces an elevation of total peripheral resistance during the early stages of exercise, followed by a decrease to the normal range in the later stages of testing.[31] Patients with fixed significant hypertension maintain an elevated systemic arterial resistance at all stages of exercise.

Boyer and Kasch[32] described a mean decrease of 11.8 mm Hg in diastolic blood pressure in 23 patients undergoing a six-month exercise training program, indicating that mild supervised exercise may be beneficial rather than harmful for the hypertensive patient. Choquette and Ferguson[33] similarly described diminution in systolic and diastolic blood pressures in borderline hypertensive patients undergoing physical training.

Until more data are available, drug therapy is still recommended for patients with confirmed hypertension, with nonpharmacologic interventions reserved for individuals with labile, intermittent blood pressure elevation.

SUMMARY

Although the application of exercise testing has not been as extensive in patients with noncoronary heart disease as in those with atherosclerotic coronary heart disease, the body of knowledge of the roles of exercise testing in these disorders is increasing. The usefulness of this extension of the clinical examination in the evaluation of patients with a variety of noncoronary cardiovascular disorders is becoming increasingly apparent.

REFERENCES

1. GILBERT, CA AND SCHLANT, RC: *Role of exercise testing in the preoperative and postoperative assessment of patients with noncoronary disease.* Cardiovasc. Clin 9(3):173, 1978.

2. BLOMQVIST, CG: *Exercise testing in rheumatic heart disease.* Cardiovasc Clin 5(2):267, 1973.

3. BRUCE, RA AND HORNSTEIN, TR, *Exercise stress testing in evaluation of patients with ischemic heart disease.* Prog Cardiovasc Dis 11:371, 1969.

4. Common Protocol: *The National Exercise and Heart Disease Project: A Collaborative Project, ed. 2.* George Washington University Medical Center, Washington, DC, 1975.

5. CHAPMAN, CB, MITCHELL, JH, SPROULE, BJ, ET AL: *The maximal oxygen intake test in patients with predominant mitral stenosis.* Circulation 22:4, 1960.

6. HUGENHOLTZ, PG, RYAN, TG, STEIN, SW, ET AL: *Hemodynamic studies: The spectrum of pure mitral stenosis in relation to clinical disability.* Am J Cardiol 10:773, 1962.

7. ALMENDRAL, JM, GARCIA-ANDOAIN, JM, SANCHEZ-CASCOS, A, ET AL: *Treadmill stress testing in the evaluation of patients with valvular heart disease.* Cardiology 69:42, 1982.

8. CARSTENS, V, BEHRENBEK, DW, AND HILGER, HH: *Exercise capacity before and after cardiac valve surgery.* Cardiology 70:41, 1983.

9. SMILEY, WH, GILBERT, CA, AND SYMBAS, PN: *Bleeding, clotting, and functional disability following Beall prosthetic mitral valve replacement.* South Med J 70:801, 1977.

10. BORER, JS, GOTTDIENER, JS, ROSING, DR, ET AL: *Left ventricular function in mitral regurgitation: Determination during exercise.* Circulation 59,60 (Suppl. II):38, 1979.

11. SCHLANT, RC, FELNER, JM, MIKLOZEK, ET AL: *Mitral valve prolapse.* Dis Month 26(10):1, 1980.

12. KLEIN, GJ, DOSTUK, WJ, BOUGHNER, DR, ET AL: *Stress myocardial imaging in mitral leaflet prolapse syndrome.* Am J Cardiol 42:746, 1978.

13. MASSIE, B, BOTVINICK, EH, SAMES, D ET AL: *Myocardial perfusion scintigraphy in patients with mitral valve prolapse.* Circulation 57:19, 1978.

14. BAILEY, IK, COME, PC, BUROW, RD, ET AL: *Thallium-201 myocardial perfusion imaging and aortic valve stenosis.* Am J Cardiol 40:889, 1977.

15. BOUCHER, CA, WILSON, RA, DANAREK, DJ, ET AL: *Exercise testing in asymptomatic or minimally symptomatic aortic regurgitation: Relationship of left ventricular ejection fraction to left ventricular filling pressure during exercise.* Circulation 67:1091, 1983.

16. KRAYENBUHL, HP, LURINA, M, HESS, O, ET AL: *Pre and postoperative left ventricular contractile function in patients with aortic valve disease.* Br Heart J 41:204, 1979.

17. HENRY, WL, BONOW, RO, BORER, JS, ET AL: *Evaluation of aortic valve replacement in patients with valvular aortic stenosis.* Circulation 61:814, 1980.

18. BORER, JS, BACHARACH, SL, GREEN, MV ET AL: *Exercise-induced left ventricular dysfunction in symptomatic and asymptomatic patients with aortic regurgitation: Assessment with radionuclide cineangiography.* Am J Cardiol 42:351, 1978.

19. DEHMER, GJ, FIRTH, BG, HILLIS, LD, ET AL: *Alterations in left ventricular volumes and ejection fraction at rest and during exercise in patients with aortic regurgitation.* Am J Cardiol 48:17, 1981.

20. FREED, MD: *Exercise testing in children: A survey of techniques and safety.* Circulation 64 (Suppl. IV):278, 1981.

21. JAMES, FW, DAPLAN, S, GLUECK, CJ, ET AL: *Responses of normal children and young adults to controlled bicycle exercise.* Circulation 61:902, 1980.

22. CUMMING, GR: *Maximal exercise capacity of children with heart defects.* Am J Cardiol 42:613, 1978.

23. GODFREY, S: *Exercise Testing in Children.* WB Saunders, Philadelphia, 1974.

24. LEWIS, AB, HEYMANN, MA, STANGER, P ET AL: *Evaluation of subendocardial ischemia in valvular aortic stenosis in children.* Circulation 49:978, 1974.

25. CONNER, TM: *Evaluation of persistent coarctation of aorta after surgery with blood pressure measurement and exercise testing.* Am J Cardiol 43:74, 1979.

26. JAMES, FW, KAPLAN, S, SCHWARTZ, DC. ET AL: *Response to exercise in patients after total surgical corrections of tetralogy of Fallot.* Circulation 54:671, 1976.

27. ABBOTT, JA, HIRSCHFIELD, DS, KUNKEL. FW, ET AL: *Graded exercise testing in patients with sinus node dysfunction.* Am J Med 62:330, 1977.

28. McHENRY, PL, FISCH, C, JORDAN, JW, ET AL: *Cardiac arrhythmias observed during maximal treadmill exercise testing in clinically normal men.* Am J Cardiol 29:331, 1972.

29. FARIS, JV, McHENRY, PL, JORDAN, JW, ET AL: *Prevalence and reproducibility of exercise-induced ventricular arrhythmias during maximal exercise testing in normal men.* Am J Cardiol 37:617, 1976.

30. CONN, EH, WILLIAMS, RS, AND WALLACE, *Exercise responses before and after physical conditioning in patients with severely depressed left ventricular function.* Am J Cardiol 49:296, 1982.

31. JULIUS, S AND CONWAY, J: *Hemodynamic studies in patients with borderline blood pressure elevation.* Circulation 38:282, 1968.

32. BOYER, JV AND KASCH, FW: *Exercise therapy in hypertension.* JAMA 211:1668, 1970.

33. COQUETTE, G AND FERGUSON, R: *Blood pressure reduction in "borderline" hypertensives following physical training.* Canad MAJ 108:699, 1973.

Exercise Training
in Noncoronary Heart Disease*

Diane Goforth, M.D. and Frederick W. James, M.D.

Exercise training has become well accepted as a measure that may aid in prevention and retard progression of coronary artery disease. In addition, exercise training appears to decrease morbidity and to enhance recovery of affected patients.[1] However, the benefits of training in the patient with noncoronary, specifically congenital or acquired, heart disease have been less well elucidated. Obviously, exercise training cannot prevent congenital or acquired noncoronary heart disease. An effect of exercise training in possibly delaying progression of cardiac lesions, such as outflow tract obstruction, valvular incompetence, systemic-pulmonary shunts, and so on is not well established and is not the subject for discussion in this chapter. Rather, it is our purpose to discuss exercise training as a means of maximizing an individual's capacity to perfom work by increasing the cardiovascular and pulmonary functional efficiency. As improvements in medical and surgical techniques continue to provide longer survival for the patient with congenital heart disease, the challenge for the cardiologist alters. We become faced with the task of providing ways in which quality may be added to the increased quantity of life. By exercise training, most patients with congenital heart disease can increase their capacity for work, recreation, and general physical activity, thereby achieving a more normal lifestyle. This discussion will present the general physiologic basis, benefits, and various techniques of exercise training in the normal individual and the means by which all of these can be applied to the patient with congenital heart disease.

Throughout this presentation, the primary goal of training in both healthy individuals and those with cardiac disease must be kept in mind, that is, to attain an individual's maximal capacity to perform work (activity) by maximizing the body's efficiency. The extent of realization of this goal depends upon four major areas of function which may vary independently: (1) muscular development; (2) neuromuscular coordination; (3) cardiopulmonary capability; and (4) psychologic state. Any of these areas may serve as a focus for a training program, and indeed great improvement in one area is usually accompanied by at least some degree of improvement in the others. However, this presentation will concentrate on the improvement of cardiopulmonary capability because in congenital heart disease this component sets a subnormal limit to the performance capacity. At the outset we would emphasize that the techniques to be discussed are not meant for use in place of medical therapy or to delay surgical intervention when it is indicated, or as a means of preventing progression of disease. Furthermore, we believe selected patients (for the most part those whose degree of illness is

*Supported in part by Grant 5 ROI HL 18454-02 and Grant 1-T32-HL07417-01 from the National Heart, Lung and Blood Institute; Grant 76 853 from the American Heart Association; and the American Heart Association Southwestern Ohio Chapter

Table 1. Exercise testing and training

Contraindications for Exercise Testing
1. Acute inflammatory cardiac disease, e.g., pericarditis, myocarditis, active rheumatic heart disease
2. Uncontrolled congestive heart failure
3. Acute myocardial infarction, initial phase
4. Acute bronchospasm (asthma) or pneumonia
5. Severe systemic hypertension (blood pressure greater than 240/120 mm Hg), uncontrolled
6. Acute renal disease (e.g., glomerulonephritis)

Special Considerations for Exercise Testing and Training
1. Severe left ventricular outflow obstruction
2. Severe right ventricular outflow obstruction
3. Serious arrhythmia
4. Coronary artery anomalies, e.g., anomalous left coronary artery, Kawasaki's disease
5. Severe pulmonary vascular disease
6. Desaturation of arterial blood (secondary to right-to-left shunt)
7. Postsurgical and post-bed rest recuperation

severe) require special considerations in exercise conditioning. In order to assess a patient's suitability for exercise training and to establish baseline capabilities, we recommend that all patients undergo a *comprehensive exercise test*[2] prior to the onset of a training program. A list of guidelines for selection of patients for exercise training is presented in Table 1. Those conditions warranting special consideration will be dealt with in further detail. The physiologic information presented is not intended to be an in-depth discussion of exercise training physiology, but rather a general foundation for the understanding of the advantages of exercise training.

PHYSIOLOGIC BASIS FOR TRAINING

The fundamental physiologic effect of training the cardiovascular and pulmonary systems is to increase the economy of the body's handling of oxygen. This change comes about by increasing the efficiency of oxygen uptake, transport, and utilization. With physical activity, it is the availability of oxygen that determines endurance.[3]

The maximal oxygen uptake (MVO_2) has been shown to increase with training both in adults[4,5] and in children.[6] The cardiac hypertrophy that occurs in trained athletes[7,8] is due to an actual increase in heart muscle mass (weight)[9-11] that accompanies the increase in heart volume.[4] This hypertrophy and increased volume may be the etiology of the "abnormal" electrocardiographic and radiologic changes seen in trained athletes.[6,8,12]

The effect of training on cardiac function is a decreased resting and submaximal exercise heart rate[3] and an increased stroke volume[5,13] at rest and at submaximal and maximal exercise both in children[14,15] and adults.[16,17] The maximal exercise heart rate seems to be unaltered by training. The results of these changes are that the trained heart provides the same cardiac output with less oxygen demand at rest and at submaximal work as compared with the untrained heart. At maximal work the trained heart provides a higher cardiac output than the untrained heart.[3]

Pulmonary changes that result from training are less striking than cardiovascular improvements, but they are significant. After exercise conditioning of healthy adolescents, an increase in tidal volume is reflected by an increase in minute ventilation at submaximal and maximal work.[18] The same study also demonstrated a more uniform ventilation/perfusion distribution during exercise, and thereby a decrease in intrapulmonary right-to-left shunting, following training, resulting in an improvement in pulmonary gas exchange efficiency.

The transport of oxygen is enhanced by an increase in total hemoglobin and total blood volume with training.[13] This increased blood volume, in addition to enhancing oxygen delivery, improves the systemic venous return to the heart, consequently improving preload and enabling the benefit of the Frank-Starling mechanism. The hypertrophy of skeletal muscle that occurs with training is accompanied by an increased capillary density and arterial collateralization,[3] providing greater surface area for exchange of oxygen, carbon dioxide, and other metabolic substrates and products in the tissues.

The efficiency of oxygen utilization is also increased by training. An increase in skeletal muscle ATP with training[19,20] reflects the increase in mitochondrial volume and concentration in hypertrophied muscle.[21,22] This change is manifested as an increased arteriovenous oxygen difference (A-V O_2 difference) at maximal work following training.

Thus the trained individual has an increased capacity to perform work and physical activity by increasing the oxygen uptake at peak work, by improving the structural and functional capacity of the heart to pump blood, by improving efficiency of pulmonary gas exchange, by expanding delivery of oxygen to the tissues, and by increasing oxygen extraction and utilization by the tissues.

PATHOPHYSIOLOGY OF CONGENITAL HEART DISEASE

The pathophysiology of congenital heart disease that affects working capacity includes four categories: (1) left-to-right shunt, (2) outflow obstruction, (3) undersaturation with oxygen (or right-to-left shunt), and (4) arrhythmia. In disorders in which there is a left-to-right shunt, the exercise capacity may be limited by decreased ventilatory capacity and in some cases by diminished stroke volume. Depending upon the amount of abnormally increased pulmonary blood flow, the pulmonary compliance and gas exchange are decreased to a varying degree. Also, if pulmonary vascular resistance is normal, the larger the amount of blood shunted left to right, the greater the decrease in left ventricular forward stroke volume. Patients who have a moderate or large left-to-right shunt will experience dyspnea at lower workloads than normal and will have an increased respiratory rate reflecting diminished gas exchange ability. They will be less capable than normal individuals of increasing cardiac output to meet exercise demands.

Moderate or severe outflow obstruction results in a greater than normal workload on the myocardium to achieve a normal cardiac output. Working capacity is limited by reduced efficiency of oxygen transport because of a decreased stroke volume and by the extent to which the body can compensate for this decrease. The heart rate rises to an inappropriate level for the particular oxygen consumption (VO_2) in order to maintain the cardiac output. This causes myocardial oxygen demand to increase. Oxygen extraction by the tissues also becomes more efficient; this is manifested as an increased A-V O_2 difference. When these compensations are inadequate, oxygen supply is exceeded by demand, and anaerobic metabolism occurs leading to higher than normal levels of lactic acid.[23]

If the blood perfusing the tissues is desaturated because of right-to-left shunting, working capacity is limited by a relative hypoxia in the tissues and by a tendency, because of decreased pulmonary flow, to accumulate CO_2 causing acidosis. In compensation for the decreased oxygen concentration an increase in hemoglobin and polycythemia occur. Hyperventilation may develop early during exercise in an attempt to eliminate CO_2. Also, oxygen extraction by the tissues is increased.

When arrhythmia prevents the heart rate from increasing normally in response to demands of exertion, maximal cardiac output may be reached at a much lower workload than normal. Some compensation may take place as an increasing duration of diastole allows for longer

245

ventricular filling times, thus improving preload, contractility, and stroke volume. However, the limiting factor, the heart rate, continues to create a ceiling on cardiac output at a lower than normal workload.

Thus each of these four abnormalities of pathophysiology in one way or another limits oxygen supply to the tissues, either by limiting the flow of blood or by limiting the concentration of oxygen in the blood. The body attempts to compensate in predictable ways to maximize its efficiency of handling the available oxygen.

METHODS OF TRAINING

There are numerous methods of training that can be used to help the body's effort to bolster efficiency in handling oxygen. However, to achieve maximal effectiveness, the training regimen must meet certain requirements. One of the most important requirements is that a training program be conducive to compliance. Surprisingly, this does not mean that the training task must be easy, but rather that the patient be comfortable. In other words, the environment in which the activity is performed, for example, outdoors vs. indoors with appropriate lighting and temperature regulation, the location of performance, that is, at home or at the hospital, the convenience of performance, and the patient's particular interests and psychologic state, must all be considered when a program is designed. Studies have determined that by varying the workload and/or the duration of work and of rest periods, training programs can be focused upon (a) increasing muscle strength with little taxing of the oxygen-handling mechanisms, (b) improving mainly the anaerobic processes, (c) developing oxygen-handling, or aerobic, efficiency without evoking anaerobic mechanisms, and (d) increasing both aerobic and anaerobic efficiency. In training the athlete who has high motivation, the last choice provides the best outcome. However, taxing the anaerobic mechanisms in patients with heart disease is undesirable. When anaerobic processes come into play, the oxygen supply to the tissues has become inadequate, CO_2 begins to accumulate as does lactic acid, and the patient experiences breathlessness and exhaustion and becomes rapidly discouraged. Inasmuch as a training effect on the oxygen handling mechanisms has been shown to occur even when $\dot{V}O_2$ is at submaximal levels,[3,17,24] there should be no need to push the cardiac patient to the point of experiencing these unpleasant sensations. As the patient trains, favorable effects of conditioning occur, permitting a gradual increase in the intensity and duration of work without experiencing exhaustion. The patient's own perception of exertion can be used as a training aid to protect against overexertion. Several rating scales have been developed for self assessment. Our laboratory has adopted the use of a numerical scale developed and updated by Borg[25,26] (Fig. 1). The numbers correspond roughly to the exercise heart rate, a rating of 14, for instance, corresponding to a heart rate of 140. Some attempts have also been made[27] to relate the training scale to levels of $\dot{V}O_2$. However, for our purposes the scale has been most helpful as an encouragement to patients who subjectively give a lower rating, after a period of training, to the same workload at which training commenced. The following section provides a general description of the methods followed in our laboratory.

All patients undergo a comprehensive exercise test before beginning exercise. Testing is performed on a bicycle ergometer according to a protocol previously described.[2] In this way, workloads corresponding to 25 percent, 50 percent, 75 percent, and 100 percent $M\dot{V}O_2$ can be determined, and heart rates, blood pressures, and cardiac outputs at the various levels can be measured. An individually tailored program in which the patient performs at corresponding workload levels on the treadmill is then outlined. Some investigators[28] have been able to supply patients with home ergometers for training, which allows for more exact standardization of the workloads performed during training according to $\%M\dot{V}O_2$. Other than in a research setting such exact standardization is probably not necessary, and the advantage of allowing the patient to perform training activity in various settings and without the expense of the ergometer is appreciated. Although some patients have a more nearly normal capacity

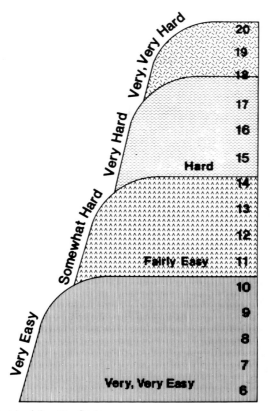

Figure 1. Modified Borg Perceived Exertion Scale.

for training than others, and some have a greater deficit at the outset than others, we have found that the choice of a workload that produces 50 percent M$\dot{V}$O$_2$ at the initiation of conditioning is one that nearly all patients can perform and corresponds fairly closely to a heart rate of 130 to 140 bpm.[3] This goal is achieved by brisk walking on the treadmill at 0 grade and is continued for 15 minutes.

Although more strict timetables for training sessions and for increasing workload have produced significant results,[28] we have preferred to divide our training schedule into stages that are flexible with regard to duration to allow for each patient's individual abilities. The patients proceed from one stage to the next only because they feel capable of doing so, not because the time of one stage is up. Our patients begin conditioning, as mentioned, with brisk walking on the treadmill for 15 to 30 minutes. This is exercise supervised by a physician and by paraprofessional personnel who watch for signs of distress and instruct the patient on proper technique, for example, foot placement, body position, and arm motion. The patient applies the subjective assessment of perceived exertion. Depending on age, a patient may learn to associate the perceived numerical rating with changes in heart and respiratory rate and with approximate percentages of M$\dot{V}$O$_2$. Programmed walking is monitored indoors for a minimum of one week and is performed a minimum of five of seven days. Thereafter, if comfortable, the patient may perform out of doors accompanied by a member of the staff and/or by a parent or spouse who has observed the previous sessions and has been instructed and tested in measuring heart rate. The patient may increase the distance walked per session during this first stage to a maximum of two miles. When this approaches a fairly easy rating (a P.E.

number 10 or 11), usually within two to three weeks, the patient may proceed to Stage II, in which running begins. This exercise takes place indoors on the treadmill at 0 grade. Running technique is taught and the patient is monitored carefully. Duration of exercise varies from 15 to 30 minutes, and a subjective P.E. rating is given at the end of each session. Again, depending on age, the patient may learn to associate the perceived exertion level with heart rate and with approximate $\%M\dot{V}O_2$. This helps in the avoidance of overexertion as training proceeds. The patient may move outdoors, again accompanied by a staff member and/or parent or spouse. The duration of running time is not stressed. The patient is encouraged to run at a rate slower than that which causes breathlessness but to cover a distance of 1.5 to 2.0 miles over a flat course. Subjectively, the exercise level is perceived as less intense at the end of a session as training proceeds, and the distance may be increased. As this takes place the distance is varied from day to day, usually with the greater distance session being followed by a much shorter, previously surpassed distance session. The maximum distance of Stage II is three miles and the average time at which a patient perceives this stage to be completed is seven to ten weeks from the onset of training. At this point the patient may proceed to Stage III. Stage III includes continuation of running on the level alternating with treadmill running with elevation. The increase in workload during Stage III takes place not in distance covered but in degree of elevation on the treadmill. Again, this exercise is closely monitored by a physician and trained personnel so that the workloads are coordinated to the individual patient's submaximal $\dot{V}O_2$ levels.

During Stage III, or after three months of conditioning, whichever comes first, a second comprehensive exercise test is performed to assess objectively the changes that have taken place in the cardiovascular efficiency. Although we and other investigators[13,28] have found detectable changes taking place in some patients earlier in training (see case examples), experience has shown much greater change after three months of conditioning. Also, we believe that retesting prematurely may have a deleterious psychologic effect upon those patients who may not yet have developed very significant objective improvement in oxygen handling economy.

Stages IV and V in our training program are not reached by all patients, and entry into them depends upon the individual's particular cardiac problem, disease state, age, and psychologic outlook. The goal of Stage IV training is to habituate the techniques learned thus far and to encourage *independent* practice sessions with running over both flat and graded courses without supervision. Again, emphasis is not placed on speed, and patients are discouraged from overexerting to breathlessness. In Stage V of conditioning, the patients are considered to have maximized their aerobic efficiency within the limits imposed by their disease. In other words, to achieve any greater efficiency would require working at a higher $\%M\dot{V}O_2$, which would be considered unwise. Thereafter, the patient persists in habitual training to maintain the level of aerobic efficiency achieved.

SPECIAL CONSIDERATIONS AND SPECIFIC EXAMPLES IN EXERCISE TRAINING

When outlining a training program for a patient with congenital heart disease, several additional factors relating particularly to the pathophysiology of the specific disease and to the existing disease state must be considered. For example, the patient with an unoperated atrial septal defect who has a normal pulmonary vascular resistance may have a decreased left ventricular stroke volume in the presence of a large left-to-right shunt. It should not, however, be assumed that surgical closure of this defect will restore normal function to the heart. It has been demonstrated that following repair of an atrial septal defect (ASD) children may have decreased cardiac output response to intense exercise owing to a subnormal stroke volume or heart rate, or both.[29,30] But it has also been shown that training can be beneficial in these patients (see Case 1). A group of unoperated but physically trained patients with ASD with normal pulmonary vascular resistance was shown to have a higher working capacity than untrained healthy control subjects.[31] This study further demonstrated that patients with unoperated atrial septal defects whose pulmonary vascular resistance was elevated had subnormal working capacities when compared with the same control subjects. Thus, when planning the conditioning regimen for a patient with an atrial septal defect, one should be aware of the presence of pulmonary vascular disease and the size of the shunt as revealed by cardiac catheterization; if the patient has undergone surgery, the comprehensive exercise test should supply information regarding the stroke volume, heart rate, and cardiac output response to exercise that will aid in the establishment of realistic goals.

The patient with postoperative tetralogy of Fallot may no longer have a problem with right-to-left shunting and undersaturation, but studies have shown that the response to exercise is often subnormal despite a good surgical result. This response also has been shown to be caused by a decreased stroke volume and heart rate response to exercise.[29,30,32] Postoperative tetralogy patients who have undergone physical training have been shown to have significantly improved exercise cardiovascular function as compared with those who have not trained.[30] Nevertheless, the development of significant conduction abnormalities that may be associated with sudden death is of great concern in these patients. Such arrhythmia (which may be absent at rest) has been shown to be induced or aggravated by exercise.[30] In the immediate post-exercise recovery period, arrhythmias are more likely to occur owing to the rapid decrease in heart rate with an increased respiratory rate and systemic venous return. This is a potentially life-threatening situation and constitutes one of the few contraindications to exercise training. However, when medical control of the arrhythmia has been achieved and proven by a repeated exercise test, we recommend initiation of a carefully monitored exercise program in which special attention is given to the avoidance of performance near the maximal $\dot{V}O_2$ and attention is also given to slow deceleration from the exercise to the resting state.

Much controversy exists regarding the advisability of exercise training of patients with moderate to severe aortic or pulmonic stenosis. As stated, the pathophysiology in these patients consists of a decreased stroke volume response to exercise. The patients are at risk of sudden death, likely as the result of arrhythmia, which may be associated with exertion. In severe aortic stenosis, the myocardium becomes ischemic with exertion because the increased oxygen demand is inadequately met by the limited coronary flow. The compensatory mechanism of increasing oxygen extraction (increasing A-V O_2 difference) does not seem to be significant in the myocardium.[33] Before considering an exercise training program for such a patient, the benefits of surgical relief of the obstruction should be evaluated. However, patients with moderate stenosis may have ST segment depression only with maximal exercise and may remain asymptomatic with a normal working capacity. Recommendation that such patients strictly limit their activity in order to avoid a maximal demand on their cardiovascular system is impractical, especially if the patient is a child or teenager. We believe that a better recommendation is to train patients to exercise more safely than they might if they were to proceed unsupervised. In other words, the patient should avoid induction of the anaerobic mechanisms by choosing activities that stress the oxygen handling mechanisms only submaximally. Specifically, in the presence of a gradient greater than 40 mm Hg or significant ST segment depression at maximal exercise, competitive sports training such as football, basketball, or wrestling should be replaced by supervised endurance training at submaximal levels, such as that described above, which will optimize aerobic efficiency. However, with a mild gradient and following completion of an aerobic training program, a patient with aortic stenosis may participate in competitive field sports, for example, baseball, that do not require maximal performance over extended time periods. We would reiterate that the improvement in cardiovascular efficiency after training the patient with aortic stenosis should not be misinterpreted as palliation or as a means of preventing progression of the disease (see Case 2).

Residual systolic hypertension is often a problem for the post-coarctectomy patient. Although regular exercise has been shown to be helpful in controlling essential hypertension,[34,35] the efficacy of training to aid in control of hypertension in the patient with coarctation is unproven. Our practice has been to control the patient's hypertension medically and then to initiate training. Workloads are maximized just below any level that produces an abnormally elevated blood pressure response.

Patient awareness is an important part of exercise conditioning in the presence of arrhythmia and an otherwise normal heart. We have found that, in some instances, the arrhythmia occurs repeatedly at approximately the same $\%M\dot{V}O_2$, and that as long as training sessions are carried out at levels below the critical $\%M\dot{V}O_2$ the training can proceed to development of maximal efficiency. The patient may or may not be aware of symptoms brought on by arrhythmia (see Cases 3 and 4), but part of the training program is to perfect the subjective perceived exertion rating so that the patient anticipates reaching the arrhythmogenic $\%M\dot{V}O_2$ level and remains below it (see Cases 3 and 4).

Avoidance of performance at maximal $\dot{V}O_2$ levels is extremely important in the patient who has a right-to-left shunt causing desaturation of arterial blood. Submaximal training aids in the increased efficiency of tissue oxygen extraction and contributes to the compensatory polycythemia by increasing the total blood volume and hence the oxygen-carrying capacity. Nevertheless, at maximal levels of exertion ($M\dot{V}O_2$) the systemic vascular resistance falls, tending to increase a right-to-left shunt. If performance at $M\dot{V}O_2$ persists and CO_2 accumulates, the patient is at much greater risk of becoming acidotic.

Special consideration must also be given to the patient who is recuperating from a surgical procedure. Most cardiac surgery, whether palliative or corrective, requires a significant period of convalescence at bed rest. The deleterious effects of bed rest on cardiovascular efficiency were investigated by Saltin and coworkers[13] in three previously sedentary and two previously active healthy young men. There was a 28 percent drop in $M\dot{V}O_2$ and a reduced submaximal and maximal cardiac output and stroke volume following a 20-day period of bed rest. Subsequently, the subjects underwent a vigorous 50-day training period. The previously sedentary men increased their $M\dot{V}O_2$ 100 percent over the post bed rest level, whereas the previously active men increased their $M\dot{V}O_2$ by 34 percent. When absolute numbers are considered, it is noteworthy that the $M\dot{V}O_2$ of the previously active men was significantly higher than that of the sedentary men at pre and post bed rest as well as post training measurements. This response demonstrates the advantage to be gained from exercise conditioning prior to surgery. The patient will benefit from a greater efficiency of oxygen handling throughout the recuperation period if efficiency is maximized preoperatively. The other important aspect of this study was the length of time required for the subjects to attain the pre bed rest levels of efficiency. The previously active men required 30 to 40 days to achieve the same level of efficiency, whereas the previously sedentary men required only 10 days. This concept should be kept in mind when training the postoperative patient. The higher degree of efficiency normally takes longer to recapture, and the patient should not become discouraged.

Case 1

A 33-year-old woman, 13 years after ASD closure, underwent a comprehensive exercise test in which she demonstrated marked exertional dyspnea, a severely depressed working capacity (67 percent below expected), a decreased cardiac output at 78 percent $M\dot{V}O_2$ (24 percent below expected), a blunted maximal exercise heart rate response, and premature development of anaerobic metabolism with an oxygen consumption of 25 cc per minute per kg, and a respiratory quotient (RQ) of 1.4 after only 4.5 minutes of exercise. After just 6 weeks of supervised exercise training, a repeated comprehensive exercise test demonstrated great improvement. Working capacity, although still depressed, was only mildly so (30 percent below expected). When working at 64 percent $M\dot{V}O_2$ the cardiac output had increased to normal. The oxygen consumption at 5.1 minutes was increased slightly to 28 cc per minute per kg and the RQ was lower, indicating a higher anaerobic threshold. These improvements occurred despite a persistence of the decreased heart rate response to maximal exercise.

Case 2

Exercise testing was performed by a 19-year-old female with mild aortic stenosis. When performing at 53 percent $M\dot{V}O_2$ the cardiac output, stroke volume, heart rate, and A-V O_2 difference were all within normal limits. However, the RQ was 1.28 at 7 minutes of exercise, and the total working capacity was markedly depressed (50 percent less than expected). A training program was begun, and two weeks later, although total working capacity had not increased, the anaerobic threshold had improved significantly, with an RQ of 0.99. Three years later the working capacity had not improved, but the disease process had progressed, as demonstrated by the presence of significant exercise-induced ST segment depression. In addition to a cardiac catheterization, continuation of training at no more than 50 percent $M\dot{V}O_2$ was recommended.

Case 3

A 39-year-old male with no history of cardiac problems had begun an unsupervised running regimen. He maximally exerted himself over a distance of one mile, at which point he repeatedly experienced dizziness, nausea, and weakness, preventing continuation of exercise. On exercise testing, multiform ventricular tachycardia (Fig. 2) appeared at a heart rate of 170 bpm and an RQ of 1.33. The perceived exertion rating was 15 to 16. The induction of ventricular tachycardia and symptoms was reproducible whenever the speed of running exceeded 6.5 mph at $\geq$ 2 percent treadmill elevation and the perceived exertion was $\geq$ 15. At a perceived exertion rating of 14, occasional multifocal PVCs were observed. Therefore, this patient was trained to exert only to the degree that induced a perceived exertion of $\leq$ 13 (approximate heart rate of 130 bpm). In this way he was able to increase the duration of training sessions and distance covered and to continue training.

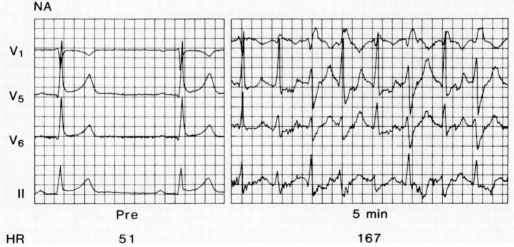

Figure 2. Symptomatic ventricular tachycardia repeatedly induced at a perceived exertion rating of 15 in an otherwise healthy 39-year-old male (see Case 3).

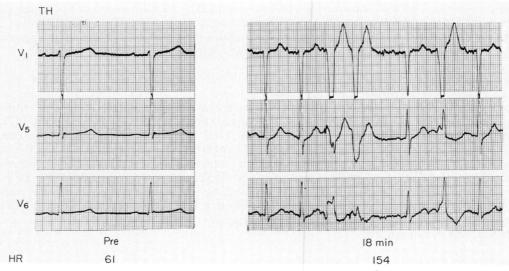

Figure 3. Asymptomatic ventricular ectopy that was reproducible at 88 percent $M\dot{V}O_2$ in a well-trained 18-year-old male competitive swimmer (see Case 4). (From James, FW,[2] with permission.)

Case 4

An 18-year-old male competitive swimmer was found to have exercise-induced ventricular ectopy (Fig. 3). He was asymptomatic and without arrhythmia at rest, but at 88 percent $M\dot{V}O_2$, he developed bursts of ventricular tachycardia, while blood pressure and cardiac output remained normal. Ectopy resolved at rest but was consistently reproducible at 88 percent $M\dot{V}O_2$, and the patient remained asymptomatic. Training was continued without alteration in this patient, and he became a competitive collegiate swimmer. Followup exercise testing three years after presentation demonstrated occasional premature ventricular beats at approximately 88 percent $M\dot{V}O_2$, and four years after presentation no arrhythmia could be elicited at submaximal $\dot{V}O_2$.

CONCLUSION

Nowadays an ever-increasing number of children with congenital or acquired heart disease survive to become teenagers and adults. These patients are more often than not limited in their abilities to perform work and recreational activities by a deficit in oxygen transport imposed by their disease. Despite these inherent limitations these patients can be offered a fuller life with greater endurance for work and play by increasing their aerobic efficiency through training. Methods for training the body's oxygen handling mechanisms lead to an increase in maximal oxygen uptake, transport, and utilization and can be performed conveniently, without pain, exhaustion, injury, or discomfort. Using special considerations based upon a patient's particular problems, the physician can recommend an exercise training program. The patient can be told with confidence to expect less fatigue with daily activities, improved ability to perform work more efficiently, more accurate perception of his or her own degree of exertion, more appropriate choice of activities suited to capabilities, and an improved sense of overall well-being. These results of training are recognized objectively by the physician as a decreased resting and submaximal exercise heart rate, increased stroke volume, increased maximal cardiac output and $M\dot{V}O_2$, and a decreased CO_2 production and RQ. Unfortunately, it is not possible for the physician to advocate exercise training as a means to alter the disease course when dealing with congenital or valvular heart disease. Nevertheless, training can be used as a means of improving the quality of patients' lives.

REFERENCES

1. NAUGHTON, JP and HELLERSTEIN, HK (EDS): *Exercise Testing and Exercise Training in Coronary Heart Disease*. Academic Press, New York, 1973.

2. JAMES, FW: *Exercise testing in normal individuals and patients with cardiovascular disease*. Cardiovasc Clin 11(2):227, 1980.

3. ASTRAND, PO AND RODAHL, K: In *Textbook of Work Physiology*. McGraw-Hill, New York, 1970.

4. EKBLOM, B: *Effect of physical training on oxygen transport system in man*. Acta Physiol Scand, Supp. 328, 1969.

5. EKBLOM, B, ASTRAND, PO, SALTIN, B, ET AL: *Effect of training on circulatory response to exercise*. J Appl Physiol 24:518, 1968.

6. DOBELN, WV: *Physical training, growth, and maximal oxygen uptake of boys age 11–13 years*. In Pediatric Work Physiology, Symp., Tel Aviv, Israel, 1972.

7. ROESKE, WR, O'ROURKE, RA, KLEIN, A, ET AL: *Noninvasive evaluation of ventricular hypertrophy in professional athletes*. Circulation 53:286, 1976.

8. VANGANSE, W, VERSEE, L, EEGLENBOSCH, W, ET AL: *The electrocardiogram of athletes: Comparison with untrained subjects*. Br Heart J 32:160, 1970.

9. SEIBERT, WW: *Untersuchungen uber hypertrophie des skelettmuschle*. Z Klin Med 109:350, 1929.

10. TORNER, W: *Neue Beitrage zur Physiologic des traininjs*. Arbeitsphysiol 14:95, 1949.

11. LIERE, E AND NORTHRUP, DW: *Cardiac hypertrophy produced by exercise in albino and hooded rats*. J Appl Physiol 11:91, 1957.

12. OAKLEY, DAG AND OAKLEY, CM: *Significance of abnormal electrocardiograms in highly trained athletes*. Am J Cardiol 50:985, 1982.

13. SALTIN, B, BLOMQUIST, B, MITCHELL, JH, ET AL: *Responses to submaximal and maximal exercise after bedrest and training*. Circulation 38 (Suppl 7), 1968.

14. EKBLOM, B: *Effect of physical training on adolescent boys*. J Appl Physiol 27:350, 1969.

15. ERIKSSON, BO AND KOCH, G: *Cardiac output and intra arterial blood pressure at rest and during submaximal and maximal exercise in 11 to 13 year old boys before and after physical training*. In Pediatric Work Physiology, Symp., Tel Aviv, Israel, 139, 1972.

16. HARTLEY, LH, GRIMBY, G, KILBOM, A, ET AL: *Physical training in sedentary middle aged and older men*. Scand J Clin Invest 24:335, 1969.

17. KILBOM, A AND ASTRAND, I: *Physical training with submaximal intensities in women*. Scand J Clin Invest 28:163, 1971.

18. KOCH, G AND ERIKSSON, BO: *Anatomical right to left shunt at rest and ventilation, gas exchange and pulmonary diffusing capacity during exercise in 11 to 13 year old boys before and after physical training*. In Pediatric Work Physiology, Symp. Tel Aviv, Israel, 151, 1972.

19. KARLSSON, J, NORDESJO, LO, AND SALTIN, B: *Muscle lactate, ATP and C.P. levels during exercise after physical training in man*. J Appl Physiol 33:199, 1972.

20. SALTIN, B AND KARLSSON, J: *Muscle ATP, CP and lactate during exercise after physical conditioning*. In PERNOW, B AND SALTIN, B (EDS): *Muscle Metabolism During Exercise*. Plenum Press, New York, 1971, p 395.

21. ERIKSSON, BO, GOLLNICK, PD, AND SALTIN, B: *Muscle metabolism and enzyme activities after training in boys 11–13 years old*. Acta Physiol Scand 87:485, 1972.

22. SJOSTROM, M: *Human muscle morphology with emphasis on the fine structure of different fiber types and effects of physical training—A review*. In BERG, K AND ERIKSSON, BO (EDS): *Children and Exercise IX*, University Park Press, Baltimore, 1980, p 208.

23. SJOSTRAND, T: *Functional capacity and exercise tolerance in patients with impaired cardiovascular function*. In GORDON, B (ED): *Clinical Cardiopulmonary Physiology*. Grune & Stratton, New York, 1960.

24. STEWART, KJ AND GUTIN, B: *Efforts of physical training on cardiorespiratory fitness in children*. The Research Quarterly, Am Assoc Health Phys Educ 47:110, 1976.

25. BORG, G: *Perceived exertion as an indicator of somatic stress*. Scand J Rehab Med 2:92, 1970.

26. BORG, G, HOLGREN, A, AND SINDBLAD, I: *Quantitative evaluation of chest pain*. Acta Med Scand, Suppl 644:43, 1981.

27. BORG, G AND NOBLE, B: *Perceived exertion.* In WILMORE, HH (ED): *Exercise and Sport Science Review.* Academic Press, New York, 1974.

28. GOLDBERG, B, FRUPP, RR, FISTER, G, ET AL: *Effect of physical training on exercise performance of children following surgical repair of congenital heart disease.* Pediatrics 68:691, 1981.

29. EPSTEIN, SE, BEISER, GD, GOLDSTEIN, RE, ET AL: *Hemodynamic abnormalities in response to mild and intense upright exercise following operative correction of an atrial septal defect or tetralogy of Fallot.* Circulation 47:1065, 1973.

30. JAMES, FW: *Exercise testing.* In ADAMS, EH AND EMMANOUILIDES, GC (EDS): *Heart Disease in Infants, Children and Adolescents.* Williams & Wilkins, Baltimore, 1979, p 107.

31. FRICK, MH AND PUNSAR, S: *Physical fitness of patients with left to right shunts.* In KARVONEN, MI AND BARRY, AJ (EDS): *Physical Activity and the Heart.* Charles C Thomas, Springfield, Ill, 1967, p 42.

32. BJARKE, B: *Oxygen uptake and cardiac output during submaximal and maximal exercise in adult subjects with totally corrected tetralogy of Fallot.* In *Functional Studies in Palliated and Totally Corrected Adult Patients with Tetralogy of Fallot.* Scand J Thorac Cardiovasc Surg, Suppl 9:116, 1974.

33. VATNER, SF AND PAGANI, M: *Cardiovascular Adjustments to Exercise: Hemodynamics and Mechanisms.* In SONNENBLICK, EH AND LESCH, M (EDS): *Exercise and Heart Disease.* Grune & Stratton, New York, 1977, p 127.

34. TZANLEOFF, SP, ROBINSON, S, AND PYKE, FS: *Physiological adjustments to work in older men as affected by physical training.* J Appl Physiol 33:346, 1972.

35. MANN, GV, GARRETT, HL, AND FARHI, A: *Exercise to prevent coronary heart disease. An experimental study of the effects of training on risk factors for coronary disease in man.* Am J Med 46:12, 1969.

Psychologic Effects of Exercise Training in Coronary-Prone Individuals and in Patients with Symptomatic Coronary Heart Disease

W. Doyle Gentry, Ph.D. and Martha A. Stewart, B.A.

In this chapter, we address the issue: Does exercise training produce psychologic effects in coronary-prone individuals and/or in persons afflicted with symptomatic manifestations of coronary heart disease (CHD) such as angina pectoris or acute myocardial infarction (MI)? The clinical import of this issue is threefold: First, as noted elsewhere,[1] persons undergoing cardiac rehabilitation typically experience fear of recurrence and death, decreased libido, and problems associated with a damaged self-concept. Persons experiencing unusual levels of mood disturbance (anxiety, depression) may also delay resumption of healthy activity in the areas of work, sex, and recreation. Second, most research studies of exercise training in patients with CHD have failed to include psychologic findings in their description of the relative successes and failures of exercise programs to affect outcome parameters such as blood pressure, weight, caloric intake, cholesterol, oxygen workload, and cigarette smoking. In other words, there has been thus far a tendency to focus narrowly on the role of exercise training in meeting the physical needs of the coronary-prone or CHD patient, while virtually ignoring its role in meeting the psychologic needs of such individuals. Psychologic needs are important not only in their own right, but also because they indirectly affect the motivation of CHD patients to comply with the prescribed medical regimen, including rehabilitative exercise training. Third, there is interest in the applicability of a nonpsychologic intervention (exercise) to psychologic needs in patients recuperating from acute episodes of CHD, as well as those at risk for the same, who all too often may resist (that is, elect not to participate in or drop out of) psychologic treatment programs designed to focus on these same needs (for example, mood disturbance). There is interest in both the preventive and therapeutic effects of exercise training on psychologic needs, hence the shared emphasis on persons at risk (coronary-prone) for CHD who are as yet free of acute MI or angina.

EXERCISE TRAINING FOR CORONARY-PRONE INDIVIDUALS

In a recent experimental study, Blumenthal and coworkers[2] demonstrated the potential psychologic benefits of supervised exercise training in healthy, albeit coronary-prone middle-aged adults. In their study of 46 persons (20 males and 26 females) recruited for an adult physical fitness program, they found that supervised exercise, consisting of a combination of stretching exercises and continuous walking/jogging three times weekly, not only led to improved physical cardiovascular function over a ten-week period (for example, decreased systolic and diastolic blood pressure, decreased body weight, increased HDL-cholesterol levels, increased plasminogen activator release, and increased treadmill performance), but also led to a significant reduction in coronary-prone behavior, as measured by the Jenkins Activity Scale.[3] The Type A or coronary-prone behavior pattern has been prospectively linked to the future occurrence of CHD in healthy persons,[4] to CHD recurrence and fatality,[5] as well as to the extent[6] and progression[7] of coronary atherosclerosis. The characteristic elements of the Type A (coronary-prone) pattern include an unusual sense of time urgency, excessive job involvement, and a hostile/competitive style of relating to others in one's immediate social environment. In their study, Blumenthal and coworkers observed that exercise produced a notable reduction not only in subjects' overall Type A scores, but also in their scores reflecting time urgency and hostile/competitive attitudes. Interestingly, the psychologic effects of exercise were observed only for Type A participants and not for Type B persons, who tended to be more relaxed and easy-going from the outset. The authors speculated that the supervised, brief exercise program may have encouraged Type A (coronary-prone) individuals to reorder their priorities in daily living, for example, taking time away from work to exercise. They also indicated that social interaction with other exercise participants may have had a therapeutic effect. Syme[8] has recently suggested that the disruption in meaningful social ties, which accompanies the Type A life-style, may well account for the differential risk for CHD seen in such persons. Exercise may, at least in part, provide one means of establishing or re-establishing a richer social (support) network for Type A individuals. Finally, it is of interest that the magnitude of the therapeutic effect (change) in Type A behavior attributable to exercise training is very comparable to that achieved by means of psychologic intervention in similar individuals, namely, anxiety management training.[9] Exercise led to a 36 percent decrease in overall Type A scores and a 35 percent reduction in Hard Driving (hostile/competitive) scores, whereas anxiety management training over a comparable time period led to a 39 percent decrease in overall Type A scores and a 23 percent decline in Hard Driving scores. In short, exercise would appear to be just as effective in ameliorating CHD risk in coronary-prone adults as would more conventional psychologic techniques.

EXERCISE TRAINING FOR PATIENTS WITH CORONARY HEART DISEASE

The clinical research evidence attesting to the psychologic effects of exercise training in CHD patients ranges from single case examples to controlled, multi-group outcome studies.*

Hackett and Cassem,[10] for example, provide an illustrative case of a 52-year-old insurance executive who benefited from exercise training after sustaining an uncomplicated MI. The patient in question had feelings of intense depression (for example, excessive sleeping, a sense of lethargy and despair, total lack of sexual interest, loss of appetite, and nightmares) and anxiety (for example about his ability to successfully return to work or drive in traffic) during the first several weeks after surviving his MI. Drug therapy was deemed unwise, and thus he was referred for a program of graduated physical exercise that involved progressive walking and mild exercises and eventually jogging under medical supervision. Depressive symptoms began to abate within 2 to 3 weeks after initiation of the exercise regimen, particularly as regards his ability to concentrate on mental tasks, interest in sex, and sleep disturbance. At a one-year followup, the patient had slimmed down to his pre-MI body weight, had stopped smoking, and gave no evidence of postinfarction mood disturbance.

Similarly, in an uncontrolled group study of 100 CHD patients, Hellerstein[11] found that feelings of depression were significantly reduced as a function of exercise training. Specifically, patients reported, and were judged by their spouses, to be better able to think and sleep, had less fatigue, were less tense, and enjoyed life more as a consequence of exercising. Exercise, which progressed gradually over a period of months to more physically demanding levels,

---

*Other studies on this topic include Hellerstein,[23] Martic,[24] McPherson and coworkers,[25] Morgan,[26] Naughton,[27] and Wrzesniewski.[28]

basically consisted of calisthenics for strength, run-walk sequences for endurance, and recreational exercise for fun.

In one of the better designed experimental tests of the issue in question, Naughton and associates[12] examined the effects of exercise training on psychologic characteristics of 14 CHD patients compared with those of 14 sedentary CHD patients and 14 additional healthy control subjects. It is difficult to appreciate their precise results with respect to an exercise effect on personality and mood disturbance, as essential data (for example, MMPI profiles at various intervals) are not reported. However, there does seem to be sufficient reason to conclude that some clinically significant, if not statistically significant, improvement in psychologic function was forthcoming. That is, 64 percent of the CHD patients undergoing exercise reported less tension, worry, and anxiety over time, as compared with only 43 percent of the sedentary CHD patients and 36 percent of the healthy control subjects. Exercising patients also reported more improvement in attitudes toward work and relationships with spouse/children, again as compared with these other two groups. Also, the exercising patients evidenced lower, albeit nonsignificant, scores on MMPI scales measuring depression and hypochondriasis; these scales are generally the ones most affected by chronic physical illness (CHD) and reflective of psychologically exaggerated sick-role, invalid behavior.

Shephard[13] recently summarized a series of experimental studies [14-17] which point out that changes in psychologic parameters (for example mood) are difficult to achieve and/or document as a result of exercise training, even over periods as long as 4 years. Again, as with the study of Naughton and coworkers,[12] these investigators place too much emphasis on statistical significance rather than clinical significance in evaluating change. For example, if one charts the MMPI profiles based on their data collected over a 4-year followup period on 44 postcoronary patients initially presenting high depression scores, it is clear that the composite profile is much healthier, psychologically speaking, after 4 years of exercise training. Patients as a group have, in fact, moved from what would be considered a mild-to-moderate level of clinical depression (requiring treatment) to a borderline level of depressed affect (not necessarily requiring treatment). These patients also moved in a more healthy direction (lower) on the MMPI scales that reflected exaggerated somatic concern/complaint (hypochondriasis), denial (hysteria), obsessive thinking (psychasthenia), and alienation (schizophrenia).

Finally, in a study by Roviaro and colleagues,[18] a comprehensive exercise-based cardiac rehabilitation program, without doubt, produced psychologic effects not observed in CHD patients who experienced what is considered routine postcoronary care. These investigators found that 28 patients, who had either sustained an MI or undergone coronary bypass surgery, reported an increase in positive self-concept, increased physical self-esteem (that is, improved physical appearance, enhanced sexuality, more positive view of body), decrease in signs of personal maladjustment, decrease in signs of personality disorder, and decreased evidence of psychosis, as compared with 20 patients not participating in the exercise program. Although the investigators failed to show significant differences in total depression scores between the two groups, they did find favorable exercise-induced changes on several aspects of depressed mood, for example, exercising patients showed improved (positive) mood, were less indecisive, felt less fatigue, and were less pessimistic in their approach to life. Interestingly, patients in the exercise group were also more self-critical and showed more irritability, as well as less guilt, than nonexercising patients. This suggests a more healthy psychologic adaptation to their coronary condition, one that reduces the probability of clinical depression. Exercising patients also showed greater improvement in terms of decreased employment-related stress, increased participation in and enjoyment of leisure-time activities, and increased sexual activity. Chronic patients (that is, those experiencing an MI or coronary bypass surgery more than 26 weeks before entry into the study) benefited as much from the exercise-based rehabilitation program as did acute patients (that is, those experiencing an MI or surgery less than 26 weeks prior to entry into the study), and treatment effects were evident both immediately after completion of the 3-month exercise program and 4 months later.

THE IMPORTANCE OF COMPLIANCE

It is clear from the reports of Hellerstein,[11] Naughton and coworkers,[12] and Shephard[13] that those CHD patients who comply with the exercise training as prescribed show more pronounced psychologic effects, for example, improved mood. In one study reported by Shephard, virtually *all* of the improvement in depression, as measured by the MMPI, occurred in those patients who complied with the postcoronary exercise regimen; noncompliers remained just as depressed 4 years later as they were at the outset of the rehabilitation effort.

Ironically, it is those individuals who would benefit the most in terms of psychologic function who are most likely to be noncompliant with exercise training. That is, as Blumenthal and associates[19] have shown, drop-outs from a postcoronary exercise therapy program tend to be more hypochondriacal, more depressed, more socially introverted, more anxious, and lacking in self-esteem as compared with those who do not drop out. Similarly, Oldridge[20] found that Type A participants were more likely to drop out of exercise training than Type B participants.

Blumenthal and associates[19] were able to successfully predict exercise compliance (90.4 percent) and noncompliance (78.6 percent) by classifying CHD patients in terms of three descriptor variables: social introversion, ego strength, and left ventricular ejection fraction (LVEF) at rest. Compliers (those who did not drop out) had lower LVEF and ego strength values, and higher social introversion scores. Blumenthal and associates[19] noted that psychologic variables had more influence on compliance than did the physiologic variable, and that the two sets of factors tended to operate independently of one another in determining whether or not a given patient would stay in the exercise training program. They further suggested that compliance might be higher in CHD patients high in social introversion if they were offered a solitary exercise program, rather than being forced to participate in a group program for which they were ill suited.

Type A individuals, either precoronary or postcoronary, are, in our opinion,[21] more likely to comply with rehabilitation efforts, including exercise training, if they are allowed and encouraged to become actively involved in goal setting (for example, number of miles walked or jogged) and if the exercise regimen is tailored to their individual needs and interests. We agree with Fuller and Eliot[22] that the latter is especially important in maintaining enthusiasm over long periods of time.

CONCLUSIONS

Exercise training (a) produces clear, well-defined psychologic effects both in coronary-prone and postcoronary individuals; (b) produces psychologic changes (for example, in Type A behavior) that are comparable to conventional psychologic treatment techniques; and (c) benefits most those who fully comply with the prescribed exercise regimen. Exercise training also provides a means of altering pathologic psychologic states (for example, depression) in postcoronary patients when drug therapy is contraindicated.[10] In some of the more severely depressed CHD patients, a combination of drug therapy and exercise training may prove most beneficial in relieving the mood disturbance,[13] as well as in keeping the patient from dropping out of the exercise program. Exercise training may appeal to postcoronary patients more than conventional psychotherapy[10] and thus may reach patients with obvious psychologic needs who, if left to their own devices, may go untreated. In some instances, for example, with socially extroverted and/or Type B individuals, group exercise programs are most beneficial in regard to changes in psychologic parameters, in large measure because of the effects of increased social support vis-a-vis the other group participants. In other instances, for example, with socially introverted and/or Type A individuals, solitary exercise programs may be more beneficial.

Some of the concern and contradictions about whether exercise training produces beneficial psychologic effects appears to come from placing too much emphasis on statistically significant changes without giving careful attention to clinical significance; as noted above, the misinterpretation of findings in the Shephard[13] studies is a case in point. Also, many patients who enter exercise training programs are not depressed or in any way psychologically disturbed at baseline, that is, point of entry. Thus, it would be unlikely that they would show any change in their psychologic state (mood) as a consequence of such a program. This, however, does not nullify the potential therapeutic effectiveness of such programs; rather, it suggests that we take into consideration the point at which a person starts in measuring change, that is, the law of initial values. With this in mind, it may not be necessary to abandon psychologic *trait* measures such as the MMPI, which tell us a great deal about an individual's total ability to cope with life stresses as well as his ongoing level of emotionality, for *state* measures, which are sensitive to influences other than mere participation in an exercise training program.[13]

REFERENCES

1. GENTRY, WD: *Psychosocial concerns and benefits in cardiac rehabilitation.* In POLLOCK, ML AND SCHMIDT, DH (EDS): *Heart Disease and Rehabilitation.* Houghton Mifflin, Boston, 1979.

2. BLUMENTHAL, JA, WILLIAMS, RS, WILLIAMS, RB, ET AL: *Effects of exercise on the Type A (coronary prone) behavior pattern.* Psychosom Med 42:289, 1980.

3. JENKINS CD, ROSENMAN, RH, AND ZYZANSKI, SJ: *The Jenkins Activity Survey for Health Prediction, Form B.* Psychological Corporation, Boston, 1972.

4. ROSENMAN, RH, BRAND, RJ, JENKINS, CD, ET AL; *Coronary heart disease in the Western Collaborative Group Study: Final follow-up experience of 8½ years.* JAMA 233:872, 1975.

5. JENKINS, CD, ZYZANSKI, SJ, AND ROSENMAN, RH: *Risk for new myocardial infarction in middle-aged men with manifest coronary heart disease.* Circulation 53:342, 1976.

6. BLUMENTHAL, JA, WILLIAMS, RB, KONG, Y, ET AL: *Type A behavior pattern and coronary atherosclerosis.* Circulation 58:534, 1978.

7. KRANTZ, DS, SANMARCO, MI, SELVESTER, RH, ET AL: *Psychological correlates of progression of atherosclerosis in men.* Psychosom Med 41:467, 1979.

8. SYME, SL: *Sociocultural factors and disease etiology.* In GENTRY, WD (ED): *Handbook of Behavioral Medicine.* Guilford, New York, 1984.

9. SUINN, RM AND BLOOM, LJ: *Anxiety management training for pattern A behavior.* Behav Med 1:25, 1978.

10. HACKETT, TP AND CASSEM, NH: *Psychological factors related to exercise.* In WENGER, N (ED): *Exercise and the Heart.* FA Davis, Philadelphia, 1978.

11. HELLERSTEIN, HK: *Exercise therapy in coronary disease.* Bull New York Acad Med 44:1028, 1968.

12. NAUGHTON, J, BRUHN, JG, AND LATEGOLA, MT: *Effects of physical training on physiologic and behavioral characteristics of cardiac patients.* Arch Phys Med Rehabil 49:133, 1968.

13. SHEPHARD, RJ: *Cardiac rehabilitation in prospect.* In POLLOCK, ML AND SCHMIDT, DH (EDS): *Heart Disease and Rehabilitation.* Houghton Mifflin, Boston, 1979.

14. KAVANAGH, T, SHEPHARD, RJ, AND KENNEDY, J: *Characteristics of post-coronary marathon runners.* Ann NY Acad Sci 301:455, 1978.

15. KAVANAGH, T, SHEPHARD, RJ, AND TUCK, JA: *Depression after myocardial infarction.* Can Med Assoc J 113:23, 1975.

16. KAVANAGH, T, SHEPHARD, RJ, TUCK, JA, ET AL: *Depression following myocardial infarction—the effects of distance running.* Ann NY Acad Sci 301:1029, 1978.

17. DOBSON M, TATTERSFIELD, AE, ADLER, MW, ET AL: *Attitudes and long-term adjustment of patients surviving cardiac arrest.* Br Med J 3:207, 1971.

18. ROVIARO S, HOLMES, DS, AND HOLMSTEN, RD: *Influence of a cardiac rehabilitation program on the cardiovascular, psychological, and social functioning of cardiac patients.* Behav Med (in press).

19. BLUMENTHAL, JA, WILLIAMS, RS, WALLACE, AG, ET AL: *Physiological and psychological variables predict compliance to prescribed exercise therapy in patients recovering from myocardial infarction.* Psychosom Med 44:519, 1982.

20. OLDRIDGE, NB: *Compliance of post-myocardial infarction patients to exercise programs.* Med Sci Sports 11:373, 1979.

21. GENTRY, WD, BALDER, L, OUDE-WEME, JD, ET AL: *Type A/B differences in coping with acute myocardial infarction: Further considerations.* Heart and Lung 12:212, 1983.

22. FULLER, EW AND ELIOT, RS: *The role of exercise in the relief of stress.* In ELIOT, RS (ED): *Stress and the Heart.* Futura, Mt Kisco, NY, 1974.

23. HELLERSTEIN, A: *Active physical conditioning of coronary patients.* Circulation 32:100, 1965.

24. MARTIC, M: *Results of psychological testing of coronary paths in a longitudinal study of the follow-up effects of training.* In STOCKSMEIER, U (ED): *Psychological Approach to the Rehabilitation of Coronary Patients.* Springer, New York, 1976.

25. McPHERSON, BD, PAIVIO, A, YUHASZ, MS, ET AL: *Psychological effects of an exercise program for postinfarct and normal adult men.* Physical Fitness 7:95, 1967.

26. MORGAN, WP: *Psychologic aspects of heart disease.* In POLLOCK, ML AND SCHMIDT, DH (EDS): *Heart Disease and Rehabilitation.* Houghton Mifflin, Boston, 1979.

27. NAUGHTON, J: *Rehabilitation for patients after myocardial infarction.* Southern Med Bull 55:29, 1967.

28. WRZESNIEWSKI, K: *Anxiety and rehabilitation after myocardial infarction.* Psychother Psychosom 27:41, 1976.

Therapeutic Exercise in Patients with Chronic Obstructive Pulmonary Disease

John G. Weg, M.D.

The easiest way of all to preserve and restore health without diverse peculiarities and with greater profit than all other measures put together is to exercise well. Mendez, C. 1552.[1]

The goal of therapeutic exercise in patients with chronic obstructive pulmonary disease (COPD) is to enhance beneficial or useful exercise performance-endurance for activities of daily living. This goal has almost invariably been achieved with a variety of exercise programs, as initially observed and then documented by pioneers in the field such as Barach, Haas, and Miller. Much unnecessary confusion has been generated, however, because of continuing difficulties in defining the mechanisms accounting for this increased endurance. Although these mechanisms are the focus of important and continuing investigations, which should clarify and refine the application of therapeutic exercise in patients with COPD, the available data amply support the value of carefully prescribed exercise training as an integral component of therapy for the patient with COPD. In addition, when exercise has been prescribed as a component of a comprehensive multidisciplinary rehabilitation program, the following benefits can be expected: (1) improved quality of life and (2) decreased hospitalization. More problematic benefits are a slowing of disease progression and a prolongation of life span (Fig. 1).

EFFECTS OF EXERCISE TRAINING

Normal Individuals

This discussion will concern itself with endurance training rather than strength of muscle training. In normal individuals, endurance training results in a 5 to 20 percent increase in maximum oxygen consumption ($\dot{V}O_{2max}$). $\dot{V}O_{2max}$ is achieved when $\dot{V}O_2$ remains stable despite increasing power; this is usually accompanied by a peak plasma lactate of 8 mmol/L. This gain in $\dot{V}O_{2max}$ results from an increased cardiac output ($\dot{Q}$) and increased arterial-venous oxygen (a-vO_2) difference. The increase in $\dot{Q}$ is achieved by an increase in stroke volume without a change in maximum heart rate. The increased oxygen extraction is attributed to an increased number and size of mitochondria, aerobic mitochondrial enzymes, and glycogen concentration in the trained muscles. An increase in muscle myoglobin content and capillary density facilitates oxygen transport. There is also an increase in maximal exercise ventilation ($\dot{V}_{E\ max}$) without an increase in maximum voluntary ventilation (MVV). At any given level of submaximal exercise, heart rate is reduced without the change in $\dot{Q}$ owing to

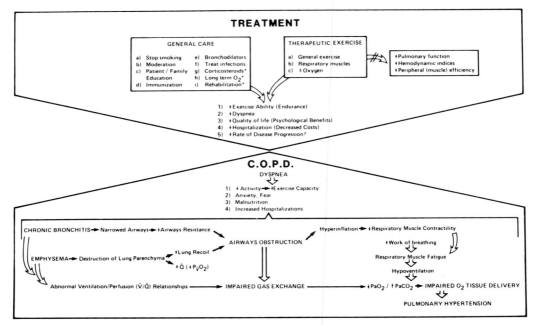

Figure 1. An overall schema of the mechanisms by which COPD results in dyspnea and exercise limitation vs. the effects of general care and therapeutic exercise (adapted from Miller, WF[93]). See text for indications

the increased stroke volume. $\dot{V}O_2$ is unchanged at any given work rate. Endurance training results primarily in improving the function of the large muscle groups that are trained, for example, upper extremity vs. lower, swimming vs. jogging, and cycling vs. treadmill running. To achieve these training effects, a certain threshold of exercise level, duration, and frequency must be achieved. In normal people, this can be accomplished by exercising at a heart rate of 60 to 70 percent of maximum or 50 percent of $\dot{V}O_{2max}$ for 30 minutes 3 or 4 times per week for a month or more.

Patients with Chronic Obstructive Pulmonary Disease

The one uniform effect noted in exercise training in patients with COPD is increased exercise performance or endurance. The effects of exercise, however, are primarily conditioned by the severity of airway obstruction, which can vary from mild to extremely severe. Individuals with mild airway obstruction will respond to exercise in a manner similar to normal individuals or those with coronary artery disease. Individuals with severe airway obstruction, however, are unable to achieve either a $\dot{V}O_{2max}$ or a sufficiently elevated exercise level and duration to obtain either the cardiac or peripheral (muscular) benefits of conditioning. Most studies focus on individuals with severe airway obstruction—a forced expired volume in 1 second (FEV_1) of 0.7 to about 1.5 (or an $FEV_1\%$) of approximately 30 percent. In such individuals, one may estimate their symptom-limited maximum oxygen consumption ($\dot{V}O_2SL$) very roughly as $\dot{V}O_2SL$ in ml STPD/0.5 min. as $= 702 + 21.76\ FEV_1\% - 10.72\ VC\%-$ where $FEV_1\%$ is percent of predicted FEV_1 and $VC\%$ is percent of predicted vital capacity. The standard error of estimate (SEE) is 102, r^2 0.78 and $p < 0.99$.[2] Vyas and coworkers also predicted the improvement in total work performed in kilogram meters (Kgm) $= 1.895 + (25.54)\ (\Delta PaO_2) - 10.52$ weight in pounds, where $\Delta PaO_2 = PaO_2$ (exercise) $- PaO_2$ rest with an SEE of 381, r^2 0.78 and $p < 0.01$.[2] Grum and associates have derived similar estimates in young adults with cystic fibrosis: $\dot{V}O_2 = 0.35$ (FEV$_1$ as % predicted) $+ 12.12$ (r $= 0.81$).[3] Less common and/or less important variables may also contribute, such as impaired left ventricular function, obesity or malnutrition, other diseases, psychologic factors independent of those related to the chronic progressive illness of COPD, and age.

Improved Endurance

Barach and colleagues in 1952 apparently were the first to note "a marked improvement in capacity to exercise (subsequently) without oxygen in two patients given a progressive walking program with oxygen."[4] Haas and associates reported a decreased $\dot{V}O_2$ with walking at 1.2 mph and with stair climbing following a general rehabilitation program including exercise with oxygen.[5,6] Subsequently, Pierce and coworkers reported the first well-documented study of the physiologic effects of exercise training on a treadmill for 2 to 20 weeks in 9 patients with severe COPD who were stable, received optimal medical therapy, and had 2 to 3 days to become familiar with a treadmill. These patients increased their mean maximal speed from 3.5 to 5.5 mph for 2.5 minutes, and "in the three patients trained to a stable level, the speed that could be tolerated for no longer than 2.5 minutes before training could be sustained for greater than 30 minutes after training." Although there was no change in pulmonary function with conditioning, there was a 24 percent decrease in heart rate, a 40 percent decrease in respiratory rate, and a 23 percent reduction in $\dot{V}O_2$ in the last minute of exercise; these returned more rapidly to baseline after exercise.[7] Christie[8] subsequently reported the results in 11 patients of a graduated outpatient exercise program consisting of a daily exercise period of 15 minutes and a ½-mile to 1-mile daily walk for an average of 10 weeks. Nine of 10 had subjective improvement in exercise tolerance, and the eleventh died of a myocardial infarction considered unrelated. These patients had significant improvements in $\dot{V}O_{2max}$, $\dot{V}_E$max, maximum work in meter kilograms/minute (mkg/min), and in $\dot{V}_E$ and $\dot{V}O_2$ at 100 mkg/min. Similar improvement in exercise performance-endurance and increased SL $\dot{V}O_2$ usually associated with a decreased heart rate, respiratory rate, and at a submaximal exercise level, a decreased $\dot{V}O_2$ and $\dot{V}CO_2$ have been reported by others[2,9-16] in studies extending 6 to 12 months,[17,18] in comparison with control subjects[19] and using the Royal Canadian Air Force 5 BX/XBX Program.[20] Similar improvement has been obtained in young people with cystic fibrosis.[21]

Walking

In 1977, McGavin and associates reported a randomized controlled trial of progressive exercise training accomplished with a 3-month outpatient, unsupervised, at least 5 days per week, stair climbing program recorded in a diary. It was evaluated by a 12-minute walking distance (12 MD) and verified by a progressive workload bicycle ergometer study. The 12 MD is the maximum distance an individual can walk in a level enclosed corridor regardless of whether it is necessary to stop for rest; the best of 2 or 3 efforts with intervening rest periods should be used for baseline. There was significant improvement in sense of general well-being, dyspnea, cough, and sputum volume, the 12 MD, length of stride (a learned and useful gain) and workload on the bicycle ergometer. More recently, a similar study[23] extending over a mean of 10.3 months with supervised exercise once per week and an unsupervised daily 12 minute walk and stair climbing resulted in a 24 percent increase in the 12 MD. The improvement of 24 vs. 6 percent in the McGavin study was attributed to ongoing supervision and longer duration of study. The increase at 6 months was 174 ± 89 m; at 8 months 185 m; and at 12 months 203 ± 77 m.[23] Another controlled study involved an initial 6 weeks in a rehabilitation center followed by simple exercises, stair climbing and walking at home, with activities recorded in a dairy. The treatment group increased 12 MD from 523 m to 643 m (19 percent) vs. the control group's increase from 564 m to 607 m.[24]

Pulmonary Function

A second common finding of most investigators has been the lack of change in most measures of pulmonary function: spirometry, including forced expired volumes; flow volume loops; lung volumes; airway resistance; static and dynamic compliance; diffusion capacity; physiologic dead space; arterial oxygen and carbon dioxide tension; and A-aO$_2$ gradients at rest and with exercise.[1,28] This is not at all surprising in a disease characterized by the fixed airway obstruction of chronic bronchitis and the parenchymal destruction of emphysema. In addition, every effort is made to provide maximal medical therapy prior to initiating an exercise program; this should remove any reversible component of the disease.

Minor and probably clinically unimportant improvements have been noted in forced inspiratory flow;[7] MVV and inspiratory capacity;[13] PaO$_2$ at rest;[11] PaO$_2$ and A-aO$_2$ gradient with exercise;[14] vital capacity;[23] FEV$_1$, DLCO, and A-aO$_2$ gradient;[20] decreased A-aO$_2$ gradient, venous admixture and increased dynamic compliance;[16] static and specific compliance;[10] and PaO$_2$ at rest.[11] Whether these changes are related to the exercise training, random variability in patients or measurement techniques, or perhaps to other aspects of treatment over time cannot be determined.

Hemodynamic Indices

As with pulmonary function, improvement in hemodynamic function is generally not achieved in patients with severe COPD. Although most achieve heart rates of 60 to 70 percent or more of their maximum, this rate is reached usually well below that of 50 percent of $\dot{V}O_{2max}$; they are unable to reach a $\dot{V}O_2$ max, but achieve only a SL $\dot{V}O_{2max}$. Thus, the increase in $\dot{V}O_{2max}$, $\dot{Q}$, and especially stoke volume that occurs in normal persons with exercise conditioning is not achieved.[10–12,16,25]

Peripheral (Muscle) Indices

No substantive data are available to support the development of increased muscle efficiency in patients with severe COPD; this is to be expected in individuals who cannot reach effective levels of exercise for conditioning. Paez and colleagues[25] studied 4 patients trained for 21 days breathing air and 4 breathing oxygen at 6 L/min on a treadmill at an equal submaximal workload on a bicycle ergometer. After training, there was a reduction in $\dot{Q}$ from 3.41 to 2.70 ($p < 0.05$) and a slight increase in arterial venous oxygen difference from 10.1 to 11.7. They attributed this to increased extraction peripherally. Degre and colleagues also noted a slight increase in the a-vO$_2$ difference from 8.2 vol % to 9.5 vol %, in the 4 patients with the largest improvement in SL $\dot{V}O_2$; however, there was no difference when all 11 patients were combined.[11] In contrast, Alpert and coworkers[10] noted a decrease from 9.1 to 7.4 vol % ($p < 0.01$). More recently, Belman and Kendregan[26] could demonstrate no increase in citrate synthase, 3 β hydroxacyl coenzyme A dehydrogenase and pyruvate kinase following a 6-week training program in either those receiving arm training or leg training. In addition, the expected decrease in heart rate attributable to improved function of peripheral muscles did not occur.[27] The difficulties concerning either the a-vO$_2$ difference or measuring muscle enzymes have recently been reviewed.[28]

Improved Mechanical Skills

In their signal study, Pierce and associates[7] attributed an important component of the increased performance to a more efficient ventilatory pattern resulting in a decreased respiratory rate. Subsequently, Paez and colleagues documented that the increased length of stride (23 percent), more efficient posture, relaxation, and economy of movement accounted for most of the increased treadmill endurance in their patients and those of Pierce and associates. Inasmuch as there was only a slight increase in $\dot{V}O_2$ and the respiratory quotient accompanied by a fall in cardiac output and slight widening of the a-vO_2 difference, it was concluded that most of the effect of training should be attributed to learned specific mechanical skills in the trained muscles. Others have also attributed the increased performance to improved specific skills.[10,12,18-20] With stair climbing and walking as the exercise, increased stride length has been found in the 12 MD.[22,23] In a group of less impaired patients with COPD (FEV$_1$ 1.48 ± 0.69 L) trained on a bicycle ergometer, the increased performance was transferred to the 12 MD.[29] It must be emphasized that improved mechanical skill, especially in a critical activity such as walking, is a worthwhile objective. It will contribute appreciably to the quality of life of the individual severely limited by COPD.

Psychologic Benefits

An improved sense of well-being has been as constant a finding as increased endurance, when it is discussed.[2,5-9,12-15,17,18,22-24] This finding has generally been reported as a global impression. However, Agle and colleagues formally confirmed this improvement using psychiatric interviews to evaluate the degree of anxiety, depression, and excessive body preoccupation along with the Minnesota Multiphasic Personality Inventory (MMPI). They found lessened depression in 8 of 16, decreased anxiety in 10 of 19, and decreased excessive body preoccupation in 9 of 15 (although 4 others developed this preoccupation.) From only 2 involved in any vocational activity at the onset, 10 were so involved at the end of the program, that is, attending college or gainfully employed, and 10 of the 21 were more actively participating in social situations and in family life. Those with fewer symptoms of depression and a better MMPI initially did better at the one-year evaluation. Although these patients have been reported to have had no physiologic improvement, that is, pulmonary or hemodynamic, they did have improved exercise performance-endurance.[9,12] It has been stated that psychologic improvement occurred in the absence of physiologic improvement, but ignoring the improved exercise performance has led to frequent misinterpretation of these data. The data indicate that improved physical performance and improved sense of well-being go hand in hand. Agle and colleagues also found that their patients exercised to extreme dyspnea while under the direct supervision (protection) of the medical care team without untoward incident. They believe this gives rise to a "desensitization of the fear of dyspnea and increased patient autonomy in the control of symptoms." Many of the studies already cited list decreased dyspnea as a subjective advantage of the exercise training.

Another important but extremely difficult to measure contributor to the improved sense of well-being is the individual empathetic caring of each member of the health care team for the patient with a (slowly) progressive chronic illness. This empathy has a powerful influence on the patient who has been ignored, shunted from physician to physician, or told with unwarranted finality, "Frankly, there is nothing more anyone can do for you." Thus the psychologic benefits of exercise are well documented. They can be attributed to the benefits of increased activity, decreased dyspnea, and more independence that can be directly related to the exercise training as well as to the nonspecific gains related to the ministrations of each member of the health care team. Although these benefits may not titillate the cardiopulmonary physiologist, they too add to the quality of life of the patient.

Oxygen

Normal individuals will increase their work capacity while breathing oxygen.[31] Barach, beginning in 1952, described the benefit of oxygen exercise training in 100 patients.[4,32,33] In 1956, Cotes and Gilson[34] reported that in 22 of 29 patients with advanced pneumoconiosis or COPD walking distance was doubled with oxygen; they considered an F_1O_2 of 0.3 as satisfactory. Cotes and colleagues[35] subsequently reported a reduction in $\dot{Q}$–7.5 percent, HR–9.6 percent, and P_{PA}–10.1 percent in a similar group while breathing oxygen. Beck and colleagues reported a lesser increase of $\dot{V}_E$ over resting with a step test while breathing an F_1O_2 of 0.4— 38 percent increase vs. 60 percent increase. Miller and colleagues[1] reported that a F_1O_2 of 0.4 maintains an adequate PaO_2, reduces $\dot{V}_E$, HR, respiratory rate, and dyspnea during and after exercise. Several investigators have reported a reduction in some patients' P_{PA} or total pulmonary vascular resistance while exercising with O_2.[1,37–39] Subsequently, Pierce and coworkers[40] described results in 4 patients, three who markedly desaturated with exercise and one who did not (but developed runs of premature ventricular contractions [PVCs]). When these patients breathed an F_1O_2 of 0.4, PaO_2 remained normal, while heart rate, $\dot{V}_E$, and $\dot{V}CO_2$ decreased; the PVCs were abolished; and there was a mean increase in $PaCO_2$ of 7 mm Hg. Woolf and associates[16] set a goal of 30 minutes of continuous walking in a study of 14 patients. Eight of their patients could walk for only 4 minutes breathing air and were then given an F_1O_2 of 0.6. Thus, one of the earliest studies used the inability to exercise as a criterion for O_2. In those who did not receive O_2, their pretraining mean values were PaO_2 rest 71, PaO_2 exercise 73; $PaCO_2$ rest 38, exercise 43; decrease in O_2 Sat with exercise 4.8 vs. those who required O_2-PaO_2 rest 56, $PaCO_2$ rest 51 and decrease in O_2 Sat with exercise of 14.9 (only one patient had determinations of resting and exercise PaO_2 77 to 62 and $PaCO_2$ 40 to 43). Those requiring oxygen were more hypoxemic and hypercarbic at rest and had almost a threefold greater fall in oxygen saturation.

Vyas and associates[2] conducted the first double-blind randomized evaluation of the effects of oxygen (F_1O_2 0.4) in an exercise training program for patients with COPD. They documented a significant increase in duration of exercise, maximal work rate, $\dot{V}O_{2max}$, and $\dot{V}CO_2$. Their patients had a mean resting PaO_2 71 mm Hg (56 to 83) with no change in the mean value with exercise. Their mean resting and exercise $PaCO_2$ was 39 and 42 breathing air vs. 40 and 46 breathing O_2. At equal workloads, O_2 reduced the respiratory rate, $\dot{V}_E$, $\dot{V}_E/\dot{V}O_2$, and $\dot{V}CO_2$, and increased $\dot{V}O_2$. There was also a tendency to increase arterial lactate level with oxygen, which would indicate an increase in anaerobic metabolism. The authors conclude: "Oxygen supplementation during exercise is a valuable adjunct in the management of these patients." It is important to note that this improvement was obtained in patients with an acceptable resting PaO_2 (71mm Hg) who did not desaturate with exercise. Most patients with severe COPD cannot reach an anaerobic threshold with increased levels of lactate. Stein and associates[41] noted improved exercise tolerance, decreased $\dot{V}_E$, and a decrease in lactate with oxygen during exercise; these findings were attributed to decreased muscle anaerobiasis. A decreased blood lactate and heart rate after training has been found by others.[42]

Recently, Woodcock and collaborators[43] in a double-blind trial, studied pink puffers (rest and exercise PaO_2 73 and 62 mm Hg; $PaCO_2$ 34 and 37 mm Hg) while breathing O_2 at 4 L/min via nasal cannula. They increased their 6 MD, maximum workload on a progressive treadmill test, and experienced less breathlessness with a quantitative scoring system. This improvement occurred whether the patient or an assistant carried the O_2 cylinder, in contrast to the findings of Legett and Flenly.[44] They had similar results with 5 minutes of pre-dosing with oxygen. They were unable to predict which patients would benefit most from O_2 by lung function, blood gases, or exercise tolerance; others also have not been able to predict this.[45] Raffestin and associates[46] studied the hemodynamic response to SL exercise breathing air in 20 patients with COPD, retrospectively placed in two groups on the basis of the response at exhaustion. Group I (8 patients) with a mean FEV_1 of 0.5 $\pm$ 0.2 L had a decrease in PaO_2, 57 $\pm$ 9 to 49 $\pm$ 6 mm Hg, an increase in $PaCO_2$ 47 $\pm$ 6 to 54 $\pm$ 6, a $P_{\bar{V}}O_2$ of 20.5 $\pm$ 3 mm Hg, a P_{PA} 54 $\pm$ 21mm Hg and oxygen delivery ($CaO_2 \times \dot{Q}$) − 65.2 $\pm$ 31 mmol min^{-1} vs. Group II with a mean FEV_1 of 1.2 $\pm$ 0.4 L in whom PaO_2 had increased slightly, $PaCO_2$ did not increase, a $P_{\bar{V}}O_2$ was 26.8 $\pm$ 6, and the P_{PA} was 39 $\pm$ 10 mm Hg and oxygen delivery 94.9 $\pm$ 31 mmol min^{-1}. The Sl workload correlated with the FEV_1, but it accounted for only about 50 percent of the variance ($r^2 = 0.48$). The $P_{\bar{V}}O_2$ in Group I was similar to that of highly trained endurance athletes. It was attributed to the decreased PaO_2 resulting in decreased oxygen transport. They concluded that (1) an inadequate ventilatory response contributed to the exercise limitation in all their patients, perhaps due to respiratory muscle fatigue; (2) inadequate O_2 delivery was a factor in Group I; and (3) individuals who hypoventilate with exercise (Group I) should receive O_2. They did not, however, study the effects of O_2 in their patients or consider the increased endurance and so forth, achieved with O_2 in patients similar to their Group II.

Oxygen also reduces hypoxia-induced bronchoconstriction, apparently acting on large airways.[47] In normal individuals breathing against high inspiratory resistance, hypoxemia (PaO_2 40 mm Hg) reduces endurance time, causes a faster rate of shift of the electromyographic power spectrum, and produces a greater rate of increase in blood lactate production.[48]

The Respiratory Muscles

Function

NORMALS. In young men the maximum static inspiratory pressure (PI_{max}) is $-$ 125 cm H_2O and the maximum static expiratory pressure (PE_{max}) is $+$ 230 cm H_2O; the value for women is about 70 percent that of men; the coefficient of variation is about 25 percent. These pressures decrease about 0.5 cm H_2O/year after age 20. Because the longer a muscle is, the greater the strength of its contraction, PI_{max} is measured from residual volume and PE_{max} from total lung capacity. With quiet or slightly increased breathing, the inspiratory muscles totally support ventilation; this is accomplished principally through the diaphragm. With increased work there is a marked increase in diaphragmatic blood flow and $\dot{V}O_2$. This increased flow permits the diaphragm to function aerobically at levels in excess of 10 times control values. The maximum voluntary ventilation (MVV), usually performed for 12 or 15 seconds, cannot be maintained for even one minute. However, normal people can sustain about 60 percent of the MVV for about 15 minutes; this is the maximal sustainable ventilation (MSV) or maximal sustainable ventilatory capacity (MSVC). Normal individuals can breathe for extended periods at up to about 40 percent of the maximum static transdiaphragmatic pressure.[49] Only 5 percent of this pressure is used in the MSV. A five-week training period of hyperpneic normocarbic breathing to exhaustion 3 to 5 times over 45 to 60 minutes in normal subjects led to a 14 percent increase in MVV and a 19 percent increase in the percent of MVV that could be maintained for 15 minutes.[50] Running over 10 to 20 weeks increased the MVV 13.6 percent and the MSV 15.8 percent.[51] Respiratory muscle function has been summarized[52-54] and reviewed in depth.[55]

COPD. In patients with COPD there is both an increased work of breathing and a compromise of respiratory muscle contractility; most of this work is borne by the inspiratory muscles. The hyperinflation characteristic of COPD shortens the fibers of the diaphragm so that it functions on an ineffective portion of its length-tension curve; the intercostals are also compromised. However, the accessory muscles, sternocleidomastoids, and scalenes are less affected.[56,57] PI_{max} and PE_{max} have been reported as normal.[58] More recently, PI_{max} and PE_{max}, as well as the rate of rise in intrathoracic pressure (dp/dt), have been reported as substantially reduced.[59,60] The reduction in PE_{max} is attributed to general muscle weakness. Zocche and associates[61] reported that patients with severe COPD can maintain 60 percent of their MVV, equivalent to the MSVC achievable by normals. With severe respiratory muscle fatigue, the ominous sign of asynchronous breathing appears; it often portends respiratory failure. It is the inward movement of the abdomen suddenly, at or near end inspiration, while the chest cage is moving outward with outward movement of the abdomen in expiration.[56,57,62] Malnutrition may contribute to muscle fatigue.[63] Hypercapneic patients, when matched for lung volumes and spirometric indices to eucapneic patients, have a significantly decreased $\dot{V}_E$

entirely explained by a decrease in tidal volume; they also have a higher residual volume/total lung capacity ratio.[64] Details of respiratory muscle function in COPD can be found in two reviews.[55,65]

Training

THE OLD. Barach again was perhaps the first to report that pursed lip breathing and breathing retraining (diaphragmatic breathing) benefited his patients with COPD.[1,32,33] Miller[66] studied 24 patients before and after diaphragmatic breathing training. It resulted in a significant increase in diaphragmatic excursion (3.0 cm); a reduction in respiratory rate (5.1/min); an increase in tidal volume (162 cc); increased $\dot{V}O_2/\dot{V}_E$ (4 cc/L at rest and 9.1/L with exercise); an increase in PE_{max} (16 mm Hg); an increase in vital capacity (600 cc, 23 percent; and increase in MVV of 26.7 percent; an increase in arterial oxygen saturation at rest (6 percent) and with exercise (8 percent); and a decrease in $PaCO_2$ at rest (4mm Hg) and with exercise (5 mm Hg). Generally, others have not been able to document objective improvement; both forms of therapy have recently been reviewed with equanimity.[67] Although subjective improvement has been generally obtained with diaphragmatic training and pursed lip breathing, the lack of reproducible physiologic gain and the observation that patients often abandon this learned form of breathing with exacerbation of disease or exercise do not permit firm recommendations. Inasmuch as no ill effects have been identified, some include diaphragmatic breathing training and pursed lip breathing as part of a general rehabilitation program.

THE NEW—RESPIRATORY MUSCLES. Remarkably soon after Leith and Bradley reported the ability to substantively increase respiratory muscle endurance with eucapneic hyperpnea in normal individuals, Keens and associates[68] reported on a group of young people with cystic fibrosis who had only mild airway obstruction—a mean FEV_1 of about 67 percent of predicted value. Before training, their patients had a 36 percent higher ventilatory endurance than normal subjects. After 4 weeks of 5 day/week breathing against increased resistive loads, the cystic fibrosis patients improved their ventilatory muscle endurance by 51.6 percent vs. 56.7 percent for other patients who had intensive swimming and canoeing for 1.5 hours/day. In a more recent study of inspiratory muscle training of cystic fibrosis patients, improvement was not obtained.[69] Andersen and colleagues trained 10 patients with "severe disabling COPD" for 30 minutes daily for 2 4-week periods against an inspiratory resistive load selected as that which caused respiratory incoordination on some but not all breaths; the resistance was increased at the end of 4 weeks, and all performed better at 4 and 8 weeks. There was a constant expiratory resistance of 7.5 cm H_2O/L/sec. At 8 weeks the tolerated resistance had increased some three- to elevenfold, vital capacity increased, and median endurance time increased from 30 seconds to 11 minutes. Subjectively, all patients said they could "do much more" and were better able to handle their secretions. Belman and Mittman[71] trained 10 subjects with severe COPD with eucapneic hyperpnea (performing an MSVC twice, with 15 minutes rest) for 6 weeks. They reported significant increase in MSVC from 32 ± 11 to 42 ± 13 L/min with concomitant increases in $\dot{V}O_2$, HR, and blood lactate. Endurance time at a constant submaximal bicycle ergometer setting increased from 7.0 to 10.8 minutes for leg exercise and from 5.8 to 10.5 for arm exercise; and the 12 MD increased from 1058 m to 1188 m; there were no significant changes in the lung volumes or spirometric measurements. Belman and Kendregan[72] reported significantly improved mean endurance workload in groups receiving arm and leg work training without improvement in their MSV. Bjerre-Jepsen and associates[73] compared 14 patients trained with inspiratory resistance to 14 control subjects who breathed through the face mask without additional resistance (similar to eucapneic hyperpnea) for 15 minutes 3 times a day for 6 weeks. Both groups increased their stair climbing ability equally by 23 percent (10 to 76 percent). Pardy and associates compared 30 minutes of daily inspiratory resistive muscle training (IMT) with 3 times a week physical therapy (PT)—exercising on a treadmill, cycle, and stairs and lifting over 2 months. The IMT group significantly increased endurance time at two-thirds maximal workload from 4.7 to 7.6 minutes (1 month) and to 7.3 minutes (2 months), whereas the PT group had no increase. Although both groups increased the 12 MD, the IMT somewhat greater, neither increase was significant. These investigators[75] also reported that 7 of 12 patients receiving 2 months of IMT had more than a 40 percent increase in endurance from 6.7 to 11.6 min; significant improvements in maximal power output, 311 to 450 kpm/min and peak $\dot{V}O_2$ from 750 to 990 cc on a progressive exercise test; and a significant increase in the 12 MD from 685 to 756 m. Six of the 7 patients who improved with IMT had pretraining electromyographic evidence of inspiratory muscle fatigue compared with none of the 5 who did not improve. One can conclude that IMT helps individuals with respiratory muscle fatigue; the effect in those without fatigue is less clear because 2 of the 5 in that group had been receiving physiotherapy. Sonne and Davis[76] reported an increased $\dot{V}O_{2max}$ of 15 percent, an increased maximum work rate of 37 percent, and an increased $\dot{V}_E$ of 17 percent with a 56 percent increase in respiratory muscle endurance after a 6-week period of inspiratory resistance and training. Several recent reviews of the entire subject are helpful.[28,67,77,78,79]

RECOMMENDATIONS

General Care

The basic components of care for patients with COPD should include:

1. *Discontinuation of Smoking.* Strong nonjudgmental physician guidance is often successful; various stop smoking plans can be helpful.[80,81] Discontinuation of smoking usually eliminates cough and sputum and will decrease the rate of decline in FEV_1 in established disease.[82] It also decreases the probability of developing COPD.[83]

2. *Moderation* in diet, drinking, temperature extremes, and excessive fatigue. Rigid restrictions have not been shown to be useful, and they severely impair the quality of life. A good diet is reasonable because malnutrition occurs in COPD.[84]

3. *Patient and family education* concerning the nature of the disease, its progression, and the limitations it imposes.

4. Influenza immunization and probably pneumococcal vaccination.

5. *Bronchodilators.* A combination of an inhaled long-acting bronchodilator, for example, metaproterenol, albuterol, or fenoterol (when released), and oral theophylline. Atropine or its derivatives appear to offer a rediscovered bronchodilator with high potential.[85]

6. *Treat infection early.* Although there is not unanimity of opinion, treatment of purulent sputum with tetracycline, ampillicin or trimethaprim-sulfa without obtaining gram stain or culture is recommended for outpatients.

7. *Corticosteroid trial.* In patients with severe COPD and marked limitation in function, despite optimal bronchodilator therapy, a trial of steroids with response monitored both clinically and with a spirogram is warranted; between 15 and 30 percent will have important and measurable physiologic improvement.[86]

8. *Long-term continuous oxygen therapy* (considered separately from O_2 with exercise training). Oxygen delivered by nasal cannula to achieve a PaO_2 of 60 to 80 mm Hg is recommended for individuals with (a) a PaO_2 of 55 mm Hg or less—this should be documented as persistent over 1 month inasmuch as 45 percent of candidates for the Nocturnal Oxygen Therapy Trial initially meeting this criterion improved in the one-month stabilization period; (b) a PaO_2 of 55 to 59 mm Hg with cor pulmonale or erythrocytosis. Such therapy clearly increases survival and 24 hours/day is better than 15 hour/day.[87–89] Nocturnal oxygen is indicated for individuals who develop serious hypoxemia, especially with arrhythmias during sleep.[90] The type of oxygen source—compressed gas in cylinders, liquid oxygen, or membrane concentrators—must be

determined individually on the basis of cost, availability in a particular location, and the mobility of the patient.[91]

9. *Rehabilitation.* The provision of total coordinated care requires the collaborative efforts of all members of the health care team in addition to the physician. The skills of one or more of the following will be needed: nurses (preferably, respiratory clinical specialists), respiratory therapists, social workers, occupational therapists, and vocational counsellors. The use of such resources will vary from the ad hoc needs of an individual patient to the organized efforts of large centers. The ability of such a team to improve overall care and quality of life and reduce hospitalizations, and thereby reduce costs, has been well described and documented;[5,6,9,92,93,94] an excellent review and monograph are available.[67,91] The statement on *Community Resources for Rehabilitation of Patients with Chronic Obstructive Pulmonary Disease and Cor Pulmonale* is a useful guide.[95]

Exercise Prescription

Mild to Moderate COPD

In the individual with mild to moderate airway obstruction and little or no limitation in normal activities, the goal may best be described as prevention of deconditioning. In addition to applicable general measures, we advise such patients to maintain all current activities, and we encourage them to regularly participate in new conditioning exercises such as walking, swimming, and so on. Whether or not they would benefit from cardiopulmonary conditioning exercises is unknown.

Severe COPD

In individuals with severe COPD who experience appreciable limitation in their usual activities and whose FEV_1 is usually 1.5 liters or less, a more structured prescription of exercise is warranted. The patient should be clinically stable and receiving the necessary general care measures described. Although a useful estimate of SL exercise can be garnered from the FEV_1, this is only a rough approximation.[2,3,46] Therefore our first step is exercise testing.

EXERCISE TESTING. We recommend the use of a treadmill although a bicycle ergometer or even a 12 min MD may be used. We monitor HR, blood pressure, electrocardiogram, $\dot{V}_E$, $\dot{V}O_2$, $\dot{V}CO_2$, PaO_2, $PaCO_2$, and Ph and their derivatives. Although ear oximetry can be substituted for arterial blood studies, useful information on $PaCO_2$ and pH will be lost. A progressive incremental workload is used. This study provides necessary information about initial exercise tolerance and the development of hypoxemia, hypercarbia, arrhythmias, or hypotension. Clinical observations should be made for persistent dyspnea, tachypnea, or incoordinated breathing after exercise—evidence of respiratory muscle fatigue.

EXERCISE TRAINING. The *simplest* form of exercise training that the patient will *regularly* adhere to is satisfactory. Thus, progressively increased walking or a 12 min MD is satisfactory for many. Patients can avoid climatic extremes by using a shopping mall. This exercise should be performed five/days a week if possible and it should be recorded. A family member can be invaluable in providing companionship and insuring compliance. Alternative nonsupervised programs include a stationary bicycle or swimming. In the severely limited individual or one in whom compliance is doubtful, training should be supervised preferably on a 5 day/week basis initially and then at regular intervals. The same modes of exercise are used. After a period of 2 to 3 months, the exercise may be reduced to 3 times per week on an indefinite basis.

OXYGEN SUPPLEMENTATION. Oxygen via cannula to maintain a PaO_2 approximately 60 mm Hg is used for all patients whose PaO_2 decreases to 55 or less with exercise with or without CO_2 retention. In addition, if the patient's exercise limitation is so severe that even modest activity cannot be maintained for 4 or 5 minutes, oxygen (approximately 4L/min) is given to evaluate its effect on exercise ability. A third kind of patient in whom oxygen should be tried is the individual who experiences overwhelming dyspnea but is able to continue the effort without hypoxemia.

Some patients who meet none of the aforementioned criteria clearly increase their exercise ability with O_2. Perhaps an exercise test with and without O_2 should be used to identify such individuals as candidates for O_2 during exercise. An alternative consideration would be the use of oxygen at least in the initial phase of exercise training in all patients with COPD to facilitate a more rapid improvement; such an approach, however, carries additional costs and adds logistical problems. Its validity has not been tested.

RESPIRATORY MUSCLE TRAINING. The precise role of respiratory muscle training is less clear. Either resistance training or eucapneic hyperpnea (requiring more complex equipment) improves respiratory muscle endurance and general exercise endurance, especially in those who develop evidence of respiratory muscle fatigue. In particular, resistive training is attractive because of its simplicity. At present, we prefer to direct our initial efforts towards training the most important large muscle groups—those required for walking. Considerably more data support this approach. If less than satisfactory improvement is obtained, we would then add respiratory muscle training.

SUMMARY

Therapeutic exercise in patients with severe COPD improves useful exercise performance-endurance. This results in an improved quality of life, decreased hospitalization, and decreased costs. Therapeutic exercise is only one modality of the general care of the patient with COPD who often requires the coordinated skills of a multidisciplinary health care team to achieve maximal rehabilitation. These benefits will accrue to most but not all patients receiving exercise therapy.

In patient with severe COPD, therapeutic exercise does not improve pulmonary, hemodynamic, or peripheral (muscle) indices. Such patients are rarely able to reach a $\dot{V}O_{2max}$ or achieve the necessary threshold of exercise level, duration, and frequency required for cardiopulmonary conditioning. Such patients do improve mechanical skills in the trained muscles and benefit psychologically.

Supplemental oxygen will improve exercise performance in patients with COPD. This is particularly evident in those who become hypoxemic or who develop overwhelming dyspnea with exercise. Others who benefit when studied cannot be otherwise identified.

The respiratory muscles in severe COPD are subject to an increased work of breathing because of increased flow resistance in the airways and a compromise in respiratory muscle contractility owing to the shortened length-tension relationship of the diaphragm because of lung hyperinflation. In addition, they are weak. As in normal persons, the inspiratory muscles are of paramount importance. The respiratory muscles in severe COPD can become fatigued. Hyperpneic eucapnea or inspiratory resistive training can improve respiratory and general exercise endurance.

Therapeutic exercise should be prescribed only after a solid general care program is instituted: (1) discontinuation of smoking; (2) moderation in activity; (3) patient and family education; (4) immunization; (5) bronchodilators; (6) early treatment of infections; (7) corticosteroids if efficacious; (8) long-term continous O_2 if indicated; and (9) general rehabilitation. In patients with mild disease and few symptoms, encouragement to participate in general conditioning activities may suffice. Individuals with severe COPD should have (1) formal exercise testing to define achievable initial exercise levels and to identify arrhythmias, hypotension, hypoxemia, hypercarbia, or evidence of respiratory muscle fatigue; (2) the simplest progressive exercise program that will be adhered to, for example, walking; individuals with severe limitation or who are unable to comply may need supervised exercise training; (3) supplemental oxygen should be given to those who became hypoxemic with or without hypercarbia during exercise, those who cannot perform even a minimal level of exercise, and those with overwhelming dyspnea with exercise training. Others who may improve with O_2 can only be identified by exercise testing with and without O_2. Once established, exercise should be continued indefinitely. (4) Respiratory muscle training is recommended for those who do not succeed with general training. However, others use it in place of general exercise.

The objective is to add life to years rather than years to life.[79]

REFERENCES

1. MILLER, WF, TAYLOR, HF, AND JASPER, L: *Exercise training in the rehabilitation of patients with severe respiratory insufficiency due to pulmonary emphysema: The role of oxygen breathing.* Southern Med J 55:1216, 1962.

2. VYAS, MN, BANISTER, EW, MORTON, JW, ET AL: *Response to exercise in patients with chronic airway obstruction. Part I and II.* Am Rev Respir Dis 103:390, 1971.

3. GRUM, CM, HALMAN, MA, WAN, D, ET AL: *Predictors of maximum exercise tolerance in adults with cystic fibrosis.* Cystic Fibrosis Club Abstracts 23:27, 1982.

4. BARACH, AL, BICKERMAN, HA, AND BECK, G: *Advances in the treatment of non-tuberculosis pulmonary disease.* NY Acad Med 28:353, 1952.

5. HAAS, A AND CARDON, H: *Rehabilitation in chronic obstructive pulmonary disease: A 5-year study of 252 male patients.* Med Clin North Am 53:593, 1969.

6. HAAS, A AND LUCZAK, AK: *The Application of Physical Medicine and Rehabilitation to Emphysema Patients.* Rehabilitation Monograph XXII. The Institute of Rehabilitation Medicine, New York University Medical Center, 1963.

7. PIERCE, AK, TAYLOR, HF, ARCHER, RK, ET AL *Responses to exercise training in patients with emphysema.* Arch Intern Med 113:78, 1964.

8. CHRISTIE, D: *Physical training in chronic obstructive lung disease.* Br Med J 2:150, 1968.

9. BAUM, GL, AGLE, D, CHESTER, EH, ET AL: *Multidiscipline treatment of chronic pulmonary insufficiency: Functional status at one-year follow-up.* In JOHNSTON, RF (ED): *Pulmonary Care.* New York, Grune & Stratton, 1973, pp 355–362.

10. ALPERT, JS, BASS, H, SZUCS, MM, ET AL: *Effects of physical training on hemodynamics and pulmonary function at rest and during exercise in patients with chronic obstructive pulmonary disease.* Chest 66:647, 1974.

11. DEGRE, S, SERGYSELS, R, MESSIN R, ET AL: *Hemodynamic responses to physical training in patients with chronic lung disease.* Am Rev Respir Dis 610:395, 1974.

12. CHESTER, EH, BELMAN, MJ, BAHLER, RC, ET AL: *Multidisciplinary treatment of chronic pulmonary insufficiency. 3. The effect of physical training on cardiopulmonary performance in patients with chronic obstructive pulmonary disease.* Chest 72:695, 1977.

13. BASS, H, WHITCOMB, JF, AND FORMAN, R: *Exercise training: Therapy for patients with chronic obstructive pulmonary disease.* Chest 57:116, 1970.

14. HOLTEN, K: *Training effect in patients with severe ventilatory failure.* Scand J Resp Dis 53:65, 1972.

15. BRUNDIN, A: *Physical training in severe chronic obstructive lung disease. Clinical course, physical working capacity and ventilation (Part I and II).* Scand J Resp Dis 55:25, 1974.

16. WOOLF CR, AND SUERO, JT: *Alterations in lung disease.* Chest 55:37, 1969.

17. MERTENS, DJ, SHEPHARD, RJ, AND KAVANAGH, T: *Long-term exercise therapy for chronic obstructive lung disease.* Respiration 35:96, 1978.

18. NICHOLAS, JJ, GILBERT, R, GABE, R, ET AL: *Evaluation of an exercise therapy program for patients with chronic obstructive pulmonary disease.* Am Rev Respir Dis 102:1, 1970.

19. AMEILLE, J, CHAMBILLE, B, ORVOEN-FRIJA, E, ET AL: *Entrainement sur tapis roulant chez des insuffisants respiratories chroniques obstructifs. (Training on a treadmill in chronic obstructive respiratory disease.)* Bull Europ Physiopath Resp 17:741, 1981.

20. MUNGALL, IPF AND HAINSWORTH, R: *An objective assessment of the value of exercise training to patients with chronic obstructive airways disease.* Q J Med, NS 49:77, 1980.

21. ORENSTEIN, DM, FRANKLIN, BA, DOERSHUK, CF ET AL: *Exercise conditioning and cardiopulmonary fitness in cystic fibrosis. The effects of a three-month supervised running program.* Chest 80:392, 1981.

22. McGavin, CR, Gupta, SP, Lloyd, EL, et al: *Physical rehabilitation for the chronic bronchitic: Results of a controlled trial of exercises in the home.* Thorax 32:307, 1977.

23. Sinclair, DJM and Ingram, CG: *Controlled trial of supervised exercise training in chronic bronchitis.* Br Med J 280:519, 1980.

24. Cockcroft, AE, Saunders, MJ, and Berry, G: *Randomised controlled trial of rehabilitation in chronic respiratory disability.* Thorax 36:200, 1981.

25. Paez, PN, Phillipson, EA, Masngkay, M, et al: *The physiologic basis of training patients with emphysema.* Am Rev Respir Dis 95:944, 1967.

26. Belman, MJ and Kendregan, BA: *Physical training fails to improve ventilatory muscle endurance in patients with chronic obstructive pulmonary disease.* Chest 81:440, 1982.

27. Clausen, JP: *Effect of physical training on cardiovascular adjustments to exercise in man.* Physiol Rev 57:779, 1977.

28. Hughes RL and Davison, R: *Limitations of exercise reconditioning in COLD.* Chest 83:241, 1983.

29. Alison, JA, Samios, R, and Anderson, SD: *Evaluation of exercise training in patients with chronic airway obstruction.* Physical Therapy 61:1273, 1981.

30. Agle, DP, Baum, GL, Chester, EH, et al: *Multidiscipline treatment of chronic pulmonary insufficiency. 1. Psychologic aspects of rehabilitation.* Psychosomatic Medicine 35:41, 1973.

31. Asmussen, E, Dobeln, W, and Nielsen, M: *Blood lactate and oxygen debt after exhaustive work at different oxygen tensions.* Acta Phys Scand 15:57, 1948.

32. Barach, AL: *Ambulatory oxygen therapy: Oxygen inhalation at home and out-of-doors.* Dis Chest 35:229, 1959.

33. Barach, AL: *Physical exercise in breathless subjects with pulmonary emphysema, including a discussion of cigarette smoking.* Dis Chest 45:113 1964.

34. Cotes, JE and Gilson, JC: *Effect of oxygen on exercise ability in chronic respiratory insufficiency.* Lancet 1:872, 1956.

35. Cotes, JE, Pisa, Z, and Thomas, AJ: *Effect of breathing oxygen upon cardiac output, heart rate, ventilation, systemic and pulmonary blood pressure in patients with chronic lung disease.* Clin Sci 25:305, 1963.

36. Beck, GJ, Nanda, K, and Bickerman, HA: *Effect of oxygen on patients with pulmonary emphysema. Changes in minute ventilation during rest and exercise.* JAMA 179:404, 1962.

37. Kitchin, AH, Lowther, CP, and Matthews, MB: *The effects of exercise and of breathing oxygen-enriched air on the pulmonary circulation in emphysema.* Clin Sci 21:93, 1961.

38. Horsfield, K, Segal, N, and Bishop, JM: *The pulmonary circulation in chronic bronchitis at rest and during exercise breathing air and 80% oxygen.* Clin Sci 43:473, 1968.

39. Burrows, B, Kettel, LJ, Niden, AH, et al: *Patterns of cardiovascular dysfunction in chronic obstructive lung disease.* N Engl J Med 286:912, 1972.

40. Pierce, AK, Paez, PN, and Miller, WF: *Exercise training with the aid of a portable oxygen supply in patients with emphysema.* Am Rev Respir Dis 91:653, 1965.

41. Stein, DA, Bradley, BL, and Miller, WC: *Mechanisms of oxygen effects on exercise in patients with chronic obstructive pulmonary disease.* Chest 81:6, 1982.

42. Mohsenifar, Z, Horak, D, Brown, HV, et al: *Sensitive indices of improvement in a pulmonary rehabilitation program.* Chest 83:189, 1983.

43. Woodcock, AA, Gross, ER, and Geddes, DM: *Oxygen relieves breathlessness in "pink puffers."* Lancet 1:907, 1981.

44. Leggett, RJE and Flenley, DC: *Portable oxygen and exercise tolerance in patients with chronic hypoxic cor pulmonale* Br Med J 2:84, 1977.

45. Bradley, BL, Garner, AE, Billiu, D, et al: *Oxygen-assisted exercise in chronic obstructive lung disease. The effect on exercise capacity and arterial blood gas tensions.* Am Rev Respir Dis 118:239, 1978.

46. Raffestin, B, Escourrou, P, Legrand A, et al: *Circulatory transport of oxygen in patients with chronic airflow obstruction exercising maximally.* Am Rev Respr Dis 125:426, 1982.

47. Libby, DM, Briscoe, WA, and King, TKC: *Relief of hypoxia-related bronchoconstriction by breathing 30 per cent oxygen.* Am Rev Respir Dis 123:171, 1981.

48. Jardim, J, Farkas G, Prefaut, C, et al: *The failing inspiratory muscles under normoxic and hypoxic conditions.* Am Rev Respir Dis 124:274, 1981.

49. Roussos, CS and Macklem, PT: *Diaphragmatic fatigue in man.* J Appl Physiol: Respirat Environ Exercise Physiol 43:189, 1977.

50. Leith, DE and Bradley, M: *Ventilatory muscle strength and endurance training.* J Appl Physiol 41:508, 1976.

51. ROBINSON, EP AND KJELDGAARD, JM: *Improvement in ventilatory muscle function with running.* J Appl Physiol: Respirat Environ Exercise Physiol 52:1400, 1982.

52. BELMAN, MJ AND SIECK, GC: *The ventilatory muscles: Fatigue, endurance and training.* Chest 82:761, 1982.

53. ROUSSOS, C AND MACKLEM, PT: *The respiratory muscles .* N Engl J Med 307:786, 1982.

54. ROCHESTER, DF AND BRAUN, NMT: *The Respiratory Muscles. Basics of RD.* American Thoracic Society, New York, Vol. 6(4), March, 1978.

55. DERENNE, JP, MACKLEM, PT, AND ROUSSOS, CH: *The respiratory muscles: Mechanics, control and pathophysiology.* Am Rev Respir Dis 118:119, 373, 581, 1978.

56. SHARP, JT, DANON, J, DRUZ, WS, ET AL: *Respiratory muscle function in patients with chronic obstructive pulmonary disease: Its relationship to disability and to respiratory therapy.* Am Rev Respir Dis 110:154, 1974.

57. SHARP, JT, GOLDBERG, NB, DRUZ, WS, ET AL: *Thoracoabdominal motion in chronic obstructive pulmonary disease.* Am Rev Respir Dis 115:47, 1977.

58. BYRD, RB AND HYATT, RE: *Maximal respiratory pressures in chronic obstructive lung disease.* Am Rev Respir Dis 98:848, 1968.

59. BRAUN, NMT AND ROCHESTER, DF: *Respiratory muscle function in chronic obstructive pulmonary disease (COPD).* Am Rev Respir Dis 115:91, 1977.

60. MARAZZINI, L, VEZZOLI, F, AND RIZZATO, G: *Intrathoracic pressure development in chronic airways obstruction.* J Appl Physiol 37:575, 1974.

61. ZOCCHE, GP, FRITTS, HW, JR, AND COURNAND, A: *Fraction of maximum breathing capacity available for prolonged hyperventilation.* J Appl Physiol 15:1073, 1960.

62. ASHUTOSH, K, GILBERT, R, AUCHINCLOSS, JH, ET AL: *Asynchronous breathing movements in patients with chronic obstructive pulmonary disease.* Chest 67:553, 1975.

63. ARORA, NS AND ROCHESTER, DF: *Effect of body weight and muscularity on human diaphragm muscle mass, thickness, and area.* J Appl Physiol: Respirat Environ Exercise Physiol 52:64, 1982.

64. PAROT S, SAUNIER, C, GAUTIER, H, ET AL: *Breathing pattern and hypercapnia in patients with obstructive pulmonary disease.* Am Rev Respir Dis 121:985, 1980.

65. ROCHESTER, DF, ARORA, NS, BRAUN, NMT, ET AL: *The respiratory muscles in chronic obstructive pulmonary disease (COPD).* Bull Europ Physiopath Resp 15:951, 1979.

66. MILLER, WF: *A physiologic evaluation of the effects of diaphragmatic breathing training in patients with chronic pulmonary emphysema.* Am J Med 17:471, 1954.

67. LERTZMAN, MM AND CHERNIACK, RM: *Rehabilitation of patients with chronic obstructive pulmonary disease.* Am Rev Respir Dis 114:1145, 1976.

68. KEENS, TG, KRASTINS, IRB, WANNAMAKER, EM, ET AL: *Ventilatory muscle endurance training in normal subjects and patients with cystic fibrosis.* Am Rev Respir Dis 116:853, 1977.

69. ASHER, MI, PARDY, RL, COATES AL, ET AL: *The effects of inspiratory muscle training in patients with cystic fibrosis.* Am Rev Respir Dis 126:855, 1982.

70. ANDERSEN, JB, DRAGSTED, L, KANN, T, ET AL: *Resistive breathing training in severe chronic obstructive pulmonary disease.* Scand J Resp Dis 60:151, 1979.

71. BELMAN, MJ AND MITTMAN, C: *Ventilatory muscle training improves exercise capacity in chronic obstructive pulmonary disease patients.* Am Rev Respir Dis 121:273, 1980.

72. BELMAN, MJ AND KENDREGAN, BA: *Exercise training fails to increase skeletal muscle enzymes in patients with chronic obstructive pulmonary disease.* Am Rev Respir Dis 123:256, 1981.

73. BJERRE-JEPSEN, K, SECHER, NH, AND KOK-JENSEN, A: *Inspiratory resistance training in severe chronic obstructive pulmonary disease.* Eur J Respir Dis 62:405, 1981.

74. PARDY, RL, RIVINGTON, RN, DESPAS, PJ, ET AL: *The effects of inspiratory muscle training on exercise performance in chronic airflow limitation.* Am Rev Respir Dis 123:426, 1981.

75. PARDY, RL, RIVINGTON, RN, DESPAS, PJ, ET AL: *Inspiratory muscle training compared with physiotherapy in patients with chronic airflow limitation.* Am Rev Respir Dis 123:421, 1981.

76. SONNE, LJ AND DAVIS, JA: *Increased exercise performance in patients with severe COPD following inspiratory resistive training.* Chest 81:436, 1982.

77. BELMAN, MJ AND WASSERMAN K: *Exercise training and testing in patients with chronic obstructive pulmonary disease.* In *Basics of RD.* American Thoracic Society, New York, Vol. 10, No 2, November, 1981.

78. PETTY, TL: *Pulmonary rehabilitation.* In *Basics of RD.* American Thoracic Society, New York, Vol 4, No. 1, September, 1975.

79. HALE, T, CUMMING, G, AND SPRIGGS, J: *The effects of physical training in chronic obstructive pulmonary disease.* Bull Europ Physiopath Resp 14:593, 1978.

80. AMERICAN COLLEGE OF CHEST PHYSICIANS: *Smoker's Cessation Kit.* Park Ridge, Illinois, 1983.

81. U.S. DEPARTMENT OF HEALTH AND HUMAN SERVICES: *The physician's guide: How to help your hypertensive patients stop smoking.* NIH Publication No. 83–1271, April, 1983.

82. FLETCHER, C AND PETRO, R: *The natural history of chronic air flow obstruction.* Br Med J 1:1645, 1977.

83. HIGGINS, MW, KELLER, JB, BECKER, M, ET AL: *An index of risk for obstructive airways disease.* Am Rev Respir Dis 125:144, 1982.

84. OPENBRIER, DR, IRWIN, MM, ROGERS, RM, ET AL: *Nutritional status and lung function in patients with emphysema and chronic bronchitis.* Chest 83:17, 1983.

85. EPSTEIN, SW AND MIDDLETON, EW, (EDS): *Advances in assessment and therapy of asthma.* Chest 82:1S, 1982.

86. MENDELLA, LA, MANFREDA, J, WARREN, MB, ET AL: *Steroid response in stable chronic obstructive pulmonary disease.* Ann Intern Med 96:17, 1982.

87. TIMMS, RM, KVALE, PA, ANTHONISEN, NR, ET AL: *Selection of patients with chronic obstructive pulmonary disease for long-term oxygen therapy.* JAMA 245:2514, 1981.

88. NOCTURNAL OXYGEN THERAPY TRIAL GROUP: *Continuous nocturnal oxygen therapy in hypoxemic chronic obstructive lung disease.* Ann Intern Med 93:391, 1980.

89. MEDICAL RESEARCH COUNCIL WORKING PARTY: *Long term domiciliary oxygen therapy in chronic hypoxic cor pulmonale complicating chronic bronchitis and emphysema.* Lancet 1:681, 1981.

90. WYNNE, JW, BLOCK, AJ, HEMENWAY, J, ET AL: *Disordered breathing and oxygen desaturation during sleep in patients with chronic obstructive lung disease (COLD).* Am J Med 66:573, 1979.

91. PETTY, TL (ED): *Intensive and Rehabilitative Respiratory Care.* Ed 3. Lea & Febiger, Philadelphia, 1982, pp 403–407.

92. HUDSON, LD, TYLER, ML, AND PETTY, TL: *Hospitalization needs during an outpatient rehabilitation program for severe chronic airway obstruction.* Chest 70:606, 1976.

93. MILLER, WF: *Rehabilitation of patients with chronic obstructive lung disease.* Med Clin North Am 51:349, 1967.

94. MOSER, KM, BOKINSKY, GE, SAVAGE, RT, ET AL: *Results of a comprehensive rehabilitation program.* Arch Intern Med 140:1596, 1980.

95. PETTY, TL, BRANSCOMB, BV, FARRINGTON, JF, ET AL: *Community resources for rehabilitation of patients with chronic obstructive pulmonary diseases and cor pulmonale.* Circulation 49:A1, 1974.

Index

A t following a page number indicates a table; an italic page number indicates an illustration.

AGING. *See* Patient(s), elderly.
Angina
  during exercise, 99, *99*
  severe
    specific problems with
      exercise therapy and, 149–151, 150t
Angiocardiography, exercise radionuclide. *See* Exercise radionuclide angiocardiography.
Antiarrhythmic agents, 140–141
Aorta
  abnormalities of
    exercise-related sudden death and, 54
  coarctation of
    exercise testing in, 238
  valve of
    congenital bicuspid, *69*
    stenosis of, *69*
Aortic regurgitation
  exercise testing and, 237
Aortic stenosis
  congenital
    exercise testing and, 236, 238
  postexcision radiogram of, *68*
Arm(s). *See* Upper extremity(ies).
Arrhythmia(s)
  atrial
    exercise-induced, 125–126
  cardiac
    distance running and
      effects of, 78–79
  exercise-induced
    hypotension and, 130
    clinical management of, 125–131
    significance of, 125–131
  ventricular
    during exercise testing, 99–100
    exercise-induced, 127–128
Arterial hypertension, systemic, exercise testing in, 240
Artery(ies)
  coronary
    anomalous origin of, *59*
    exercise-related sudden death and, 51–52

    frequency of
      in exercise-related sudden death, *60, 61, 62, 63*
    trauma to
      exercise-related sudden death and, 53, *66*
    tunneled epicardial
      exercise-related sudden death and, 52, *64, 65*
Atherosclerosis, coronary, exercise-related sudden death and, 51
Atrial fibrillation, exercise-induced, 126
Atrial flutter, exercise-induced, 126
Atrial septal defect, large, exercise testing in, 237
Atrioventricular (AV) block
  exercise testing and, 239
  first degree
    exercise-induced, 126
  second degree
    exercise-induced, 126
  third degree
    exercise-induced, 126

BED rest, physiologic effects of, in elderly patients, 208–209
Beta adrenergic blocking drugs, 137–139
Blood pressure response, abnormal, during exercise testing, 100
Bone(s), in elderly patients, 208
Borg Perceived Exertion Scale, *247*
Bundle branch block
  left
    exercise and, 126–127
  right
    exercise and, 126–127

CALISTHENICS, warm-up, *212, 213*
Cardiac patient(s), exercise prescription for, 159–162, *160*, 161t
Cardiac rehabilitation
  community based, 170–171
  current status of, 185–191
  effect of
    evaluation of
      exercise radionuclide angiocardiography and, 117

Cardiac rehabilitation—*Continued*
  exercise therapy and
    medical problems with, 167
    supervised vs nonsupervised, 193–199
  future possibilities of, 190–191
  inpatient, 162, *163–165*
  myocardial revascularization surgery and
    morbidity associated with, 171
    mortality associated with, 171
    physiologic factors associated with, 171
  outpatient, 167–170, 168t
  physical conditioning programs and, 188–190,
    189t, 190t
Cardiomyopathy, hypertrophic, exercise testing in,
  239
Cardiovascular disease, unmasking of, exercise and,
  54, 56t–57t, *67*
Cardiovascular disorders, miscellaneous, exercise
  testing in, 239–240
Cardiovascular drugs
  antianginal, 135–140
  antiarrhythmic, 140–141
  antihypertensive, 141
  beta adrenergic blocking, 137–139
  calcium entry blocking, 139–140, 139t
  exercise testing and, 133–142
    clinical application of, 135
  exercise training and, 133–142
    clinical application of, 135
  myocardial oxygen demand and, 134t
Cardiovascular system
  effects of training on
    in elderly patients, 209
  functional changes in
    elderly patients and, 205–206
  in elderly patients, 204–205, *204*
  structural changes in
    elderly patients and, 205
Catecholamines, 141
Cholesterol, high-density lipoprotein, exercise and,
  146, 147t
Chronic obstructive pulmonary disease (COPD)
  exercise training in
    effects of, 262–263, *262*
    recommendations for, 269–271
  mild to moderate
    exercise prescription in, 270
  respiratory muscles in, 267–268
  severe
    exercise prescription in, 270–271
  therapeutic exercise in, 261–272
Coarctation of aorta, exercise testing in, 238
Conduction disturbances
  exercise-induced, 126–127
  exercise testing and, 238–239
Coronary artery(ies)
  anomalous origin of, *59*
    frequency of
      in exercise-related sudden death, *60, 61, 62, 63*
  major
    anomalous origin of
      exercise-related sudden death and, 51–52
  tunneled epicardial
    exercise-related sudden death and, 52, *64, 65*

Coronary artery bypass grafting, left ventricular
  response to, prediction of, exercise radionuclide angiocardiography and, 117
Coronary artery disease. *See also* Heart disease.
  atheromatous
    exercise conditioning and, 2t
  atherosclerotic
    prevention of
      primary, 3–4
      secondary, 4–6
      studies of, 6t
  diagnosis of
    exercise radionuclide angiocardiography for,
      115–116
  evaluation of
    exercise nuclear imaging in, 105–119
  exercise and
    epidemiologic studies of, 5t
  extent of
    exercise radionuclide angiocardiography and,
      116
  genesis of
    epidemiologic studies and, 2–3
  lowered risk of
    characteristics of, 7
  myocardial perfusion in, 105–106
  severity of
    exercise radionuclide angiocardiography and,
      116
Coronary atherosclerosis, exercise-related sudden
  death and, 51
Coronary heart disease. *See also* Heart disease.
  individuals prone to
    exercise testing in, 255–259
  longitudinal echocardiographic studies in, 93
Coronary ostium(a), high take-off of, exercise-related
  sudden death and, 52–53
Coronary risk factors, leisure time activity and, 2t
Coronary spasm, exercise-induced, sudden death and,
  53

DEATH
  sudden
    atherosclerotic plaques in, *50*
    causes of
      in old conditioned subjects, 28, 31t
      in young conditioned subjects, 10–11, *25,
        26*
    congenital coronary anomalies associated with,
      27
    exercise-related
      anomalous origin of coronary artery and, 51–
        52
      aortic factors in, 54
      cardiovascular structural abnormalities and,
        51–54
      comparison of
        in old and young conditioned subjects,
          29
      coronary arterial trauma and, 53, *66*
      coronary atherosclerosis and, 51
      coronary ostia and
        high take-off of, 52–53
      exercise-induced coronary spasm and, 53

in young conditioned subjects, 9–11, 12t–13t
    demographic data and, 10
        known cardiac disease and, 54–55, 58t
        mitral caged-ball prosthesis and, *70*
        morphologic observations in, 18t–23t
        myocardial factors in, 53
        postmortem findings in, *32, 33, 34, 35, 36, 37, 38, 41, 42, 43, 44, 45, 46, 47*
        tunneled epicardial coronary arteries and, 52, *64, 65*
    in old conditioned subjects, 28–29
    valvular factors in, 53–54
Depression, myocardial infarction and, exercise therapy and, 154t
Digitalis, 141
Diltiazem, 139, 139t
Disopyramide, 140
Drug(s). *See also* Cardiovascular drugs.
    antianginal, 135–140
    antiarrhythmic, 140–141
    antihypertensive, 141
    beta adrenergic blocking, 137–139
    calcium entry blocking, 139–140, 139t
    cardiovascular. *See* Cardiovascular drugs.
    nitrate, 135–136
    vasodilator, 136–137

EBSTEIN'S anomaly, *24*
Echocardiogram(s)
    post-exercise, *88*
    pre-exercise, *88*
Echocardiography
    altered cardiac functions and, 90, *90, 91,* 92
    altered cardiac structure and, 90, *90, 91,* 92
    animal data and, 89
    exercise and
        myocardial effects of, 87–94
        in trained subjects, 88–89
    longitudinal studies with
        in coronary heart disease, 93
        in normal subjects, 89–90
    methodologic considerations in, 87–88
    minimal cardiac changes and, 92–93
Elderly patients. *See* Patient(s), elderly.
Electrocardiogram
    exercise
        inconclusive, 109
        positive
            in asymptomatic patient, 109
        in conditioned subject, *42*
    resting, *48*
        in conditioned subject, *39*
    treadmill test and
        in conditioned subject, *40*
Encainide, 140
Ethmozine, 140
Exercise
    atherosclerotic heart disease and,
        prevention of
            primary, 3–4
            secondary, 4–6
    atrial arrhythmias and, 125–126
    combined static and dynamic
        upper extremity and, 180
    conduction disturbances and, 126–127
    distance running as
        adaptive cardiovascular changes produced by, 79–80
        cardiovascular adaptations and, 77–81
        cardiovascular benefits of, 75–84
        cardiovascular risks of, 75–84
        effects of
            on cardiac arrhythmias, 78–79
        myocardial damage and, 82–84
    dynamic
        upper extremity and, 176–180, *177,* 178t, *179*
    hypotension induced by, 128–131, *129*
        etiology of, 129t
    isometric
        upper extremity and, 175–176, *176*
    jog-walk regimen for, *214*
    left ventricular function and
        evaluation of
            exercise radionuclide angiocardiography and, 117
    marathon runners and
        characteristics of
            sedentary controls compared with, 79t
        lipoprotein levels in, 80–81
    nonfatal cardiovascular disease and
        unmasking of, 54, 56t–57t, *67*
    premature ventricular contractions and, 127–128, *127*
    static
        upper extremity and, 175–176, *176*
    sudden death and
        anomalous origin of coronary artery and, 51–52
        aortic factors in, 54
        atherosclerotic plaques and, *50*
        cardiovascular structural abnormalities and, 51–54
        causes of, *16, 17, 25, 26*
            in old conditioned subjects, 14t–15t, 28, 31t
            in young conditioned subjects, 9–11, 12t–13t, 16t
        congenital coronary anomalies associated with, *27*
        coronary arterial trauma and, 53, *66*
        coronary atherosclerosis and, 51
        coronary ostia and
            high take-off of, 52–53
        exercise-induced coronary spasm and, 53
        in known cardiac disease, 54–55, 58t
        in marathon runner, 30
        in old conditioned subjects, 28–29
        mitral caged-ball prosthesis and, *70*
        morphologic observations in, 18t–23t
        myocardial factors in, 53
        postmortem findings in, *32, 33, 34, 35, 36, 37, 38, 41, 42, 43, 44, 45, 46, 47*
        tunneled epicardial coronary arteries and, 52, *64, 65*
        valvular factors in, 53–54
    therapeutic
        in chronic obstructive pulmonary disease, 261–272
    warm-up, *212, 213*
Exercise conditioning, effects of, beneficial, 2t

Exercise nuclear imaging
  coronary anatomy and
    assessment of, 109–110
  coronary artery disease and
    evaluation of, 105–119
  interpretation of, 106–108, *107*
  procedure for, 106
  severity of disease and
    assessment of, 109–110
  thallium-201 for, 108–109, *108,* 110
  tomography and, 111–112, *112, 113,* 114
  quantification and, 111
Exercise radionuclide angiocardiography (RNA),
    114–118
  assessment of therapy and, 117–118
  cardiac rehabilitation and
    evaluation of, 117
  clinical use of, 115–118
  coronary artery bypass grafting and
    left ventricular response to
      prediction of, 117
  future directions in, 118
  interpretation of, 115
  left ventricular function and
    evaluation of, 117
  myocardial infarction and
    assessment of patient following, 116–117
  procedure for, 114–115
Exercise radionuclide studies, 100–101
Exercise radionuclide ventriculography, 101
Exercise testing
  abnormal blood pressure response during, 100
  abnormalities during
    reproducibility of, 100
  angina during, 99, *99*
  aortic regurgitation and, 237
  aortic stenosis and, 236
  atrioventricular block and, 239
  cardiovascular drugs and, 133, 135
  conduction disturbances and, 238–239
  early, 186–186, 186t
  elderly patients and, 201, *202, 203*
  evaluation of
    following myocardial infarction, 98t
  general principles of, 185
  hypertrophic cardiomyopathy and, 239
  in coarctation of aorta, 238
  in congenital aortic stenosis, 238
  in congenital heart disease, 237
  in large atrial septal defect, 237
  in mitral regurgitation, 235–236
  in mitral stenosis, 235
  in mitral valve prolapse, 236
  in myocarditis, 240
  in noncoronary heart disease, 233–240, *234,* 234t,
    244t
  in severely depressed left ventricular function,
    239–240
  in systemic arterial hypertension, 240
  in tetralogy of Fallot, 238
  in valvular heart disease, 235
  in ventricular septal defect, 237–238
  late, 187–188, 187t, 188t
  methods of, 96–97

physical conditioning programs and, 188–190,
    189t, 190t
postinfarction
  timing of, 100
predischarge
  diagnostic value of, 97–98, *97*
  therapeutic implications of, 101–102,
    102
  prognostic significance of, 98–100
  radionuclide studies in, 100–101
  radionuclide ventriculography in, 101
rationale for
  myocardial infarction and, 95
sinus node dysfunction and, 238–239
supraventricular tachyarrhythmias and, 239
tomography and, 111–112, *112, 113,* 114
upper extremity, 175–182
ventricular arrhythmias during, 99–100
ventricular ectopy and, 239
Exercise therapy
  cardiac rehabilitation and
    medical problems with, 167
  contraindications to
    myocardial infarction and, 154–155
  following myocardial revascularization surgery,
    159–171
  intense
    following myocardial infarction, 148–149
  myocardial infarction and, 145–157
    body composition with, 146t
    daily energy expenditure with, 146
    depression following, 154t
    endurance training and, 146, *147*
    HDL cholesterol levels and, 146, 147t
    stroke volume following
      endurance training and, 148, *148*
  myocardial revascularization surgery and
    morbidity associated with, 171
    mortality associated with, 171
    physiologic factors associated with, 171
  prescription for,
    in cardiac patients, 159–162, *160,* 161t
  supervised vs nonsupervised
    cardiac rehabilitation and, 193–199
    cost of, 196–197
    guidelines for, 197–199
    patient evaluation and, 194–195
    relative safety of, 195–196
  rationale for 145–149
  response to, 151–155
  severe angina and
    specific problems with, 149–151, 150t
Exercise training
  asymptomatic ventricular ectopy and, *252*
  cardiovascular drugs and, 133–135
  compliance with
    importance of, 258
  effects of, 180–181
    in chronic obstructive pulmonary disease, 262–
      263, *262*
    in normal individuals, 261–262
    reversing physiologic deterioration and
      elderly patients and, 208–210
    in coronary-prone individuals, 255–259

elderly patients and, 201, *202, 203,* 211–214, *212, 213, 214*
in heart failure, 225, *226,* 227
in noncoronary heart disease, 243, 244t
in symptomatic coronary heart disease, 255–259
in symptomatic ventricular tachycardia, *251*
limitations to
in ventricular dysfunction, 220–225, *222, 223,* 223t, *224*
methods of
in noncoronary heart disease, 246–248, *247*
myocardial oxygen demand and, 134t
physiologic basis for
in noncoronary heart disease, 244–245
rationale for
in ventricular dysfunction, 219–220
recommendations for
in chronic obstructive pulmonary disease, 269–271
special considerations in
in noncoronary heart disease, 248–253, *251, 252*
exceeding anaerobic threshold and, 130
ischemic left ventricular dysfunction and, 130
upper extremity, 175–182
Extremity(ies)
upper
exercise and
combined static and dynamic, 180
dynamic, 176–180, *177,* 178t, *179*
isometric, 175–176, *176*
static, 175–176, *176*
exercise testing and, 175–182
exercise training and, 175–182

FRAMINGHAM Study, 3, 5t

HEART disease. *See also* Coronary artery disease.
cardiovascular
unmasking of, 54, 56t–57t, *67*
congenital
exercise testing in, 237
pathophysiology of, 245–246
coronary
individuals prone to
exercise testing in, 255–259
longitudinal echocardiographic studies in, 93
symptomatic
exercise training in, 255–259
noncoronary
exercise testing in, 233–240, *234,* 234t
exercise training in, 243–253
methods of, 246–248, *247*
physiologic basis for, 244–245
valvular
exercise testing in, 235
Heart failure, exercise training in, 219–230
Hydralazine, 136
Hypertension, systemic arterial, exercise testing in, 240
Hypotension
exercise-induced, 128–130, *129*
arrhythmias and, 130
etiology of, 129t

exercise-induced arrhythmias and
clinical management of, 125–131
significance of, 125–131

INFARCTION, myocardial. *See* Myocardial infarction.

JOG-walk regimen, *214*
Joint(s), in elderly patients, 207–208

LIPOPROTEIN, levels of, in marathon runners, 80–81
Lorcainide, 140

METOPROLOL, 138
Mexilitine, 140
Mitral regurgitation, exercise testing in, 235–236
Mitral stenosis, exercise testing in, 235
Mitral valve prolapse, exercise testing in, 236
Muscle(s), in elderly patient, 207
Musculoskeletal system
effects of training on
in elderly patients, 210
in elderly patients, 207–208
Myocardial infarction
absence of
mortality with
exercise therapy and, 151t
assessment of patient after
exercise radionuclide angiocardiography and, 116–117
depression and
exercise therapy and, 154t
exercise therapy following, 145–157
body composition with, 146t
daily energy expenditure with, 146
endurance training and, 146, *147*
evaluation of, 98t
HDL cholesterol levels and, 146, 147t
intense, 148–149
methods of, 96
predischarge
diagnostic value of, 97–98, *97*
prognostic significance of, 98–100
rationale for, 95–96, 145–149
reproducibility of abnormalities and, 100
timing of, 100
multivessel disease following
thallium perfusion and, 110
recurrence of
fatal
exercise therapy and, 152–153, 153t
nonfatal
exercise therapy and, 152–153
risk factors and, 150t
stroke volume following
prolonged endurance training and, 148, *148*
Myocardial perfusion
for evaluation of coronary artery disease, 105–106
thallium-201
radionuclide ventriculography and
comparison of, 118–119
Myocarditis, exercise testing and, 240
Myocardium
damage to
from distance running, 82–84

Myocardium—*Continued*
  ecnocardiography and, 87–94. *See also*
    Echocardiography.
  structural abnormalities of
    exercise-related death and, 53

NATIONAL Exercise and Heart Disease Project, 5
Nifedipine, 139, 139t
Nitrate preparations, 135–136
Nitroglycerin, 135–136
Nuclear imaging. *See* Exercise nuclear imaging.

OLD age. *See* Patient(s), elderly.
Ostium(a), coronary, high take-off of, exercise-
    related sudden death and, 52–53

PAROXYSMAL atrial tachycardia (PAT), exercise-
    induced, 125
Patient(s)
  elderly
    bed rest and
      effects of, 208–209
    cardiovascular system of, 204–205
      effects of training on, 209
      functional changes in, 205–206
      structural changes in, 205
    exercise prescription for, 211–214, *212, 213,*
      214
    musculoskeletal system of
      bones in, 208
      effects of training on, 210
      joints in, 207–208
      muscles of, 207
    physiologic deterioration in
      effects of exercise on, 208
    physiologic function in, 202–204
    respiratory system of, 206–207
      effects of training on, 210
Physical conditioning programs, cardiac rehabilita-
    tion and, 189–190, 189t, 190t
Physiologic function, aging and, effects of, 202–203
Prazosin, 136
Premature ventricular contractions (PVCs)
  elimination of
    exercise and, 128
  exercise-induced, 127–128, *127*
Procainamide, 140
Propranolol, 138
Prosthesis, mitral caged-ball, exercise-related sudden
    death and, *70*

QUINIDINE, 140

RADIONUCLIDE angiocardiography. *See* Exercise
    radionuclide angiocardiography.
Radionuclide studies, during exercise, 100–101
Radionuclide ventriculography, thallium-201 myo-
    cardial perfusion and, comparison of,
    118–119
Respiratory muscles, function of, chronic obstructive
    pulmonary disease and, 267–268

Respiratory system in elderly patients, 206–207
Risk factors
  coronary
    leisure time activity and, 2t
  lowered
    characteristics of
      in coronary artery disease, 7
Runner(s)
  marathon
    characteristics of
      sedentary controls compared with, 79t
    lipoprotein levels in, 80–81
Running
  distance
    cardiovascular adaptations and, 77–81
    cardiovascular benefits of, 75–84
    cardiovascular risks in, 81–84
  effects of
    on cardiac arrhythmias, 78–79
    myocardial damage and, 82–84

SCINTIGRAPHY, thallium-201, in exercise testing, 100–
    101
Sick sinus syndrome (SSS), exercise-induced, 125–
    126
Sinus node dysfunction, exercise testing and, 238–
    239
Spasm, coronary, exercise-induced, sudden death
    and, 53
Stenosis
  aortic, *69*
    postexcision radiogram of, *68*
Sudden death. *See* Death, sudden.
Surgery
  myocardial revascularization
    exercise regimens following, 159–171
      guidelines for, *163–165*
      intensity of, 166–167
    rehabilitation and
      morbidity associated with, 171
      mortality associated with, 171
      physiologic factors associated with, 171

TACHYARRHYTHMIA(S), supraventricular, exercise
    testing and, 239
Tachycardia, ventricular, symptomatic, exercise
    training and, *251*
Tetralogy of Fallot, exercise testing in, 238
Thallium-201 imaging
  clinical use of, 108–109, *108*
  in exercise testing, 100–101
  multivessel disease and
    evaluation of, 110
  radionuclide ventriculography and
    comparison of, 118–119
  stress
    nonexercise, 114
Tocainide, 140
Tomography, exercise testing and, 111–112, *112,*
    113, 114
Trauma, coronary arterial, exercise-related sudden
    death and, 53, *66*

UPPER extremity(ies)
  exercise and
    dynamic, 176–180, *177,* 178t, *179*
    isometric, 175–176, *176*
    static, 175–176, *176*
  exercise testing and, 175–182
  exercise training and, 175–182

VALVE(S)
  aortic
    congenital bicuspid, *69*
    stenosis of, *69*
  cardiac
    abnormalities of
      exercise-related sudden death and, 53–54
Vasodilator(s), 136–137
Ventricular arrhythmia(s). *See* Arrhythmia(s), ventricular.

Ventricular dysfunction
  exercise training in, 219–230
    limitations to, 220–225, *222, 223,* 223t, *224*
    rationale for, 219–220
Ventricular ectopy
  asymptomatic
    exercise training and, *252*
  exercise testing and, 239
Ventricular function, left, severely depressed, exercise testing in, 239–240
Ventricular septal defect, exercise testing in, 237–238
Ventricular tachycardia, symptomatic, exercise training and, *251*
Ventriculography, exercise radionuclide, 101
Verapamil, 139, 139t

WALKING, exercise training and, in chronic obstructive pulmonary disease, 263
Wolff-Parkinson-White (WPW) syndrome, exercise and, 126